£6.75

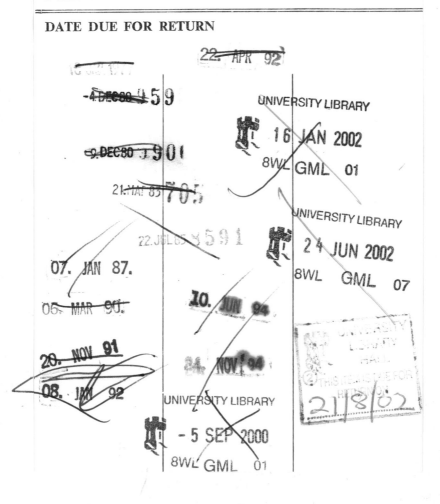

A History of Poliomyelitis

Yale Studies in the History of Science and Medicine, 6

A HISTORY OF POLIOMYELITIS

by John R. Paul, M.D.

New Haven and London: Yale University Press

1971

Designed by John O. C. McCrillis,
set in Baskerville type,
and printed in the United States of America by
Connecticut Printers, Inc., Hartford, Connecticut.

Distributed in Great Britain, Europe, Asia, and
Africa by Yale University Press Ltd., London; in
Canada by McGill-Queen's University Press, Montreal; and
in Mexico by Centro Interamericano de Libros
Académicos, Mexico City; in Australasia
by Australia and New Zealand
Book Co., Pty., Ltd., Artarmon,
New South Wales; in India by
UBS Publishers' Distributors
Pvt., Ltd., Delhi; in Japan
by John Weatherhill, Inc.,
Tokyo.

To
those past and present colleagues of the
Yale Poliomyelitis Study Unit who during
forty years gave loyal and tireless service
to this Unit—and to the cause of poliomyelitis

The author and the Yale University Press gratefully acknowledge grants given by Lederle Laboratories; Merck, Sharp & Dohme; Parke, Davis & Co.; Pfizer Inc.; and Smith Kline & French, to help defray publication costs of this book.

Contents

Illustrations

Tables

Preface

As with other histories of pestilence and disease there can be no real understanding of the relative values involved without an appreciation of various attitudes which have been held in earlier centuries. Changing philosophies, new biomedical discoveries, even ever-changing climates of a political, sociological, and religious nature—all have had their impacts, and all have reflected different points of view about the nature of illness. A prime example has been the various goals and philosophies which have influenced the approach to infantile paralysis in different eras and cultural settings not only in the nineteenth but particularly in the twentieth century.

It is difficult to imagine that anyone, in any population, could regard a child having to start life under the fearful handicap of a crippling deformity with anything but dismay, yet early ideas were that paralysis during infancy was just something to be accepted as the price one sometimes had to pay for "teething" or a "simple fever," or sitting on the damp ground, and accordingly, there was nothing that could be done about it except to bolster the limbs of these cripples by the use of splints and braces.

However, the turn of the twentieth century and the flowering of scientific medicine brought a new point of view, an era of sudden and incredible hope that something might be done after all. This hope soon ripened into eager optimism. By the 1940s and 1950s the compassion and interest of the American people and indeed of the world had been aroused to such a pitch that in a scientific age of almost unbelievable accomplishments it seemed possible that infantile paralysis might actually be conquered at last. As the crusade heightened, the world looked on expectantly. This new attitude, which in the United States was particularly fostered by the National Foundation for Infantile Paralysis, had a profound influence on ethical values attributed to the disease. Much as our grandparents had contributed during the nineteenth century to missionary societies, our dimes and dollars went to another "religious" cause, signalized by efforts to stamp out this pestilence and to alleviate the suffering and tragedy that it inflicted. Resignation gave way to activism directed against a preventable evil. And, in due time, the disease was abruptly scotched by means of vaccination. It was to all intents and purposes finished. The crusade has been described as one of the greatest technical and humanistic triumphs of the age. It was one of those rare achievements which the world greeted as an example of what could be done when science and technology were directed to good use for mankind. Even if the dread picture of poliomyelitis still lingers in the minds of some of us, many individuals, particularly parents of growing families, would be happy enough if they never were to hear about polio-myelitis again.

With such a background, the temptation to write this account as a complete success story has been almost irresistible. The events during the first half of the twentieth century which led up to the eventual conquest of poliomyelitis and the almost unbelievable decline in epidemics as a result of vaccination have the makings of a dramatic story with a triumphant ending—a story that has been, and will be, written several more times.

But granted that the success story is the familiar one, it is not the whole history of the disease, nor should I place the main emphasis there. What of the disease itself? What of its biological nature, regardless of its disastrous implications? Little appreciation of what this book stands for is possible until the image of poliomyelitis as an unmitigated evil is dispelled and the story of poliovirus as a cause of a common viral infection is brought into perspective. For some, this approach may seem to miss the whole point and therefore be totally unrealistic; for others it will be absolutely unwarranted. To understand my point of view it is necessary to emphasize that although the specter of the paralyzed child has dominated the image of poliovirus infection for a long time, other aspects have been of enormous importance for medical scientists and those who have striven to understand the nature of the disease. Indeed, the fruits of concentration on these various features were what made the conquest of poliomyelitis possible. Wordsworth has said: "We murder to dissect" in "The Tables Turned," but in the telling of this history it is essential that we commit what would be described in poetic nineteenth-century terms as wholesale massacre.

One facet of the story includes the researches brought to bear on poliomyelitis in the twentieth century. The frequent almost agonizing efforts by individual scientists to achieve something which they felt would contribute to knowledge and to the ultimate defeat of the disease; the determination in the face of frustrating delays and frequent backtracking; the almost frantic attempts to do anything about paralytic poliomyelitis—to portray these aspects is the major purpose of this story. The struggle was one of trial and error, and many a doughty investigator was to succumb. Yet it was only by this means that eventual control of the disease was made possible.

It may be too soon still to judge these events in their proper perspective. However, they can at least be documented. My intention has not been to startle with new material, which is sparse, but to give a convincing account of the old. In so doing, I have described landmarks and intimate events in terms of those individuals who have contributed most to this history. And I confess that I have related these events from a highly personal point of view, simply because this is the aspect of the story which is best known to me. For the many who are not mentioned I apologize and lamely plead the necessity of conserving space, for the book is long indeed. But accounts of contributions and careers of individual investigators tell only part of the story, and it would be foolish, even specious, to maintain that an accurate history could not have been written from other points of view.

So it is clear that by trying to tell the story from the standpoint of the natural history of the disease and of those individual scientists personally known to me who made valiant efforts to conquer it, to the neglect of the sociological and psychological points of view, I can be blamed for a failure to worship a multiplicity of ideologies.

It now sounds as if I were writing a rhapsodic review of this book instead of a preface—and in the course of these efforts I may have overshot the mark. For it was with the crippling disability and the withered limb that, from the start, the history of poliomyelitis has been identified. Thus, if I am to give a meaningful account it will have to be based first on the acute disabling paralysis as a focal point.

The following acknowledgments should be recorded: I am particularly grateful to Dr. Dorothy M. Horstmann of the Yale University Medical School for reviewing the entire manuscript; and to Dr. Saul Benison from whom I have received many helpful suggestions. Also, my wife has been of infinite help to me throughout the whole of this project. Another who has reviewed the entire manuscript is Mr. Stuart Stone of Guilford, Connecticut, to whom I am extremely grateful.

Others who have supplied much valuable information, whose names should be mentioned, have been included in the footnotes in the appropriate places and in the chronological order in which their help with regard to this manuscript has been given.

Among institutions or agencies which have graciously given permission to allow quotations and illustrations to be reproduced, the *Journal of the American Medical Association,* the *Journal of Experimental Medicine,* the *American Journal of Hygiene,* the Rockefeller Institute Press, and the National Foundation for Infantile Paralysis should receive special mention.

To Mrs. Anne Wilde of the Yale University Press I am indebted for much helpful criticism.

I am grateful also to Mrs. Virginia M. Simon for redrawing some of the charts used in the illustrations, and to Mrs. Mara Wenzel, Mrs. Frances Larvey, and particularly Mrs. Evelyn Ball for typing the manuscript.

Publication was assisted by grants ROL LM00068 01–4 from the National Library of Medicine, National Institutes of Health, Bethesda, Maryland.

J. R. P.

Guilford, Connecticut
1970

CHAPTER 1

The Disease Itself

A definition of poliomyelitis which went through several editions of a prominent American medical textbook in the 1940s and 1950s was:

> Poliomyelitis is a common, acute viral disease characterized clinically by a brief febrile illness with sore throat, headache and vomiting, and often with stiffness of the neck and back. In many cases a lower neuron paralysis develops in the early days of illness.[1]

This description falls far short of the usual picture which this disease has conjured up in the minds of most people. For whenever an individual who has suffered from poliomyelitis is mentioned, one generally visualizes a young person who has had to drag his way through life—perhaps totally confined to a wheelchair. Indeed, this image dates from the time the disease was first recognized. Interest during the nineteenth century was centered entirely on the paralytic aspects, and it has actually been only within the last two generations that the image of the cripple has given way to an appreciation of the underlying infectious process. The twentieth century witnessed a realization that the disease is a common, contagious, epidemic viral infection, not wholly confined to infants but also affecting children, adolescents, and occasionally young adults. In keeping with other viral infections, it gradually became apparent that there was more to it than the occasional patient who suffered from myelitis and the resulting paralysis.

In order to make this changing concept intelligible to the reader at the start and to dispel the idea that the disease inevitably has only calamitous effects, a biological view is necessary, somewhat in the sense that Sir Macfarlane Burnet[2] advocated more than twenty-five years ago and has continued to advocate since. His principles are consistent with attempts to bring poliomyelitis into focus with the overall scheme of nature, i.e. in terms of its demographic, environmental, and sociological features. To some this

1. J. R. Paul: "Poliomyelitis (Infantile Paralysis)," in *A Textbook of Medicine,* ed. by R. L. Cecil and R. F. Loeb, 10th ed. Philadelphia, Saunders, 1959, pp. 60–70.

2. This point is developed in two books with different titles, one a second edition of the first: F. M. Burnet: *Biological Aspects of Infectious Disease.* New York, Macmillan, 1940; and Sir Macfarlane Burnet: *Natural History of Infectious Disease.* London, Cambridge University Press, 1953.

may seem unnecessary, although perhaps the recent wide use of poliovirus vaccines has mitigated the image of the acutely paralyzed child and made the task easier than it was a generation ago. Yet the overall picture of poliomyelitis infection is still incomplete as of 1970. We have come a long way, some might say practically all the way, but here I would not agree, for the story is still unfinished.

In order to appreciate any view which takes in the whole disease and the world in which it exists, one should start appropriately with the *virus* that causes poliomyelitis—poliovirus.[3] This agent is extremely widespread throughout most inhabited portions of the world, in this respect almost like the viruses of measles, influenza, and mumps, except that these infections behave in their own particular way and have their own seasons. But in considering the manner in which poliovirus seemed to have been almost universally distributed in prevaccinal days, it is a wonder that any susceptible child escaped infection for long. Generally, contact with the agent resulted in *inapparent* infections which far outnumbered the forms that were recognizable by either symptoms or physical signs. Gradually it was learned that this hidden universality of infection was actually one of the main traits of poliomyelitis. The agent spreads, if given a chance, from one susceptible child to another, almost in the same manner that air rushes into a vacuum or water seeks its own level. But fortunately, as already mentioned, most of the infections are silent, inapparent and harmless, and, more fortunate still, have the capacity to immunize the person infected.

So much for a sketch of circumstances under which poliovirus infection prevails. It is a totally inadequate description of course, but the major part of this story will be developed later on. Now what effect has the agent on the individual if and when it succeeds in entering the body?

Although it was a matter of great controversy for years, by far the commonest mode of spread is by personal contact with an already infected person, and by far the commonest portal through which the virus gains entrance to the body is the mouth. Once in the wall of the alimentary tract it becomes implanted and multiplies there for longer or shorter periods of time, generally a matter of weeks. Particularly it seeks to establish itself in the lymphatic tissue which lines the intestinal tract. In the mouth and throat (oropharynx) it is apt to settle in the tonsils and cervical nodes; in the lower intestines it settles in the lymphoid follicles and regional (mesenteric) lymph nodes. These sites, although the first to be attacked, might also be called the first line of defense, since fortunately in the majority of infections the virus seems to be stopped there and progresses no farther in

3. The abbreviated name *poliovirus* has been adopted for popular and scientific usage since the term was first introduced in 1955. See H. von Magnus, J. H. S. Gear, and J. R. Paul: A recent definition of poliomyelitis virus. *Virology, 1*: 185–89, 1955.

the body. It is an extraordinary fact that the virus apparently does no appreciable damage in the alimentary tract and its immediate and adjacent lymph nodes, where its effects seldom amount to more than slight swelling of these structures. By far the majority of infections are of such limited nature. Most individuals have no symptoms at all, while others experience only the *minor illness of poliomyelitis,* a brief, mild, febrile episode that might ordinarily be disregarded and does not go on to paralysis. Such illnesses have been variously estimated as amounting to from 5 to 25 percent of the total number of infections induced by poliovirus during an epidemic. In the unlikely event of an abdominal operation being performed at this point, the mesenteric lymph nodes are likely to be found enlarged, the main visible evidence of what might be called extraneural lesion, for which poliovirus can be incriminated during this so-called minor illness.

But when the virus has actually penetrated into the central nervous system and has caused lesions there, the early clinical signs are quite different. They include, usually, a stiff neck and back, and when the lesions are extensive, weakness of the muscles which are dependent for their motor nerve supply on the brain stem and spinal cord. It is most unfortunate that the one place where poliovirus causes its most destructive and irreparable damage in the body should be in the central nervous system,[4] particularly the gray matter of the spinal cord. For motor nerve cells, once destroyed, do not have the property of regenerating themselves as do cells of the skin, the liver, or other organs. This is why paralysis, once established, is often permanent.

Meanwhile, to return to the virus for a moment, after establishing itself in the intestinal tract it has probably been doing its best to get a further foothold in the body of the susceptible child.[5] But in the earliest days of the infection there has been an automatic reaction to the virus by its host. The body has marshaled its natural defense mechanisms consisting of cellular reactions and the production of specific antibodies. Provided such defenses are adequate, which usually is the case, the virus can be destroyed or stopped in its tracks. The net result is a lasting immunity which protects the child from future infections with poliovirus. It is an internal drama of which the majority of nineteenth-century physicians were almost totally unaware. Outward manifestations of the struggle, in the form of mild symptoms, may become evident, but usually there are no indications which would in any way attract attention to the central nervous system. This is the *minor illness* of poliomyelitis that the Swedish epidemiologist Wick-

4. The term *central nervous system* (CNS) ordinarily includes the anatomical srtuctures of the brain, brain stem, medulla, and spinal cord.

5. If the child is *insusceptible* (already immune), the chances are that antibodies and other defense mechanisms from a previous poliovirus infection block the virus.

man recognized early in the twentieth century as being crucial to the solution of the poliomyelitis puzzle. The concept proved to be one of the most important ones of all time concerning the disease.

The minor illness starts after an incubation period[6] of from two to five days. It usually represents the entire recognizable course of the infection, sometimes known as *abortive poliomyelitis.*[7] But the first sign of real trouble comes when the minor illness is transformed into or followed by the *major illness,* in which there is clear-cut central nervous system involvement and occasionally paralysis. Even though this is estimated to occur in less than 3 to 4 percent of all poliovirus infections, the toll of disabled persons in a sizable epidemic can reach tremendous proportions. No wonder that this disability was the first to be emphasized. For instance, in the United States alone, the annual incidence of poliomyelitis reached a high during several epidemic years in the 1930s and 1940s of more than 10,000 paralytic cases. It is fair to assume that in almost half of these the muscle weakness subsided within six months or more and was not the cause of serious disability; but even if a third of the patients remained permanently paralyzed, this would mean that more than 3,000 were left with crippling deformities in the wake of a given epidemic year.

Thus it is not surprising that the paralytic form eventually came to be known as the "true polio." It is natural that our story should begin with this characteristic feature.

At the start I shall try to list the past and present names and terms under which the disease was known. These terms shifted almost from one generation to the next, particularly in the nineteenth century, for inevitably nomenclature kept pace with changing concepts about the disease.

The first name applied in the late eighteenth century sounds vague and nonspecific: "debility of the lower extremities." Inasmuch as the affliction was given this label by a pediatrician, it can be assumed that the debility applied to infants and children. Yet the term was considered an adequate description for the next fifty years. But it was as if one described pulmonary tuberculosis in infants under the blanket term: "weakness of the chest."

From 1840 to 1875, however, a variety of terms was introduced, some of which only contributed to the existent confusion about the disease and its

6. The *incubation period* is that period between the time when the virus actually enters the body until it has multiplied sufficiently to give rise to symptoms, which in poliomyelitis is frequently 2–4 days.

7. *Abortive poliomyelitis* is a term descriptive of either the minor or major illness, in which the patient escapes without paralysis. This is not to be confused with the inapparent infection, which has no symptoms. Throughout this book the terms *abortive* and *nonparalytic* poliomyelitis have been used loosely and more or less interchangeably. Their meaning would seem clear enough.

nature. The following incomplete tabulation carries most of the dates and a list of the men who suggested the names:

Debility of the lower extremities
Underwood, 1789[8]

Lähmungszustände der unteren Extremitäten
Heine, 1840[9]

Morning paralysis
West, 1843[10]

Paralysie essentielle chez les enfants
Rilliet, 1851[11]

Paralysie atrophique graisseuse de l'enfance
Duchenne de Boulogne, 1855[12]

Spinale Kinderlähmung
v. Heine, 1860[13]

Tephromyelitis anterior acuta parenchymatose
Charcot, 1872[14]

Poliomyelitis anterior acuta
Kussmaul (quoted by Frey), 1874[15]

Heine-Medin disease
Wickman, 1907[16]

Infantile paralysis

Poliomyelitis

Polio

In the mid-nineteenth century physicians and pathologists were unde-cided about the real seat of the damage that caused the paralysis. French authors thought there might be no physical injury whatsoever and even in-

8. M. Underwood: *A Treatise on the Diseases of Children with General Direction for the Management of Infants from the Birth,* new ed. London, Mathews, 1789.

9. J. Heine: *Beobachtungen über Lähmungszustände der unteren Extremitäten und deren Behandlung.* Stuttgart, Köhler, 1840.

10. C. West: On some forms of paralysis incidental to infancy and childhood. *London. med. Gaz., 32:* 829, 1843.

11. F. Rilliet: De la paralysie essentielle chez les enfants. *Gaz. méd. Paris,* 3rd s., *6:* 681, 704, 1851.

12. Duchenne de Boulogne: *De l'électrisation localisée et de son application à la physiologie, à la pathologic et à la thérapeutique.* Paris, Baillière, 1855.

13. J. v. Heine: *Spinale Kinderlähmung.* Stuttgart, Cotta, 1860.

14. J.-M. Charcot: Groupe des myopathies de cause spinale; paralysie infantile. *Rev. phot. hôp. Paris, 4:* 1, 36, 1872. (Charcot was in favor of the term tephromyelitis instead of polio-myelitis. He derived this from a Greek word meaning ash gray. Also, it is said that Charcot was the first to use the term myelitis.)

15. A. Frey: Ein Fall von subakuter Lähmung Erwachsener, wahrscheinlich Poliomyelitis anterior acuta. *Berl. klin. Wschr., 11:* 549, 566, 1874.

16. I. Wickman: *Beiträge zur Kenntnis der Heine-Medinschen Krankheit (Poliomyelitis acuta und verwandter Erkrankungen).* Berlin, Karger, 1907.

troduced the ill-conceived term *essentielle* to mean that the paralysis was not caused by an organic lesion. But Heine in Germany soon reversed all this when he correctly observed that the seat of the trouble was in the spinal cord. After that, with the development of histological methods, it was only a step for members of Charcot's clinic in Paris to pinpoint in the 1870s the exact location of the lesions in the anterior part of the gray matter of the spinal cord.

A hundred or more years later the extent of involvement was illustrated in Bodian's schematic anatomical diagram which shows the whole human brain and includes the medullary portion of the spinal cord (see fig. 1).

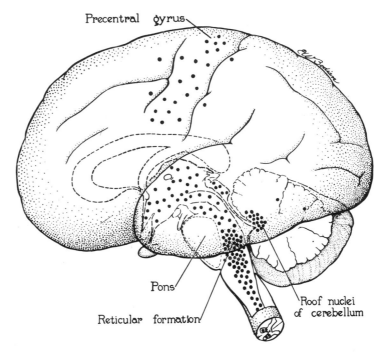

FIG. 1. **Bodian's schematic view of the human brain which includes the upper portion of the spinal cord. The solid dots show the general distribution of lesions of poliomyelitis (from Bodian, n. 17). Reproduced by permission of the National Foundation for Infantile Paralysis.**

This drawing indicates the location of scattered lesions which extend beyond the spinal cord to the medulla and midbrain and even penetrate the precentral gyrus of the cortex.[17]

Terminology based on the location of lesions within the spinal cord has been ascribed to Adolph Kussmaul (1822–1902), who is given credit by

17. D. Bodian: "Virus and host factors determining the nature and severity of lesions and of clinical manifestations," in *Poliomyelitis; Papers and Discussions Presented at the Second International Poliomyelitis Conference.* Philadelphia, Lippincott, 1952, p. 65.

ANTERIOR

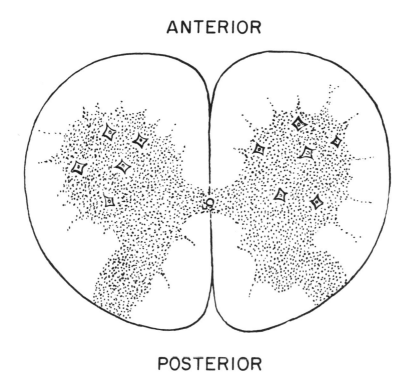

POSTERIOR

⬦ = Most likely sites of neuropathological lesions in poliomyelitis

FIG. 2. Schematic diagram of a cross section of the human spinal cord (cervical level). Stippled areas denote the gray matter within which the motor nerve cells are diagrammatically shown.

Frey in 1874 for first using the term *poliomyelitis anterior acuta;* the derivation is from the Greek words πολιός, gray, and μυελός, marrow (the gray marrow of the spinal cord). The suffix *itis* is derived from the Latin, meaning inflammation of. In this complicated name, anterior refers to the anterior horns of the cord. *Acuta,* sometimes supplanted by *subacuta,* is self-explanatory.

To illustrate these anatomical relationships a schematic diagram of a cross section of the human spinal cord, transected in its upper (cervical) portion, is shown in figure 2.[18] Actually, except in the most fulminating of cases, when gross abnormalities can be seen, the microscope is necessary

18. Further neuroanatomical features of the human spinal cord should be described here even though they may be familiar enough to many. Briefly, a cross section of the cord reveals it to be divided into two portions: a central inner portion of *gray* matter and its surrounding *white* matter. These areas are visible to the naked eye. The difference in color stems from the fact that the gray matter is occupied mostly by large nerve cells, whereas the white matter consists almost entirely of nerve fibers.

to detect the characteristic histological changes in the large motor nerve cells.

French authors were also the originators of the term "fatty atrophic paralysis of infancy," soon anglicized and shortened to "infantile paralysis." The adjective atrophic referred to the eventual withered state of affected limbs and was not particularly appropriate. But the label, infantile paralysis, has remained for many years and is still used. It was a name with a descriptive appeal that few others had. That it has persisted and is eminently respectable is proved by its adoption by such reputable organizations as the Harvard Infantile Paralysis Commission and the National Foundation for Infantile Paralysis. Yet the term is no longer generally applicable, for in most highly developed countries the disease has ceased to be infantile, having come to be recognized as a recurrent scourge afflicting children of school age, even adolescents and young adults; and in only a tiny fraction of poliovirus infections is there paralysis.

So the very multiplicity of names under which poliomyelitis has gone has proved to be primarily of historical value—first the debility of limbs about which pediatricians, orthopedists, and trussmakers had their say; next the pathologists peering through their crude early microscopes to locate the exact anatomical site of lesions in the spinal cord. Pathology was almost the only basic medical science in the 1870s, so its adherents were eminently justified in taking themselves seriously. Hence came the use of impressive Greek and Latin terminology for a disease which might have, even should have, been given a simpler name, which it eventually acquired—*poliomyelitis anterior acuta*, inevitably shortened to poliomyelitis.

For a time, however, it looked as if the term poliomyelitis was going to be superseded by "Heine-Medin disease." This eponym was introduced in 1907 by Wickman, who was anxious to immortalize the names of two notable figures who had contributed mightily to the history of the disease— Jacob von Heine (1799–1878), a German orthopedist, and Wickman's teacher, Oskar Medin (1847–1927), a Swedish pediatrician, both of whom we shall hear more about in subsequent chapters. The term Heine-Medin disease became popular both in Europe and in America for a time. As a matter of fact, it was the only name under which I first came to know the disease in 1915, as a medical student in Baltimore. It is now fortunately outmoded. *Poliomyelitis* has stood the test of time and seems to be the designation of choice today. Nevertheless, the term has been largely restricted to the medical profession; unlike appendicitis and hepatitis, poliomyelitis has proved too lengthy or perhaps too erudite a word for common usage. It was inevitably abbreviated to "polio," which, although really a slang word, caught on and became a common term for parents and science writers alike. One reason perhaps that *poliomyelitis* never attained general acceptance is that it seems to reflect the physician's desire to appear learned and, at the same time, to cloak his ignorance with a Greco-Latin word whose meaning is judiciously obscure. Such usage harks back to the past when learned physicians held their consultations over an understandably frightened patient in Latin. Be that as it may, "polio," although colloquial, has not quite reached the stage when it can be accepted into the scientific vocabulary.[19]

By the time the virus had come into the picture, *poliomyelitis* had become too fixed to allow changes. The causative agent has also suffered its own evolution of terms, and its story will be reviewed in due time. When discovered in 1908, it was referred to as the *virus of poliomyelitis*. Forty years later, this terminology was reduced to one word, *poliovirus;* and still later, the polioviruses were absorbed into the huge and growing membership of the family of *enteroviruses*. It was a long and tortuous journey for the causal agent of "debility of the lower extremities."

19. However, the term *polio* appears in Webster's seventh Collegiate edition as a shortened form of poliomyelitis.

CHAPTER 2

Ancient Records

Poliomyelitis is unique in that it is almost the only *common* disease in which sudden paralysis in a previously healthy infant or young child can occur. This characteristic behavior alone might be considered sufficient to enable one to trace its identity through the past. And yet, actually, the search has proved disappointing. There are many examples dating from biblical or Homeric times of lameness, or a withered limb in a child, but these descriptions are apt to be so brief that it is well nigh impossible to tell whether the deformity was actually the result of poliomyelitis. To some students of medical history this dearth of unequivocal early cases has been sufficient reason to characterize the disease as a recent one—a reasonable assumption, particularly when one seeks in vain for a pre-nineteenth-century description of anything resembling an epidemic of poliomyelitis. Also the enormous increase in incidence of recognized cases that occurred during the first half of the twentieth century might be another reason for branding it as a disease of the twentieth century.

But from the opposite point of view, it is altogether probable that some of the recorded examples of lameness and withered limbs dating from ancient times did actually represent the aftermath of sporadic cases of poliovirus infection. Indeed this probability is strong enough to convince the majority of authorities that poliomyelitis has existed since the dawn of written history, and even before. No one can really say that poliovirus did not undergo certain mutations during this period, but this is pure speculation. What did undoubtedly undergo a recent evolution that profoundly influenced both the clinical and epidemiological behavior of the disease at the turn of the twentieth century were man's changing ways of life. Especially did the introduction of modern sanitation, with its impact on bacterial enteric infections, bring about pronounced changes in the behavior of poliomyelitis. Thus, an increasing frequency of recognized cases did not necessarily mean that the disease was actually new, considering the kind of infection that poliomyelitis eventually turned out to be. On the contrary, it could mean that changing times and customs had exerted their effects not only on the dissemination of the virus but also on human immunity. These two influences were in all probability responsible for bringing a disease to the surface which had been in existence long before, although more or less hidden.

To enlarge upon this theme for a moment is is fair to speculate that man's very earliest habitations did not swarm with viruses. But this situation was bound to change as villages and towns became larger and more crowded, and traffic in and out became heavier. Presently such communities became hotbeds of infection, and if we are to judge from historical evidence they were plagued by pestilences and epidemics of many kinds during the Dark and Middle Ages—right through the eighteenth century.[1] Apparently it took an inordinately long time for man to learn to adapt to an urban environment; and he has by no means learned his lesson even now. Yet in the age just past, pollutants were of a different kind. Bacteria and parasites galore must have thriven in the filthy urban environment of not so long ago. Records of constantly recurring outbreaks of plague, smallpox, and "distempers" of various kinds bear ample witness. Added to all these was an astronomically high infant mortality rate, which is usually a measure of the prevalence of endemic diarrheal diseases. More than likely, poliovirus, which also is a highly infectious agent, must have invaded urban communities, but considering its nature it could have been easily overshadowed by other infectious agents.

The estimates are that once introduced, poliovirus became established and survived for centuries on end in an *endemic* fashion, as opposed to its later characteristic of causing periodic epidemics.[2] Considering that most infantile infections were—and are—*subclinical* or inapparent, the great bulk of them could have escaped recognition completely. Indeed a similar state of affairs prevails today in many South American, African, and Middle and Far Eastern cities and villages, where polioviruses are prevalent but the disease is uncommon. In such situations the virus has come more or less into equilibrium with the population; a continuous supply of new susceptible infants being born into the community regularly provides for the uninterrupted circulation of the virus. As a result of this extensive exposure and infection, some few infants develop paralysis, some even succumb to the disease, but the great majority are silently infected and thus immunized at an early age.

Under such endemic conditions, paralytic poliomyelitis could have remained under cover for centuries in populations in which infant mortality was high. Naturally it was regarded as not of much importance, considering the many more serious diseases that ancient (and modern) civilizations had to face. Only later when infantile paralysis emerged as a disease of slightly older children did it come into its own, and the buildup of susceptibles in the population was sufficient to invite epidemics.

1. H. E. Sigerist: *Civilization and Disease*. Ithaca, Cornell University Press, 1943; C.-E. Winslow: *The Conquest of Epidemic Disease*. Princeton, N.J., Princeton University Press, 1943.

2. The word epidemic has been derived from two Greek words 'επι and δεμός which implied that something, presumably a blight, has been thrust upon the people. The word *endemic* has a similar implication, meaning something that is already in the people.

But to get back to the ancient history of poliomyelitis, it has been the general consensus of medical scientists, historians, and other authorities that sporadic cases of the endemic disease are at least as old as written history. Archaeological evidence of one of these is shown in a familiar illustration (fig. 3) depicting a deformity so characteristic of the aftereffects of poliomyelitis that the diagnosis is practically assured. This picture of an Egyptian stele dating from the Eighteenth Dynasty (1580–1350 B.C.) has been reproduced countless times. It is now in the Carlsberg Glyptothek at Copenhagen. We owe its original medical interpretation to the Danish physician Ove Hamburger.[3,4] Here the crippled young man, apparently a priest, is pictured with a withered and shortened left leg, with his foot held in the typical *equinus* position characteristic of flaccid paralysis; his staff is apparently being used as a support. Hamburger rightly concluded that the most probable cause of the priest's deformity was infantile paralysis, and few physicians with appropriate experience who have examined this picture carefully during the more than half century since its publication have doubted the significance of his historic diagnosis. Of course it is only a single case, and one might argue that the wasted limb could be due to a variety of causes (even a variety of neurotropic viruses), but the fact remains that by far the most likely explanation is that the deformity resulted from paralytic poliomyelitis.

Also, there have been occasional descriptions of abnormalities of skeletons dating from earliest times in which the claim has been made that poliomyelitis was the cause, but on these I will not dwell.

Descriptions of what could be paralytic poliomyelitis have come down from biblical and Greco-Roman times. However, the next milestone in this story occurred in ancient Greece where there began to be an appreciation of what might be termed a "scientific" attitude toward disease, as opposed to a supernatural or magical one. The chief mentor of this era was, needless to say, Hippocrates, the so-called father of medicine. Hippocrates was supposed to have been born in 460 B.C. His very existence has been questioned, but there are excellent reasons for believing that he was more than a legendary figure and that he had headquarters on one of the Greek islands in the Aegean. Also, there seems to be little doubt that he traveled widely and during his wanderings acquired great knowledge of peoples,

3. The argument that poliomyelitis is an old disease is not presented to indicate that no new noninfectious diseases have "arisen" in recent times. On the contrary, many new diseases have appeared on the current scene—some of them literally in epidemic form. In some of these, just as in the case of poliomyelitis, the infectious agent is not new but its means of spread has undergone a transition or its patterns of immunity in certain human populations have been upset and this is the reason that the new menace has burst upon the scene.

4. O. Hamburger: A case of infantile paralysis in ancient times. *Ugeskr f. laeger., 73*: 1565, 1911; extracted in *Bull. Soc. franc. hist. Med.*, Paris, *11*: 407–12, 1911.

A translation into English has been made by E. Hansen: A probable case of infantile paralysis in ancient Egypt. *Hosp. Bull. Univ. Maryland, 8*: 192, 1912–13.

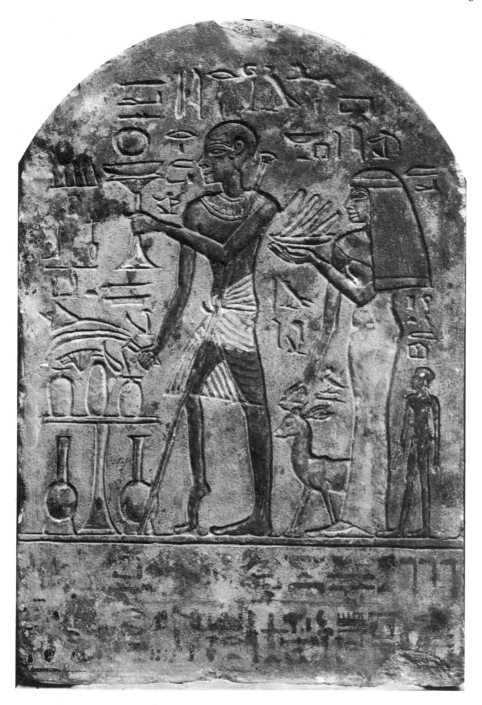

FIG. 3. Egyptian stele, dating from the eighteenth dynasty (1580–1350 B.C.) now in the Carlsberg Glyptothek, Copenhagen. Kindness of the National Foundation for Infantile Paralysis.

places, and things. He was neither prophet nor magician, but an observant physician—almost in the modern sense. And he was even more than that; he saw that disease varied in type under different conditions of climate and race. In short, he was not only a physician but also an epidemiologist.

It would be surprising that as astute a medical observer as Hippocrates would have omitted from his two volumes, *Of the Epidemics,* a description of a bona fide epidemic of poliomyelitis if there had been any in that age. The absence of such a description must have reflected a situation which continued for centuries, the logical conclusion being that before and after classical Greco-Roman times, even up to the mid-nineteenth century, outbreaks were rare. So in the absence of epidemics, the most likely explanation is that Hippocrates' descriptions of paralytic poliomyelitis were limited to sporadic cases.

Pertinent here is his account of cases of *clubfoot,* for which I have used the Adams translation.[5] Adams, a mid-nineteenth-century surgeon and student of Hippocrates, used the term in the sense that it was commonly applied during his time and for some years thereafter,[6] rather than in the specific manner of inherited deformities in which we interpret it today. According to Adams, "clubfoot" covered most, if not all, deformities involving the ankles and the feet, including flail-like conditions of the lower legs and subluxations of the ankle joints leading to abnormal positions of the feet.[7] Nevertheless, it seems probable that the Greek word which Hippocrates employed in his text, κυλλός, means "crooked, crippled, or with legs bent outward by disease." The ancients apparently made no distinction between one kind of crookedness and another, except that a different term, βλαισος, was used to mean "having the legs bent out and the feet in." We will have occasion in chapter 6 to refer to a somewhat similar use of the term clubfoot by nineteenth-century American surgeons.

In recording the section of Hippocrates' works which deals with articulations, Adams has the following comments:

> But in all the works in ancient surgery, I verily believe there is not a more wonderful chapter than the one which relates to *Club-foot.* In it he has not only stated correctly the true nature of the malformation, but he has also given very sensible directions for rectifying the deformity in early life.[8]

5. Among numerous translations of the complete works of Hippocrates I have chosen the one by Francis Adams done in London in 1849. *The Genuine Works of Hippocrates,* trans. by F. Adams, American ed. New York, Wood, 1886, vol. 2, pp. 137–39.

6. *Complete Works of Hippocrates,* trans. by W. H. S. Jones and E. T. Loeb, Classical Library, 4 vols. London, 1923–31.

7. I am indebted for these comments and the translation of the text of Hippocrates to Professor Edward T. Silk of the Department of Classics, Yale University.

8. See n. 5, p. 78.

In the passage referred to, Hippocrates himself comments:

Most cases of club-foot are remediable, unless the declination be very great, as when the affection occurs at an advanced period of youth . . . and before the deficiency of the bones of the foot is very great, and before there is any great wasting of the flesh of the leg. There is more than one variety of club-foot, the most of them being not complete dislocations, but impairments connected with the habitual maintenance of the limb in a certain position.[9]

Five centuries after these words were supposedly written, Galen (138–201), that Roman physician and indefatigable student of the rules and the art of medicine as laid down by Hippocrates, was also to preempt the broad field of medicine. In fact some medical historians maintain that Galen was perhaps the greatest medical figure of all time: "He has been much abused because his works held despotic authority over European medicine for thirteen centuries after his death, with all their error as well as truth accepted as medical gospel. It is hard to see how this is Galen's fault."[10] His comments have been inserted in the Adams translation in a footnote which reads as follows:

Galen remarks, in his Commentary on this passage, that it is clear our author treats of the cure both of congenital club-foot, and of the club-foot which occurs in early infancy.[11]

My own estimate of these statements by the two ancient physicians is that Hippocrates and Galen were familiar with both congenital and acquired "clubfoot." It seems reasonable to suspect that some of the latter cases were due to paralytic poliomyelitis. Also, the accuracy of Hippocrates' observations on these deformities and his familiarity with their treatment testify to his having a certain amount of experience in handling them. This might lead to the conclusion that he had frequently met various forms of club-foot in his travels through Greece and Asia Minor and among his surgical patients at the Temple of Aesculapius on the Island of Cos. The same might be said of Galen, who followed Hippocrates by some 500 years, first in Asia Minor and eventually in Rome. The conclusion that sporadic cases of paralysis of one or both legs, occurring at an early age, did exist in the Mediterranean area in Greco-Roman times is based on the above considerations. There is reason to speculate that such deformities were not rare.

To attempt to follow poliomyelitis through the Dark and Middle Ages is an unrewarding task. It is not surprising that this was a sterile period in the

9. Ibid., pp. 137–38.
10. E. R. Long: *A History of Pathology*. Baltimore, Williams & Wilkins, 1928, p. 28.
11. See n. 9, p. 137.

annals of clinical medicine because physicians even as late as the fifteenth century continued to search for knowledge in the writings of Greek, Roman, and Arabic authorities instead of recording their own observations.

For a continuation of the story of deformities we must skip a full millennium and a half to the seventeenth century. Both Garrison[12] and Hutchins[13] mention a passion for portraying the abnormal during the latter era. Both authors had little doubt that there was a high proportion of the maimed, halt, blind, and imbecile in the population of that period. Hieronymus Bosch and Pieter Breughel the younger depict crippling deformities due to paralysis and amputated limbs. It is said that some of the paralytic gaits depicted in *The Procession of Cripples* by Bosch are possibly the results of poliomyelitis.

Thus we may speculate that paralyses due to poliomyelitis must have existed sporadically as a grim oddity. As to where and whence the infirmity arose, no one in that era had the slightest idea.

In any event, it was not until the end of the eighteenth century that paralytic poliomyelitis was described with any degree of accuracy; nor was it observed that fever often precedes the appearance of weakness of the limbs.

12. F. H. Garrison: *An Introduction to the History of Medicine,* 3rd ed. Philadelphia, Saunders, 1922.

13. E. F. Hutchins: "Historical summary," chap. 1, in *Poliomyelitis.* International Committee for the Study of Infantile Paralysis, Baltimore, Williams & Wilkins, 1932, p. 4.

CHAPTER 3

The Eighteenth Century

Early eighteenth-century references, either literary or medical, to what may have been isolated examples of paralytic poliomyelitis seem to be of dubious validity and hardly of sufficient importance to warrant listing here.[1] Recognizable sporadic cases could certainly have existed in Europe and America in the seventeenth and early eighteenth centuries, although only the scantiest of descriptions have come down to us. The medical historian Dr. Ernest Caulfield has succeeded in collecting a number of references to possible cases in colonial America, but one cannot say whether or not they represent paralytic poliomyelitis.

A typical description can be found in the medical papers of Governor John Winthrop, Jr., of Connecticut, who practiced medicine along with politics. One item, which dates from the years 1657–60, states: "young Mr. Fowler's daughter—4 years old, paralytical on one side."

Dr. Caulfield's investigations also show that more than a century later the lame distemper was prevalent in New England (in 1771–72). It seems to have been a winter malady (unlike poliomyelitis) and something akin to acute rheumatic fever which affected adolescents and young adults alike.

Of vastly more significance is an arresting, late eighteenth-century item, which is the account of Sir Walter Scott's lameness. It is more than reasonable to suspect that this was due to poliomyelitis. As such, it probably amounts to the earliest case on record in the British Isles—or possibly anywhere.

Sir Walter was born in Edinburgh in 1771. It is recorded that an attack of fever in infancy left him permanently lame. But we are fortunate in having an autobiographical account of his own illness as it was recounted to him by his family. The quotation is derived from Lockhart's memoirs:

> I showed every sign of health and strength until I was about eighteen months old. One night, I have been often told, I showed great reluctance to be caught and put to bed, and after being chased about the room, was apprehended and consigned to my dormitory with some difficulty. It was the last time I was to show much personal agility. In the

1. A listing of these questionable cases appears in E. F. Hutchins: "Historical summary," chap. 1, in *Poliomyelitis*. International Committee for the Study of Infantile Paralysis, Baltimore, Williams & Wilkins, 1932, pp. 4–5.

morning I was discovered to be affected with the fever which often accompanies the cutting of large teeth. It held me three days. On the fourth, when they went to bathe me as usual, they discovered that I had lost the power of my right leg. My grandfather, an excellent anatomist as well as physician, the late worthy Alexander Wood, and many others of the most respectable of the faculty, were consulted. There appeared to be no dislocation or sprain; blisters and other topical remedies were applied in vain.

When the efforts of regular physicians had been exhausted, without the slightest success, my anxious parents, during the course of many years, eagerly grasped at every prospect of cure which was held out by the promise of empirics, or of ancient ladies or gentlemen who conceived themselves entitled to recommend various remedies, some of which were of a nature sufficiently singular . . .

The impatience of a child soon inclined me to struggle with my infirmity, and I began by degrees to stand, to walk, and to run. Although the limb affected was much shrunk and contracted, my general health, which was of more importance, was much strengthened by being frequently in the open air, and, in a word, I who in a city had probably been condemned to helpless and hopeless decrepitude, was now a healthy, high-spirited, and, my lameness apart, a sturdy child—*non sine diis animosus infans.*[2]

From this subjective account it seems clear and understandable that neither the therapeutic efforts of the worthy Dr. Wood[3] nor those of the other skilled and respectable members of the faculty of the University of Edinburgh were effective. These consultants also seem to have experienced considerable difficulty in the matter of diagnosis except in the elimination of other conditions. Their explanation, however weak it sounds today, was an acceptable one at that time—that the lameness of the patient was due to a kind of paralysis which sometimes follows a fever and occasionally accompanies the cutting of teeth.

2. J. G. Lockhart: *Memoirs of the Life of Sir Walter Scott, Bart.,* 2 vols. Philadelphia, Carey, Lean & Blanchard, 1837, vol. 1, pp. 23–27.

3. A number of biographical sketches exists of Alexander Wood (1725–1807), surgeon. The one I have used, for which I am indebted to Mr. Whitfield Bell, librarian of the American Philosophical Society, appears in Kay's Portraits (J. Kay: *A Series of Original Portraits and Caricatures; Etchings with Biographical Sketches and Illustrative Anecdotes.* Edinburgh, Hugh Paton, Carver and Gilder, 1837, vol. 1).

From this sketch one gets the impression that Mr. Wood, who was popularly known to the students of Edinburgh University as "lang Sandy Wood," was an eminent surgeon and a beloved figure in Edinburgh. John Bell, brother of Sir Charles Bell, both of whom we shall hear more about in this account, was a pupil of Mr. Wood and dedicated the first volume of his *Anatomy* to him. Thus the opinion of Wood's granddaughter regarding his knowledge of anatomy seems to have been well founded.

Did this mean that sporadic cases of poliomyelitis were accepted as the inevitable accompaniment of some childhood fevers and were common in Scotland in 1772? This certainly seems to have been the accepted view. Yet despite a lack of precision in diagnosis which characterized medicine in the greater part of the eighteenth century, physicians actually *did* at last begin to notice cases of "infantile paralysis" in various parts of the British Isles in the late 1700s and early 1800s. The usual situation was that the acute short fever had been disregarded by the parents, and only after some days or weeks was the lameness noted. Here was a situation demanding aftercare, not diagnosis of a particular kind of fever. It was not until a century later that sizable epidemics appeared in Europe, making the task of the diagnostician much simpler than it was when only sporadic cases were encountered. Furthermore, it was not until 1789 that the first clinical description of poliomyelitis appeared in a medical text.

In order to appreciate the long road to be traveled before poliomyelitis was recognized as a distinct clinical entity, it is necessary to know something of the medical climate in which this landmark was achieved. During all of the seventeenth and most of the eighteenth century, physicians did not consider matters of exact diagnosis to be of great moment except perhaps in "really important" diseases of epidemic potential, such as smallpox, yellow fever, and the plague. Apparently, few doctors of this era disagreed with this orthodox position. One who did was a London practitioner without academic position or pretensions but with an extraordinary degree of clinical discernment. This was Thomas Sydenham (1624–89),[4] who has been sometimes characterized as the first "modern" clinician—sometimes as the father of epidemiology. Coming from a background dominated by speculations of the school of iatrochemists, who sought to apply their crude notions of contemporary chemistry to the treatment of disease, he chose to emphasize clinical observation instead, thus renewing the Hippocratic method, which had gone out some two thousand years before. Sydenham relied upon observations made at the bedside, correlating symptoms and signs as seen in the sick patient with an occasional pathological examination of a fatal case. Against considerable opposition he proposed that the individuality of certain maladies was sufficiently manifest to allow a classification of diseases. But Sydenham was far in advance of his time, for during most of the eighteenth century, doctors continued to have a fine and utter disregard for diagnosis, except in the crudest sort of manner. Fevers, for instance, were recognized and given names only if accompanied by certain gross lesions such as spots or a rash on the skin, the spotted fever for instance, or the scarlet fever; or if the fever was accompanied by visible inflammation of some part of the body. But there seemed to be no reason for

4. D. Riesman: *Thomas Sydenham.* New York, Hoeber, 1926.

assuming that fevers for which there was no obvious cause could be classified other than as: short fevers, intermittent fevers, or continued fevers. Indeed, such a temporal classification of fevers held sway for more than a century. Nevertheless Sydenham did prepare the way for a new era which demanded that many individual diseases be named, recognized, and identified.

A century after Sydenham, other scholars in France, Scandinavia, Germany, and England began to devise their own enumeration of diseases and their own systems of classification and nomenclature.[5] This proved to be the start of a never-ending task, considering the ideas and concepts which inevitably accompanied questions as to how to differentiate symptoms, such as fever, cough, and malaise, from the diseases and the lesions which caused them. But at least it was a start in the right direction.[6] Indeed, during all of the seventeenth and most of the eighteenth century in Europe and England exact diagnosis of a trivial illness was probably considered a prolix and inconsequential matter. It was not worthy of the attention of a practicing doctor, who was supposed to do something "useful" for his patients, such as purgings or bleedings, or the giving of powders and concoctions, instead of bestowing names upon the diseases from which they suffered. In other words physical diagnosis was in a crude state; even such simple procedures as counting the pulse and taking the temperature were not currently practiced, although Galileo had measured both. And yet, if diagnostic procedures were primitive, treatment was even more so. But that is another story.

It was this prevailing attitude of resistance toward precise diagnosis that kept poliomyelitis from being recognized as a disease, sui generis, for such a long time. Yet lameness, coming on suddenly and unexpectedly in a child, often after a short bout of fever, must have been a not infrequent occurrence. As mentioned, the probable reason poliomyelitis had failed to achieve a definite name at this time was that the doctor was not called early enough, but was consulted only after the child had been lame for some weeks or even months. Lameness might be due to a fall, a chill—anything. The same situation often exists even today, particularly in developing countries. It took a London physician who specialized in obstetrics and pediatrics to recognize the relationship between the fever and the onset of the lameness—and to put them together.

This man was Michael Underwood (see fig. 4), who very likely was the first physician to give an intelligible clinical account of poliomyelitis. His

5. K. Faber: *Nosography in Modern Internal Medicine.* New York, Hoeber, 1923, pp. 20–27.

6. With almost every decade in the twentieth century an ever-increasing number of new diseases has been added and old terms occasionally eliminated. For instance, a *Standard Nomenclature of Diseases and Operations,* 5th ed. Chicago, Amer. med. Ass., 1961, lists more than 16,000 diagnoses.

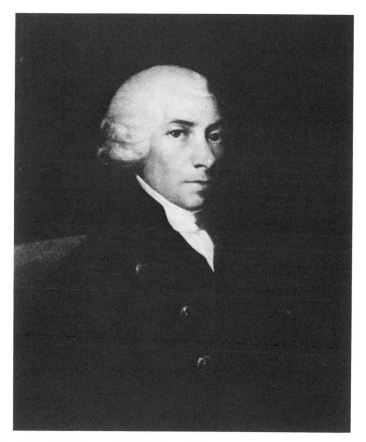

Fig. 4. Michael Underwood (1738–circa 1810). Portrait attributed to Zoffany. Reproduced through the kind permission of J. E. Scatcherd of London.

description included both the inconsequential febrile features of the early stage and the spectacular and flagrant character of the paralysis which dominates late phases of this disease.

Michael Underwood, besides being a London pediatrician, a specialty hardly recognized at that time, was apparently the first to become a licentiate in midwifery of the College of Physicians. His license was granted in 1784, the same year that the first edition of his *Treatise on Diseases of Children* was published. It was a successful book, for it is said that it went through at least twenty-five editions, including several American ones, and was translated and republished several times in Germany. Originally trained as a surgeon, Underwood had received, in 1764, a diploma admitting him to the Company of Surgeons. He obviously must have acquired a huge practical experience in children's injuries and ailments to have been able to write such a book in the early years of his practice. Later he proved himself to be a skillful and popular *accoucheur*—an accomplishment that enabled him to continue as an expert in the field of maternal and child welfare.

The first edition of his *Diseases of Children* contained no mention of anything resembling poliomyelitis, but the second edition (1789) contains an unmistakable description of the disease. Under the heading of "Debility of the Lower Extremities," he writes:

> The disorder intended here is not noticed by any medical writer within the compass of my reading, or is not so described as to ascertain the disease. It is not a common disorder, I believe, and seems to occur seldomer in *London* than in some parts. Nor am I enough acquainted with it to be fully satisfied, either, in regard to the true cause or seat of the disease, either from my own observation, or that of others; and I have myself never had opportunity of examining the body of any child who has died of this complaint. I shall, therefore, only describe its symptoms, and mention the several means attempted for its cure, in order to induce other practitioners to pay attention to it.
>
> It seems to arise from debility, and usually attacks children previously reduced by fever; seldom those under one, or more than four or five years old.[7]

The clinical picture thus described by Underwood in eighteenth-century terms was doubtless characteristic of the disease as it then existed in England. He mentioned nothing about epidemics. But his emphasis on the limitation of cases to the infantile age group is consistent with the endemic pattern of age distribution which was subsequently observed in practically all the countries of the world in the early nineteenth century. In fact, this infantile pattern still persists in areas where the sanitary practices have remained distinctly primitive.

This description by Underwood suggests that he had seen a number of children with paralysis, notwithstanding that the disease had previously received so little attention from others. Although he says that he is "not fully satisfied, either in regard to the true cause, or seat of the disease," in subsequent editions of the work there is the added unhelpful comment: "except in the instance of teething and foul bowels."

Underwood's account of his treatment in dealing with this condition, which he said called for brisk purges, follows:

> When only one of the lower extremities has been affected, the above means, in two instances out of five or six, entirely removed the complaint; but when both have been paralytic, nothing has seemed to do

---

7. M. Underwood: *A Treatise on the Diseases of Children with General Directions for the Management of Infants from the Birth,* 2nd ed. London, Mathews, 1789; American ed. printed at Philadelphia, Dobson, 1793.

any good but irons to the legs, for the support of the limbs, and en-enabling the patient to walk. At the end of four or five years, some have by this means got better, in proportion as they have acquired general strength; but some of these have been disposed to fall after-wards into pulmonary consumption, where the debility has not been entirely removed.

Underwood seems to have increased his clinical experience with these cases so that in the fourth English edition (1799), a description is added which gives a somewhat clearer picture of poliomyelitis than he had written in 1793.

Under a section on paralysis, or palsy, he said:

> The Palsy is a more common disorder in infants and young children than writers seem to have imagined, being confined to no age (having been seen as early as the third day after birth), and attacking children in very different degrees, in the manner it does adult persons. It, accordingly, sometimes seizes the upper, and sometimes the lower, extremities; in some instances, it takes away the entire use of the limbs it has attacked, and in others, only weakens them.[8]

Again in speaking of treatment during the first few days or weeks of the disease, as well as prognosis, Underwood has the following to say:

> The palsy in young subjects being usually attended with costiveness, calls for brisk purges in the first instance, and a repetition of opening medicines throughout the course of the complaint. And, indeed, if cathartics and blisters do not soon afford relief, the disorder usually becomes chronical, and the child sinks gradually in the course of a few months, or drags on a miserable life for ten or twelve years, with more or less debility of the arms or legs; but very rarely arrived at manhood.
>
> Besides teething infants, whom it has been said to attack, I have seen it in others who are older, and the finest children, . . . In any case, the only remedies I have found necessary, have been calomel or some other purgative; sometimes an emetic, and volatile embrocation[9] to the limbs. Electricity, I am told, has been advised in one instance; and if the complaint should not otherwise yield, may be properly had recourse to. . . .

It is a fair assumption that the great majority, but not all, of Underwood's infantile cases were examples of poliomyelitis. As was customary in

8. *Ibid.*, 4th ed. London, Mathews, 1799.

9. *Embrocation*, meaning to moisten or soak in. "The application in a fluid form, of volatile and spirituous ingredients, mostly used to relieve pains, numbness and palsies." *The American Medical Lexicon*. New York, T. and J. Swords, 1811.

textbooks of the eighteenth and early nineteenth centuries, orthodox methods of treatment and claims to their effectiveness are stressed at great
length. It would have been medical heresy in this era to have admitted that
a child had recovered by himself, so to speak, i.e. due to his own powers of
recuperation. Underwood doubtless believed that his methods of medical
treatment, in addition to the use of irons (braces), actually were beneficial.

To Underwood goes the credit for being the first physician to consider
poliomyelitis as an entity, and he recorded his observations accordingly. As
for a characteristic name, although he may have recognized "debility" or
"palsy" of infants as a special kind of affliction, he described it in loose
terms. Specific names were to be bestowed later.

According to Maloney,[10] who made an extensive study of Underwood's
life, he was apprenticed in 1754, at the age of sixteen, to one of London's
leading surgeons, a Caesar Hawkins who was "Serjeant Surgeon to George
II." He also served on the staff at St. George's Hospital for eight years, and
his name appears as the hospital house surgeon in 1761. He received the
Grand Diploma of the Company of Surgeons in 1764 and was duly registered as a member. That same year, at the age of twenty-seven, he began
practice in London but subsequently changed his line of activities, having
evinced skill as a physician accoucheur. He gradually rose to prominence
in the latter field, thus managing to receive the high appointment of Physician to the Princess of Wales.

One of the curious features about Underwood's career is that nowhere
among the several accounts of his life is his skill and experience as a children's doctor emphasized! Starting out life as a surgeon his attention was
concentrated on that specialty for a decade or more, especially upon the
cure of ulcers and sores. Indeed, in 1783 he issued a tract entitled: *A Treatise upon Ulcers of the Legs.*[11] It is said that "his business in ulcers may
have brought him more beggars than baronets," and, perhaps because of
this, in 1784 he applied for and was granted a license in midwifery from
the College of Physicians. By this move he lost the surgeon's franchise to
treat ulcers—"he was not supposed to touch them." For this breach, Underwood not only forfeited his membership in the Company of Surgeons, but
was fined twenty guineas as well. Later on, between 1800 and 1810, he suffered from a "severe indisposition, that in an instant almost precluded me
for several years from any attention to business." But his recovery from this
ailment enabled him to bring out in 1810 the sixth London edition of his

10. W. J. Maloney: Michael Underwood; A surgeon practising midwifery from 1764 to
1784. *J. Hist. Med.,* 5: 289–314, 1950.
11. It is recorded by Maloney that the Public Advertiser of November 19, 1783, announced:
This day is published/dedicated to Sir Caesar Hawkins, Bart./*A Treatise upon Ulcers of the
Legs* by Michael Underwood.

revised text, *Diseases of Children,* which proved to be an erudite work indeed—for that particular era.

Coincidentally with the period of Underwood's greatest reputation, in the final decade of the eighteenth century, there appeared in London another remarkable man, who was a mechanic by trade but an astute orthopedist by interest. Apparently he was the first person in eighteenth-century England to have had the vision to set about collecting and documenting a series of cases of deformities involving the foot and ankle. This was one Timothy Sheldrake, trussmaker to the Westminster Hospital in London. His interest seems to have developed as a result of his truly wide experience in handling crippling deformities in children, to which his ability to maintain a handsome shop in London testifies.

Sheldrake made an effort, unique at that time, to classify various kinds of deformities of the foot into some sort of order. In his first book, published in 1794, he described six cases of what seem to be orthodox examples of congenital clubfoot.[12] Late cases of paralytic poliomyelitis are not included. In his second book, however, published in 1798, trussmaker Sheldrake, besides enlarging the series to thirty-one cases, described other deformities as well, some of which were acquired in infancy and in all probability were cases of paralytic poliomyelitis. As indicated in the title of this second book he differentiated clubfoot from other distortions in the legs and feet of children.[13] And he also resigned himself to the belief that some deformities were not amenable to the best he could do in the way of mechanical support. In other words, he left no doubt that he sometimes failed. This is an example of the humble mechanic or artisan forging ahead of learned eighteenth-century doctors who were understandably loathe to document in writing their failures in therapy—except as their patients went down with the consumption.

Whether Sheldrake ever had the opportunity to see Underwood's popular book on diseases of children, the second edition of which had been published in 1789 (nine years before his own second book appeared), is not clear. Anyway, he was probably the first to collect and document a *series* of paralytic poliomyelitis cases. It was indeed a pioneer effort and a notable landmark in the history of the disease.

12. Modern usage has generally limited the use of the term clubfoot to a congenitally acquired deformity—so-called *pes talipes.*

13. T. Sheldrake: *A Practical Essay on the Club Foot and Other Distortions in the Legs and Feet of Children Intended to Show Under What Circumstances They are Curable or Otherwise, with 31 cases.* London, Murray & Highly, 1798. This went into two editions, the second published in 1806.

CHAPTER 4

The Beginnings of Clinical Recognition

Underwood's description of debility of the lower extremities in his *Diseases of Children* must have been brought to the attention of many physicians in Europe and America from 1793 to 1820, but there were few who took advantage of it. It was more or less typical of medical affairs in an age when "practitioners of medicine" kept their carefully guarded trade secrets, their medicines, and even their knowledge to themselves. It was an age when medical communication was none too good, and so probably it is not remarkable that it took some forty or fifty years for this affliction to begin to be recognized as anything other than a curiosity even in the most informed medical circles.

The vague name which Underwood gave to the disease did not help the cause along either. This casualness regarding medical nomenclature, which was also in keeping with current medical fashions, perhaps contributed to the obscurity that spelled failure for the early and universal recognition of infantile paralysis.

As a matter of fact, for the twenty-five years following Underwood's account, with the exception of a description by the Italian surgeon Monteggia, we hear very little about either debility of the lower extremities or paralysis in infants following fever. It was just as if the disease did not exist or had never been described. None of thirteen classifications of illnesses published between 1793 and 1818, which listed all the diseases known to the medical world, included a reference to it.[1] As far as the term paralysis was concerned, in the thirteen lists of diseases, descriptions were

1. A system of terminology of diseases which was published in 1818 by David Hosack of New York City included twelve other nosological systems by different European and British authors. His own represented the latest, but paralysis of infants fails to appear in any of the thirteen lists.

D. Hosack: *A System of Practical Nosology to which is prefixed the Systems of Sauvages, Linneaeus, Vogel, Sagar, MacBride, Cullen, Darwin, Crichton, Pinel, Parr, Swediaur, and Young with references to the best Authors on each Disease.* New York, C. S. Van Winkle, Printer to the University (of the State of New York), 1818.

After mentioning three anatomical types of "idiopathic paralysis," Hosack lists a number of references in an extensive footnote (on p. 216) to which the reader may be referred, including John Clarke's: *Commentaries on Diseases of Infants*, part the first. London, Longman, Hurst, Rees, Orme & Brown, 1815, whose mention of paralysis does not include anything remotely resembling poliomyelitis. But neither Underwood nor Monteggia receives any recognition from Hosack or Clarke.

limited to mention only of the anatomical parts involved, such as paralysis of one limb or two, or paralysis of one side of the body. There was nothing to indicate the age groups afflicted, and certainly nothing to indicate differences in regard to the cause of such paralysis, even allowing for the crude notions about etiology prevalent at that time.

One man who produced a detailed and accurate description of the disease in the early nineteenth century was the Italian physician and surgeon Giovanni Battista Monteggia (1762–1815), shown in figure 5. For a long

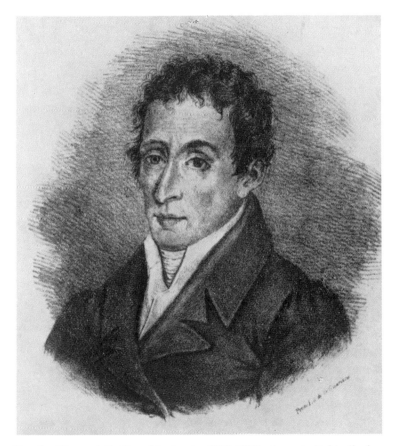

Fig. 5. Giovanni Battista Monteggia (1762–1815). A portrait kindly furnished by Dr. A. Giovanardi of Milan.

time the vivid description which appeared in the second edition of his *Instituzione Chirurgicale,* published in 1813,[2] seems to have received little notice outside of Italy. Monteggia mentioned that he had not yet found this kind of paralysis described in the literature, which certainly would in-

2. G. B. Monteggia: *Instituzione Chirurgicale,* 2nd ed., 8 vols. Milano, Guiseppe Maspero, 1813, vol. 1.

dicate that his observations were made independently. Suffice it to say that his was a more vivid account of poliomyelitis than that made by Underwood.

A translation of three passages from Monteggia's book follows:

Case IX. Paralysis and Atrophy

558. In this connection should be mentioned a certain kind of paralysis limited to one or the other of the lower extremities which I have observed several times in practice but have not yet found in the literature. It occurs in children who are nursing, or not much later; it begins with two or three days of fever, after which one of these extremities is found quite paralyzed, immobile, flabby, hanging down, and no movement is made when the sole of the foot is tickled. The fever ceases very soon, but the member remains immobile and regains with time only an imperfect degree of strength. I knew such a person who even when adult remained dragging a weak leg, for it had not become cured by time.

559. Likewise it often happens that the disease shows itself simultaneously in both the lower extremities, but this does not last long, since in one or two days the paralysis is reduced to one only.

560. I am not very certain as to the cause of this disease, but having observed that it comes with fever, and having recently seen it in a child accompanied by symptoms of dysentery makes me suspect that it comes from colic or rather a rheumatic affection.[3]

This creditable description leaves little doubt that the cases were examples of poliomyelitis. It also stamps Monteggia as a keen observer, certainly keener than most physicians and surgeons of his time. He must have had wide clinical experience to enable him to describe the clinical course from onset through late residual effects; furthermore he was apparently the first to record that the paralysis was flaccid and that there was no muscular response to sensory stimulation, no withdrawal of the foot when "the sole of the foot is tickled." His ideas as to the nature of the illness are vague, but it is to his credit that he makes no mention of teething as a possible cause.

As to events in Monteggia's short but busy life, these will be given only briefly.[4] He was born in 1762 in the small village of Laven on Lake Maggiore. At the age of seventeen he was admitted as a pupil at the Ospedale Maggiore of Milan, to be trained in medicine and surgery. He obtained his

---

3. A translation of paragraphs 558–60 in vol. 1 of the *Instituzione Chirurgicale* appears in: *A Bibliography of Infantile Paralysis, 1789–1949*. Prepared under the auspices of the National Foundation for Infantile Paralysis, ed. by Morris Fishbein, Ella M. Salmonsen (with Ludvig Hektoen), 2nd ed. Philadelphia, Lippincott, 1950.

4. I am indebted to Dr. A. Giovanardi, Instituto d'Igiene, University of Milan, Italy, for certain details of Monteggia's life.

surgical degree at the ancient University of Pavia in 1785 and his medical degree there three years later. He became a professor of surgery at the Ospedale Maggiore in Milan, and later professor of surgery and obstetrics at the "Pia Casa della Partoriente di S. Catarina della Ruota" in that city. Thus both Underwood and Monteggia were obstetricians who absorbed maternal and child health into their respective activities.

Monteggia was clearly a prodigious and able worker and accomplished a tremendous amount in a short life. He wrote a number of books[5] and as a member of the Commission of Health supervised the recently introduced program of smallpox vaccination. His concern was not only with surgery but also with *medicine* in all of its branches—pathology, internal medicine, pediatrics, obstetrics, and public health. It was probably this universality of interests that prompted him to include in his surgical text such a discerning account of poliomyelitis. The manner in which he was able to cope with such a multiplicity of interests in his eight-volume *System of Surgery* leaves one aghast. Happily he was rewarded in his own time by being elected to many academies and scientific institutions.

Although it is not my intention to document all medical writers of the first third of the nineteenth century who described an illness which might have been poliomyelitis, John Shaw, a London surgeon, is worthy of mention. His contribution appeared in a curious little book, published in 1823, which deals especially with distortions of the spine.[6] Here, besides giving a clinical description of paralysis and wasting of the limbs during infancy "which frequently produce distortion of the spine," he also refers to patients who acquired this affliction outside of England. He says: "I have been told that such sudden attacks are common among children in India and that strong and healthy children are more frequently affected than those of a weakly constitution." Shaw also mentions an English child that came under his treatment "who, during his childhood had lost power over one leg in the course of a single night." India might seem to be an exotic source of poliomyelitis, but this is not the case. It is probable that even in the early nineteenth century susceptible English children transported to India were exposed to an environment in which different strains of polioviruses existed and where the sanitary conditions were even more primitive than in England. This is reminiscent of similar occurrences which received attention some 120 years later—actually during World War II. Between 1941 and 1945 British troops in India, who had recently come out from

5. At the age of 27, Monteggia published his *Fasciculi Pathologici*. In 1791 he translated from German to Italian Fitze's *Compendium on Venereal Diseases,* and in that year published his own *Annotazioni sui Mali Venerei.* In this book he was the first to propose the surgical removal of uterine cancer.

6. J. Shaw: *On the Nature and Treatment of the Distortions to which the Spine and the Bones of the Chest are Subject.* . . . London, Longman Hurst et al., 1823.

England, suffered a relatively high incidence of poliomyelitis, much higher
than the rate in England during those years. This is thought to have been
due either to their having encountered new and different strains or types
of poliovirus or simply to greater exposure because of the poor sanitary environment into which they came as "susceptible immigrants." Apparently
geographic and environmental factors in the spread of this disease were
operative even at the beginning of the nineteenth century, although more
than 120 years were to pass before their significance was appreciated.

After Monteggia and Shaw, subsequent writers gradually added bits of
information to the clinical picture of poliomyelitis and attempted to explain its various features. Some authorities had the extraordinarily advanced view that the seat of the trouble was mainly in the spinal cord;
others were less impressed by this possibility. It remained for Abercrombie,
a Scottish neurologist, to surmise in 1828,[7] from neurophysiological information alone, that only a part of the gray matter of the cord was involved; namely, the *anterior* segment. This characteristic localization was
the reason, it may be recalled, that one of the names subsequently attached
to the disease was acute *anterior* poliomyelitis. That Abercrombie was able
to make this remarkable discovery was due to his awareness of the separate
functions of different parts of the spinal cord. Earlier in the century the
neurophysiological researches of Charles Bell of London and Magendie of
Paris had demonstrated a division of sensory and motor functions—the motor ones being controlled by nerve cells in the anterior part of the central
gray matter and the sensory ones by neurons in the posterior segment of the
cord. Abercrombie deduced that if the lesions of poliomyelitis were in the
spinal cord, they must be confined to the anterior part which controlled
motor nerves, since sensation, which depends on the posterior segment, was
not abolished in the paralytic case. This is one of the characteristic features
of paralytic poliomyelitis, and indeed it is used today as a diagnostic point.

However, the main historical landmark in the first half of the nineteenth
century was the appearance of a monograph by Jacob Heine (see fig. 6) in
1840.[8] It was the first proper study to which poliomyelitis had been subjected. The work was more than a review of cases. It was a meticulous, systematic, and discerning investigation which stemmed from long personal
experience of this German orthopedist and exponent of physical medicine.
Moreover it was a book devoted to all the features of the disease which
Heine felt were important—as of 1840. Indeed the Swedish pediatrician
Wickman, who was to come after Heine by more than half a century, felt
justified in naming the disease after him—obviously not because Heine had

7. J. Abercrombie: *Pathological and Practical Researches on Diseases of the Brain and the
Spinal Cord*. Edinburgh, Waugh and Innes, 1828.
8. J. Heine: *Beobachtungen über Lähmungszuztände der unteren Extremitäten und deren
Behandlung*. Stuttgart, Köhler, 1840.

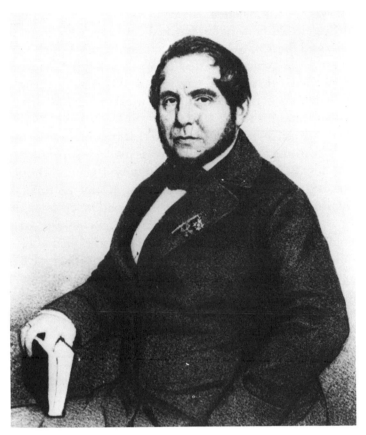

FIG. 6. Jacob von Heine (1800–79). From the Historical Library of the Yale University School of Medicine.

any claim or priority, but because he had made the earliest adequate study of it. Poliomyelitis went under the name of Heine-Medin disease for a dozen or more years.

The Heines were a family whose various members were intimately connected with orthopedic surgery.[9] Jacob's father, an ex-farrier, was the inventor of an extension bed; another member of the family, Bernard, was the first to use osteotomy in straightening bones. Jacob himself (1800–79) was a distinguished orthopedic surgeon of Cannstadt, a suburb of Stuttgart. His son Karl, later a professor at Prague, also became noted for his orthopedic writings.

Jacob Heine was prompted to report his own experiences with a series of paralyzed young patients after reading an account of four cases published by Badham in England in 1836. The small outbreak of English

9. J. Ruhräh and E. E. Mayer: *Poliomyelitis in All Its Aspects.* Philadelphia and New York, Lea & Febiger, 1917.

cases (which will be discussed in detail in the next chapter) had occurred
in 1835. Although Badham had described his cases accurately, he was at a
loss to understand their nature or how to treat them.

Heine's first monograph consisted of a seventy-eight-page volume with
seven lithographed full-page plates, mostly illustrating the condition of
affected limbs before correction and afterward as well as the types of apparatus used in rehabilitation. His abiding interest seems to have been in
long-term therapy with his own improved forms of braces and supports
and his own directions for the use of exercise machines for the development
of weak muscles. But Heine did not, as many a good orthopedist might
have done, confine his attention solely to improvements furnished by this
type of long-term care. In his series of fourteen juvenile cases of flaccid
paralysis he was also concerned with the early febrile stage of the disease
which preceded paralysis of limbs. He listed some characteristics which
were "prominent in almost every case." These points may have been noted
previously, but with Heine's report of such an impressive series of cases, the
clinical picture of poliomyelitis, at long last—after some fifty or more years
—began to take recognizable shape. His unusual list of prominent features
of the acute disease included the following:

1.   The age of the patient, viz. 6 to 36 months.
2.   The good general health preceding the illness and the strong, "blooming"
     bodily constitutions of the patients before the illness struck.
3.   The congestive, febrile, irritative, and convulsive manifestations which, in the
     majority of cases, immediately precede the paralysis.
4.   Pain, recognized in small children by their crying.
5.   In most of the cases the primary result of this affliction was paralysis of both
     lower extremities. There were almost no cerebral symptoms.

Heine concluded that, all in all, these symptoms "point to an affection of
the central nervous system, namely the spinal cord." He had intricate explanations to account for the transitory nature of the paralysis in some
cases, but it is unnecessary to dwell on these. His recommendations on the
subject of therapy were eminently sensible. He lived in an era when purges,
emetics, blisters and bleedings, and similar drastic treatments were the order of the day, but he apparently steered clear of these fashionable remedies. For the aftercare of his patients he preferred instead to use exercise,
baths, and various simple surgical procedures, followed by the application
of braces and apparatus which were well illustrated in his monograph.
Considering the degree to which the handling of a given disease is wont to
change over a period of 125 years, Heine's treatment of paralyzed limbs
and the resulting deformities and disabilities of children has undergone
remarkably little alteration.

In addition, a feature which distinguished and dignified Heine's effort is that he did his best to answer the questions that had greatly concerned the young British physician Dr. John Badham,[10] of whom we shall hear in the following chapter. There is no suggestion of an attempt to display his own knowledge in order to give the impression that he was a great authority or knew more about the disease than anybody else. He was just trying to be helpful. Indeed a very real contribution which he made rests in no small measure on this attitude.

In 1860, a second edition of Heine's book appeared, this time under the title of *Spinale Kinderlähmung*.[11] He had evidently become more convinced in the twenty-year interim that the seat of the trouble was in the spinal cord. This time the author appears as Jacob von Heine, and the name is followed by a considerable list of titles and honors that had been bestowed upon him.

However, in spite of Heine's substantial contribution in 1840, knowledge was to proceed at a snail's pace. Isolated cases or small groups of cases were reported in several different countries, but little was added to an understanding of the nature of the illness. Henry Kennedy, a prominent Irish physician, described the disease in a series of two papers,[12] the second of which was promptly translated into French and German. He does not mention Heine in his first article, and it is fair to presume that he did not know of his work. Kennedy observed that in certain instances the paralysis disappeared promptly and cure was complete; such cases he classified as "the temporary paralysis of early life." He believed that there was no organic lesion in many cases and deplored the tendency of the day to relate nervous diseases accompanied by paralysis to lesions within either the brain or cord. This was a step decidedly in the wrong direction. Yet such a view was taken up enthusiastically by the French observers De Nancy[13] and Rilliet,[14] who were definitely opposed to Heine's hypothesis of a spinal origin of the disease. One of the reasons that the term "essential infantile paralysis" was suggested was the apparent absence of gross pathological lesions in either the brain or cord in fatal cases on which autopsies had been performed. Not until some years later were the cord lesions of poliomyelitis, invisible to the naked eye, revealed by the microscope.

At this time, in 1843, the Englishman West, who was responsible for

10. J. Badham: Paralysis in childhood; four remarkable cases of suddenly induced paralysis in the extremities occurring in children without any apparent cerebral or cerebrospinal lesion. *Lond. med. Gaz., 17*: 215, 1834–35.

11. J. v. Heine: *Spinale Kinderlähmung*. Stuttgart, Cotta, 1860.

12. H. Kennedy: Observations on paralytic affections met with in children. *Dublin med. Press, 6*: 201–04, 1841; On some of the forms of paralysis which occur in early life. *Dublin, Quart. J. med. Sci., 9*: 85, 1850.

13. Richard de Nancy: Un mot sur la paralysie essentielle chez les enfants. *Bull. gén. Thérap., 36*: 120, 1849.

14. F. Rilliet: De la paralysie essentielle chez les enfants. *Gaz. méd. Paris, 6*: 681–704, 1851.

coining the clinical term "morning paralysis," wrote about poliomyelitis[15] and described it in his *Diseases of Children*. It was a term quite appropriate for that era.

At least one account, published by A. G. Walter in 1840, carries with it the suggestion that the disease had occurred in America, in Ohio, as early as 1810.[16] Walter was a surgeon from Pittsburgh, and something of a specialist in orthopedics. In the tradition of Timothy Sheldrake of London and Heine of Cannstadt, he had had the opportunity of seeing a sizable group of patients who might be described as "the lame and the halt," but, unlike Heine, he was not interested in the whole disease—only in the surgical treatment of its late effects. Walter's motive in publishing a large series of cases was apparently to further a special form of operative treatment at which he was adept. His story begins at the time that operations for clubfoot[17] first became popular in America.[18]

In 1833 the Hanoverian surgeon Strohmeyer had announced an operation for partially relieving the deformity of clubfoot.[19] The procedure consisted of subcutaneous section of the Achilles tendon. Such an operation had been performed previously, but Strohmeyer seems to have developed and improved it. As a result it was immediately and enthusiastically taken up by European surgeons, as is evident from reports from France and England. Surgeons in the United States soon followed suit, the first report[20] appearing in 1838; during the next four or five years there were several papers in American medical literature dealing with results of cutting tendons in clubfoot. Walter's paper describing his results in a large number of patients appeared in 1840, the same year in which Heine's first monograph was published. He had only arrived in Pittsburgh in 1837 but had

15. C. West. On some forms of paralysis incidental to infancy and childhood. *London med. Gaz., 32*: 829, 1843.

16. A. G. Walter: Observations of tenotomia and myotomia, for the cure of deformed members; anatomically, physiologically and therapeutically considered. With seventy-four cases. *Select med. Library and Eclectic J. Med., 4*: 385, 421, 1840.

A note on Walter's series of cases was published by the writer in 1936. J. R. Paul: A note on the early history of infantile paralysis in the United States. *Yale J. Biol. Med., 8*: 643–48, 1936.

17. It will be recalled that in the mid-nineteenth century the term clubfoot was not limited to deformities of congenital origin (see chap. 3).

18. I am indebted to Dr. W. McD. Hammon of the University of Pittsburgh for certain details regarding A. G. Walter's biography and particularly to Dr. Thomas G. Benedek of the Department of Medicine, School of Medicine, University of Pittsburgh, who was able to locate for me a chapter on Walter, in *Pioneer Medicine in Western Pennsylvania,* by Theodore Diller, New York, Hoeber, 1927, pp. 139–64.

19. L. Strohmeyer: Die Durchschneidung der Achillessehne, als Heilmittel des Klumpfusses, durch zwei Fälle erläutert. *Mag. ges. Heilk., 39*: 195, 1833.

20. W. Detmold: Report of several cases of successful operation for clubfoot by the division of the tendo achilles, with remarks. *Amer. J. med. Sci., 22*: 105–16, 1938.

immediately set up shop there as an orthopedic surgeon. Since he was pre-pared to carry out the new operation for clubfoot, it is likely that many patients in whom this had been an old problem flocked to him, eager for the new treatment. This, rather than an "epidemic of clubfoot," accounted for his ability to collect such a large series of cases in so short a time.

Walter described seventy-four tenotomy or myotomy operations per-formed between September 1837 and February 1840. The majority were on patients with congenital clubfoot, but about a third were for deformities resulting from acquired lesions. The case histories are brief, and it is evi-dent that the author was not particularly interested in the circumstances under which his patients had developed deformities. A brief extract from one of his five case reports is transcribed:

> *Case XII.* Everted clubfoot in a very aggravated state, consequent on paralysis of the muscles of the front and inner side of the leg.
>
> Miss Anne Long, of Bloomsfield, Jefferson County, Ohio, thirty years of age, was operated on May 15, 1839, for everted clubfoot of the left extremity. The deformity commenced after an attack of fever when she was a year old, and grew worse as she advanced in years.

Six other such cases are included in Walter's series. Furthermore, a few similar ones may be found in other contemporary reports of the treatment of deformed extremities, notably two described in 1841 by Chase of Phil-adelphia.[21]

Walter's brief case reports seem to represent examples of poliomyelitis. The ages of the patients at the time of onset are typical, the muscles affected are those commonly involved in poliomyelitis, and there are other sugges-tive details. One gathers therefore that paralysis acquired during infancy was not regarded by either Walter or Chase as an unusual event; the earli-est of Walter's cases (no. XII) occurred in 1810; others are listed as having onsets between 1817 and 1835, the period in which fragmentary accounts of the disease appeared in England and Italy. Walter seems to have accepted "teething" as a cause, thus agreeing with the opinions of his time. From these reports it would seem probable that during the early part of the nine-teenth century, poliomyelitis was not uncommon in this country, at least not in Pennsylvania.

Confirming the idea that early nineteenth-century cases of paralysis in infants were not rare in America is an item which appeared in an Ameri-can edition of Underwood's *Diseases of Children,* published in Philadel-phia in 1818, with notes supplied by a "physician of Philadelphia." This

21. H. Chase: Report of cases of deformed feet, treated by mechanical means, with a description of the apparatus employed. *Amer. J. med. Sci.,* n.s., *1:* 88–99, 1841.

physician, commenting on Underwood's text describing the treatment of acute palsy, saw fit to insert the following footnote:

> The plan of treatment here detailed, is very similar to that adopted by the best practitioners in the United States. It is only requisite for me to make one farther observation, which is, that in addition to cathartics and blisters, we use the lancet without hesitation, wherever circumstances seem to demand it.[22]

From the dates of Walter's cases we can add little to the early history of epidemics of poliomyelitis in the United States. One cannot say whether a small outbreak occurred in the 1830s in the Pittsburgh area, which enabled him to collect a series of such cases, although four or five of his patients suffered their attacks sometime between 1832 and 1835. It is perhaps far more reasonable to assume that these were sporadic cases.

22. M. Underwood: *Diseases of Children; Notes by a Physician of Philadelphia,* 6th London ed., 3 vols. in one. Philadelphia, James Webster, 1818, vol. 1, p. 82.

CHAPTER 5

Outbreaks of Paralysis in the
Mid-Nineteenth Century

Up to this point I may have given the impression that no one who described poliomyelitis had seemed very concerned about its epidemiological nature. Nor had anyone thought it was contagious. An occasional physician surely must have pondered the question why a healthy child should suddenly become paralyzed in one or both lower limbs, with the added tragedy that this paralysis was apt to last throughout life. But physicians and laymen alike were beset by so many imponderables about illness in the mid-nineteenth century and before that they accepted these tragedies as inexplicable episodes which occurred in the natural course of man's journey through life. Pestilences, high infant mortality, and all manner of diseases whose causes and natures remained totally obscure to physicians and laymen alike were routine before 1850.

Two common ailments, smallpox and measles, had been recognized as contagious for centuries, having been described by the Arabian physician Rhazes[1] as early as the year 900, but beyond that all was apt to be confusion. By the eighteenth and early part of the nineteenth centuries physicians were indulging in endless speculations on the questions of contagion and infection (certainly the line between them was very fine indeed),[2] and it must be admitted that such speculations were often, although not always, far from illuminating. Europe was plagued at this time with all kinds of devastating epidemic diseases. These were variously attributed to comets, earthquakes, storms, and other absurd causes, and even to the poisoning of wells by Jews.

Nevertheless, it is small wonder that these intricate puzzles regarding infection and the genesis of epidemics, which still pose real problems today,

1. Rhazes: *A Treatise on the Small-pox and Measles,* trans. by W. A. Greenhill. London, Sydenham Soc., 1848.

2. Early nineteenth-century definitions of these two terms were:

"*Contagion* . . . a secreted humour from a living vascular surface of a poisonous quality and capable of exciting disease . . ."

"*Infection* is that manner of communicating disease by some effluvia, or particles which fly off from distempered bodies, and mix with juices of others which occasion the same disorders as in the bodies they came from." *The American Medical Lexicon.* New York, T. and J. Swords, 1811.

defied even an attempt at solution in the eighteenth century. Was a certain disease contagious? Or could it be attributed to poisoning similar to the kind Thomas Cadwalader of Philadelphia described in his *Essay on the West-Indian Dry-Grippes* (published by Benjamin Franklin, 1745)? This was an account of a veritable "epidemic" of chronic lead poisoning from the drinking of rum distilled in coils of lead pipe. Certainly the high incidence of the "dry-grippes," particularly among some social classes, must have suggested contagion. Even in modern times the question of deciding whether a given disease is infectious or not can be most difficult. In addition one may be reminded that it was not until the mid-nineteenth century that those who pondered the cause of epidemic disease had anything but the most primitive ideas of contagion or of the meaning of *contagium vivum* (except perhaps in relation to vaccination with cowpox). How one could have comprehended the concept of infection in the eighteenth or early nineteenth century, considering the then current ideas, is difficult to imagine.

The vitriolic arguments which ensued over the causes of the outbreaks of yellow fever that swept Philadelphia in the· 1790s were an example of the extent to which the general public could become embroiled in such questions. Could the disease be spread from person to person? Or was the whole place infected by a polluted atmosphere? Or was it as Rush (1745–1813), that outstanding Philadelphia physician, maintained, from piles of rotting coffee? Or as that amateur American epidemiologist Noah Webster claimed, defending his concept of contagion—a kind of "septic acid" which operated at a maximum distance of ten paces?[3]

In any event, there was no idea in the eighteenth and early nineteenth centuries that poliomyelitis was contagious. It is reasonable to imagine that the clustering of half a dozen cases of paralysis in infants in time or place, i.e. within half a mile or so of each other, would not have been regarded by the rank and file as an epidemic or indeed as an ominous occurrence. Had there been larger outbreaks in the early or mid-nineteenth century it seems highly unlikely that they would have gone unnoticed.

Actually it was not until the mid-1830s that physicians began to report small groups of poliomyelitis cases which had occurred almost simultaneously. Probably the earliest of these on record is the well-known outbreak recorded by Badham in England in 1835.[4] Badham's outbreak occurred in the midland town of Worksop, which is in Nottinghamshire and near the

3. N. Webster: *A Brief History of Epidemic and Pestilential Diseases; with the Principal Phenomena of the Physical World which precede and accompany them,* 2 vols. Hartford, Hudson & Goodwin, 1799.

4. J. Badham: Paralysis in childhood; four remarkable cases of suddenly induced paralysis in the extremities, occurring in children, without any apparent cerebral or cerebro-spinal lesion. *London med. Gaz.,* n.s., *17*: 215, 1834–35; J. Badham: Paralysie chez les enfants. *Gaz. méd. Paris,* 1835, p. 825.

city of Sheffield. The four cases described reflect the extent of his keen observations and a mood of understandable puzzlement and anxiety. It was
an example of how a well-trained, conscientious, and sensitive physician,
faced with an emergency, went all out to meet it—as best he could:

Case I. Ann Hare, aged 2 years, was brought to me by her mother, on
the 14th of August, with paralysis of the right leg. Her account of this
seizure was as follows:

The child had enjoyed uninterrupted health to the evening of her attack, with the exception (if, indeed, it can be so-called) of slightly
augmented thirst and some drowsiness, not remembered by the
mother to have preceded the seizure by two days. On the evening of
the 13th the child was put to bed, having run about and amused herself as usual during the day. On the following morning her mother's
attention was first attracted, in dressing her, to an unusual appearance
of the eyes, which as she said, appeared to be turned inwards. A new
cause of apprehension presented itself in putting the child on her feet,
when it was found she could not stand. Medical advice being immediately sought for, it was thought sufficient, I understand, to keep the
bowels open and to employ a warm bath. No advantage, however, being procured under this treatment, she was brought to me on the
14th; a week after her attack. Her *appearance* at this time did not
denote *any* disease—she was playing in her mother's lap; but on accurately examining the two limbs, it was found that *motion* in the right
was completely destroyed, and in the left somewhat diminished;
while *sensation,* perfect in the left limb, was impaired, without being
suspended, in the other. At this period there was neither wasting of
the limb nor diminution of temperature. Strabismus[5] very decided;
the pupil drawn to the inner canthus, and the eyeball fixed there, as I
found in attempting to direct the vision outwards, and the pupil on
the same side as the palsied limb was dilated. No disturbance of constitution could be traced from teething, or from torpor of the bowels;
nor on examining the spine attentively, could I detect any tenderness
on pressure.

I directed calomel in repeated doses, cold applications to the head,
blisters to the spine, and cataplasms[6] to the affected limb. Under this
treatment the drowsiness was removed in five days. On the fourth, indeed, from its adoption, the ball of the right eye became suddenly
liberated from its constrained position; the other eye recovered more
slowly, a few days afterwards. The limb now shows (on the 15th of October) some return of sensibility, but the temperature is considerably

5. Strabismus: squinting (Footnotes to this quotation are mine.)
6. Cataplasms: poultices.

below that of the other, and loss of substance has proceeded to a considerable extent. The exercise of the will over the affected extremity though entirely abolished at first, has now partially returned, inasmuch as she no longer drags the limb after her, as she at first did, but projects or flings it forward with a jerk, the direction and force of which she seems not to have the slightest power to moderate or control.

Badham's other three cases which occurred a few days after the fourteenth and were all in infants under three years of age were described with similar meticulous detail. In one he went on to give his treatment but says that the limb remains "perfectly palsied and useless though sensation has been somewhat restored"; in another, "The limb is now after a lapse of nearly two months, hopelessly paralyzed, and swings like a suspended object attached to the body." In his discussion Dr. Badham comments on:

1. The extreme youth of these patients.
2. The fact that in each case the paralysis was ushered in by some apparent cerebral symptoms, i.e. drowsiness and an abnormal state of the pupils of the eye.
3. The remarkable fact "that in no instance has the health of the child been in any degree impaired."
4. Derangement of eye muscles in one case which leads us "to suspect a cerebral complication, rather than a spinal one."[7]

Badham promptly wrote up his four cases of paralysis and submitted them for publication within six to eight weeks of their onsets, thus allowing himself little time for a long-term follow-up of his patients. This prompt submission of the report for publication was made in an apparent effort to seek immediate advice from as wide an audience as he could muster. Particularly with regard to treatment was he anxious to obtain ideas.

He went on to say:

> The above cases (of which the first was seen some time ago by Dr. Outram,[8] and three of the four subsequently by my father, Professor Badham),[9] may probably suggest analogous ones in the experience of some few of your readers, who may also be able to help me to a treatment from experience; for we know nothing of the intimate character of any species of palsy, so as to manage it philosophically, and to adopt a medication without a defined object.

7. The muscles of the eye and face are commonly affected in poliomyelitis when the inflammatory lesion involves the base of the brain or brain stem.

8. It has been suggested that the Dr. Outram mentioned above may have been Sir Benjamin Fonseca Outram (1774–1856) who was closely associated with the navy as a surgeon to the royal sovereign's yacht, and in 1841 was inspector of fleets and hospitals (Munk's *Roll*, 3: 90–91).

9. The elder Badham was Professor Charles Badham, professor of medicine at the University of Glasgow, who in 1808 gave the first description of chronic bronchitis, even before that of Laennec.

A view which admits of being stated in intelligible language, is scarcely medicine. Some would doubtless in these cases recommend issues; some would counsel electricity; others would put me in mind of Arnica, or other *soi-disant* remedies for palsy; but I am unwilling to disturb the digestive and nutritive functions in such young subjects and would rather count on these important processes as my auxiliaries, than venture on equivocal remedies which may, or rather must, depress them. I shall be thankful, however, for any suggestion, for it is lamentable indeed to witness one of the most humiliating infirmities of age inflicted on infancy! Perhaps one may reasonably expect some of the little patients to outgrow their disastrous conditions, unless it shall be concluded that palsy in such instances is only an unusual and early evidence of deeply latent cerebral mischief.

Even though these cases of infantile paralysis apparently occurred within a few days or weeks of one another in the same community, Badham makes no suggestion regarding the possibility of contagion. Considering the views of his time, he was justified in this.

An abbreviated French review of Badham's paper, which he must have been glad to see, appeared promptly in the *Gazette médicale de Paris* (see n.4):

This paper reports four remarkable cases of paralysis of the lower extremities which appeared suddenly in infants, without any apparent evidence of a cerebral or cerebro-spinal lesion.

As none of these four cases was fatal, it will be impossible to say whether the lesion was in the neck or the spine, as the title seems to indicate.

The French reviewer went on to point out that, as observations of this kind were rare, particularly in infants as young as the ones described, the attention of those readers who might be able to throw some light on the questions Dr. Badham has raised was solicited.

If this French report is accurate, it emphasizes the *uniqueness* of the situation, not only in England but also on the Continent. Luckily, Badham's report had the desired effect of attracting the attention of Jacob Heine in Germany, who responded handsomely by making the most important contribution to the cause of infantile paralysis which had been made so far, although Badham did not live to see it.

Reasons for the occurrence of Badham's summer outbreak are certainly not clear. Possibly it was just a cluster of cases which came along at a time when and where a young conscientious physician was ready with a mind prepared to recognize the significance of the cases and to report the incident. There is little to suggest that a shift in environmental sanitation had occurred just at that particular time in the little town of Worksop. Nor was there evidence that the infection spread elsewhere throughout the countryside.

Fortunately we have some information[10] about John Badham. He was born in 1807 and graduated from the University of Glasgow in 1828. Before his graduation he had begun to suffer from tuberculosis, which caused his death at an early age. There is an extract from the university minutes of October 1828 that refers to John Badham as having had a degree conferred on him "without personal examination as severe illness renders it necessary to leave this country for a warmer climate without delay."

A section from an obituary note that appeared in 1840 is given, in part, below:

> The fatal disease (phthisis) to which at length he fell a victim, began to develop itself in its least equivocal signs fourteen years ago, at which period it consigned him, as apparently his only chance, to the solitude of a small West India Island, from which, after a few years' residence, and a fallacious truce, he, perhaps unfortunately, returned to settle in England. Soon after his arrival, he was induced . . . to undertake the medical charge of the Duke of Newcastle's family at Clumber, and settled in the neighboring town of Worksop; but in the course of two or three winters, finding his complaints aggravated . . . it became necessary to give up his post, and to place himself in a less inconstant climate, and admit duties at once more grateful and more easily performed.[11]

Subsequently he sought relief in the more salubrious climates of Touraine, southern France, and Italy. He died in his thirty-third year in Nice, in 1840.

It was in the period of the "fallacious truce" and after his return from the West Indies to England that Badham encountered his poliomyelitis "epidemic," and was able to describe the cases accurately and to voice his apprehension about the seriousness of the situation. His prompt action in publishing an account of the puzzling cases in order to seek a wider audience and to benefit from the advice of someone more experienced with the disease than himself was a manifestation of the real concern of an anxious physician.

But there was another appealing side to young Dr. Badham's life which was also brought out in the obituary note:

10. I am indebted for this information to Prof. C. H. Stuart-Harris of the University of Sheffield, and to Dr. C. E. Newman, Harveian Librarian of the Royal College of Physicians, London.

11. W. I. Addison: *Roll of the graduates of the University of Glasgow, 1727–1897*, 1908, p. 26; also obituary note on Dr. John Badham. *London med. Gaz., 26*: 559–60, 1840.

Several pages . . . on the diseases of the West Indies, have scarcely been overlooked by the readers of the MEDICAL GAZETTE; his extensive knowledge of the moral and social condition of the negro was exhibited in a series of Letters, . . . was sufficient to show the lively interest he took in public affairs, and the possession of much more than ordinary insight into what was going on in the world in questions which affect the improvement and the happiness of mankind.

One cannot help feeling a twinge of sadness over the premature demise of this capable and conscientious young physician. It was a pity he did not live to see Heine's significant work on the subject of poliomyelitis, prompted by his own report. This would have been a rewarding experience for him and perhaps others, including the editors of the *Gazette médicale de Paris*.

The next recorded outbreak was to occur far afield and under totally different circumstances, on the island of St. Helena. An account is given by Sir Charles Bell (1774–1842), the distinguished British neurologist. It may indeed have been a first, superseding Badham's outbreak, but Bell did not give the exact date; even the time of his consultation on one of its victims is unspecified. It is more than probable however that he saw the patient after 1830 but before 1836. Circumstances under which the St. Helena cases occurred are a bit more understandable than the Worksop "epidemic."

The transcription of Bell's account is as follows:

Case 183. A lady, whose husband was the English Clergyman at St. Helena, consulted me about her child, who had one leg much wasted in its growth. In conversing about the illness which preceded this affection in her little girl, she mentioned that an epidemic fever spread among all the children in the island about three or five years of age; and her child was ill of the same fever. It was afterwards discovered that all the children who had the fever, were similarly affected with a want of growth in some part of their body or limbs! This deserves to be inquired into.[12]

---

12. C. Bell: *The Nervous System of the Human Body as Explained in a Series of Papers Read Before the Royal Society of London,* 3rd ed. London, H. Renshaw, 1844, pp. 434–35.
I can find no record of any second edition of this work. It may have been simply a reprinting. It seems obvious that the third edition must have been printed at least two times, once in Edinburgh in 1836, and again in London in 1844. The Edinburgh printing of 1836 contains an account of the St. Helena outbreak, but there is no mention of it in the first edition, which appeared in 1830 and included far fewer cases in its appendix than did the third. It was in the third edition that the St. Helena case appears as case no. 183. Although Bell sometimes arranged his cases in chronological order, he often did not; yet it is pertinent to mention that case no. 182 may have been seen very shortly after 1832, and definitely before 1836.

The first important thing that can be learned from this brief account is that the outbreak occurred on an isolated island. This is reminiscent of the circumstances which surround remote populations in the Pacific today, where many such islands have experienced devastating poliomyelitis epidemics even within recent times. In other words, it is natural and understandable that one of the earliest recorded outbreaks should have been in a community where juvenile visitors from the outside were not the rule. Another feature is that children, presumably native-born children, over the age of three years were afflicted, i.e. those of "3 or 5 years of age." This slight increase in age, even though almost insignificant, suggests that a population of susceptible young children had reached the age of three to five years without having been exposed to or infected with poliovirus. Thus an interval of supposedly not over five years had elapsed since poliovirus had last been introduced and circulated on the island of St. Helena.

Another incidental feature is the implication that the epidemic had taken place some years before the child was brought to London for consultation. Mention that her leg "was much wasted in its growth" is evidence for this, because it usually takes some time for "a want of growth" in a child's limb to become clearly evident. Since the case was reported in 1836, it dates the outbreak to some time before that year; not that this is important, except perhaps as a matter of priority.

But a most significant statement in Bell's report of case no. 183 is his final comment, "This deserves to be inquired into." Coming from one of the most distinguished neurologists of his time, and one with a wealth of experience, this clearly sounded a note of concern. Sir Charles was interested not only in how to treat the disease, but also in its nature and in the circumstances under which it occurred. Certainly, Bell's question should have aroused some sort of inquiry, but there is no evidence that it did. And yet it was a milestone in the history of the disease—it marked the beginning of that period when physicians, apart from treating the disease, recognized a situation or circumstances that deserved to be looked into.

Charles Bell (1774–1842) was born in Edinburgh and educated at the University of Edinburgh. While there, he devoted himself briefly to the study of anatomy under the direction of his brother John. Like John, Charles was an artist of talent and one of the medical men who illustrated his own books with distinction. In 1804, like so many Scottish physicians, he went to London, where his main reputation as a neurologist was made. He was appointed professor of anatomy, physiology, and surgery in the College of Surgeons, and surgeon to the Middlesex Hospital in London. In the course of his experiments and observations of neurologic problems he discerned that different nerve functions are related to different parts of the brain. In 1811 he made the first recorded reference to experiments which indicated the differential functions of the spinal nerve roots. It is said, however, that he failed to recognize the significance of his discovery, believing that all nerve roots were to some extent sensory. The crucial experiments in this field remained to be performed by the Parisian neurophysiologist François Magendie (1783–1855), who in 1822 demonstrated that the anterior roots of the spinal column are motor and the posterior ones sensory.[13]

In 1815, Bell enormously enhanced his experience with nerve injuries by going to Brussels to treat the wounded who were arriving there from the battle of Waterloo, an example to be followed by the distinguished American neurologist Weir Mitchel some fifty years later, whose treatise, *Injuries of Nerves and their Consequences* (1872), dealt largely with wounded soldiers in the American Civil War. Bell's name is sufficiently distinguished to maintain a place in history, if only from his description of Bell's palsy or facial paralysis, which is a common variety of unilateral paralysis of the muscles of the face due to involvement of the seventh cranial nerve in its peripheral course. It is said that Sir Charles was a genial, unaffected, kind-hearted man with a captivating twinkle behind his eyeglasses (see fig. 7).

The last of the three important early poliomyelitis outbreaks was reported from Louisiana, in the United States. It had more cases than either of the two mentioned above, and the claim has been made that it was the first "real epidemic." It was described by Colmer in a short note which appeared in a leading American medical journal, but because of the brevity of clinical details, it is the least important report of the three which occurred between 1835 and 1841. The Louisiana account has often been quoted:

Medical Notes. By George Colmer.

Paralysis in Teething Children.—Whilst on a visit to the parish of West Feliciana, La., in the fall of 1841, my attention was called to a child about a year old, then slowly recovering from an attack of hemiplegia. The parents (who were people of intelligence and unquestionable veracity), told me that eight or ten other cases of either hemiplegia or paraplegia, had occurred during the preceding three or four months within a few miles of their residence, all of which had either completely recovered, or were decidedly improving. The little sufferers were invariably under two years of age, and the cause seemed to be the same in all—, namely *teething.*[14]

13. F. Magendie: Expériences sur les fonctions des racines des nerfs rachidiens. *J. Physiol. exp. Pathol.,* 2: 276–79, 1822.

14. G. Colmer: Paralysis in teething children. *Amer. J. med. Sci.,* n.s., 5: 248, 1843.

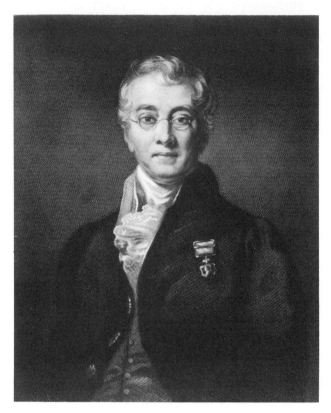

Fig. 7. Charles Bell (1774–1842). From the Historical Library of Yale University School of Medicine.

This sounds like an epidemic of poliomyelitis cases in a setting in which the infection was normally endemic. As is usual under these circumstances, the cases involved infants—all were "invariably under two years." But Dr. Colmer seems to have reported this outbreak somewhat belatedly, and rather as a newspaper item.

Thanks to Dr. Casey of Birmingham, Alabama, we have details of Dr. Colmer's life.[15] He was born in London in 1807 but eventually settled in Springfield, Louisiana, which is about thirty miles from West Feliciana. Apparently Dr. Colmer had many activities besides the practice of medicine. He served as a justice of the peace, published a local newspaper, and was active in various real estate transactions as well as in civic duties. His diaries, which have been preserved, include numerous records of who caught the largest fish, who got prizes at the local flower and vegetable show. It would seem that the West Feliciana epidemic was reported in this

15. A. E. Casey and E. H. Hidden: George Colmer and the epidemiology of poliomyelitis. *Southn. med. J., 37*: 471–77, 1944.

same vein and not as an event which aroused his medical curiosity or in which he felt the need of exercising much clinical or scientific judgment.

These three small outbreaks in England, St. Helena, and Louisiana were the harbingers of things to come. There must have been many more unreported ones like them, before and immediately afterward. It was not, however, until the 1860s, when larger outbreaks were observed in Scandinavia, that any opinions for or against contagion in this disease began to appear.

CHAPTER 6

New Approaches in Medicine, Pathology, and Bacteriology
The Beginnings of Neuropathology

The second third of the nineteenth century saw the emergence in Europe of a new type of medicine which attained its stature largely through advances in physiology and pathology. A sudden burst of interest in these fields, coupled with a rapid growth of research activities, had a large share in raising clinical medicine to the dignity of a science.

Paris became the early and flourishing center for pathology, largely through the influence of Pierre-Charles-Alexandre Louis (1787–1872), who ardently pursued the subject as an essential adjunct to clinical medicine. At the start, mentors of the school of pathology were not without opposition, particularly from those who advocated that more weight should be attached to symptoms exhibited by patients than to the demonstration of anatomical alterations caused by disease. These opponents argued from the inescapable position that all diseases are abstract entities created by man. Indeed, they had a point there. But what spurred on the early pathological anatomists was that they had discovered, and were in possession of, the necessary evidence—the lesions, which are the basis of symptoms and signs of a given disease. These were firm hooks to which concepts of disease could be attached. Such an approach was fundamental to accurate clinical diagnosis. Ultimately the tide turned in favor of the pathologists and their more scientific approach.

Places where the new teaching in medicine prevailed somewhat later were Dublin and London. In London the "great men of Guy's" Hospital contributed mightily. Thus French and British physicians became workers in the same fruitful vineyard, sharing similar points of view and laying the foundations of a new kind of clinical medicine. This revolution, due to an abrupt mutation in ideas, took place in a few decades. It continues to remain one of the wonders of medical history.

During this same period of the nineteenth century German medicine had been floundering in the jungles of romantic speculation and natural philosophy. Vienna was the first place in the Germanic world where the new approach was adopted. Here the pathologist Rokitansky became a leader as Professor of Pathological Anatomy in Vienna, in 1844. His department became a famous gathering place for young physicians. Also into the German arena came the remarkable figure, Rudolf Virchow (see fig. 8). Virchow's primary influence in medicine was in the field of cellular pathology, but he was three-dimensional in stature—practically a universal genius. As an exponent of microscopic pathology he gave impetus to this

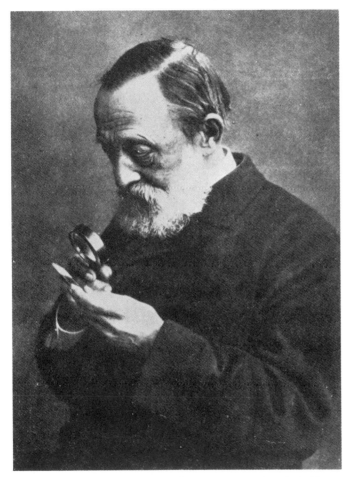

FIG. 8. Rudolph Virchow (1821–1902). From the Historical Library of the Yale University School of Medicine.

science. In addition he was a statesman and a student of anthropology and archaeology.[1] It is said that it was he who guided Schliemann in his discovery of Troy and its excavation. Together they made several archaeological expeditions to the Near East.

Yet it was in the field of cellular pathology that Virchow was supreme. He was lucky here. The magnifying power of microscopes had been

1. E. H. Ackerknecht: *Rudolf Virchow; Doctor, Statesman, Anthropologist.* Madison, Univ. of Wisconsin Press, 1953.

brought to such a degree of perfection by the early nineteenth century that cellular and tissue changes which had long been invisible could now be detected. German medicine, after languishing for so long, awoke to vigorous activity which was soon to give it a leading position in the world.

Coincidentally the science of physiology began to assume its rightful place. One physiological institute after another sprang up in the various German universities. These two major branches of medical science, physiology and pathological anatomy, set clinical medicine free to develop its own scientific potential. Germany thus emerged as a tardy pioneer in the medical sciences, following France and England.

In the meantime, how did the concept of the specificity of diseases fare in this upsurge of new ideas? At first German physiologists were loud in their condemnation of the view that a disease could be construed as a definite entity, claiming that such an interpretation mistook abstract concepts for realities. This view was not without justification considering that sometimes the newly created diseases masqueraded in different clinical forms as a result of involvement of different organs. What was evidently lacking in the argument put forth by the proponents for the specificity of diseases was the concept of etiology. That too was to come in due time, indeed quite promptly, for bacteriology soon joined the other disciplines as an emerging science. But pathologists had at least been on the right track.

It may be almost impossible for us to imagine the incredulity with which the "germ theory" of disease was greeted when first proposed as a general doctrine in the latter part of the nineteenth century. Many of the older and more staid members of the medical profession greeted it sullenly. Some remained unconvinced to the end of their days. In fact, the size of the reaction against the new discoveries was a measure of their novelty—and significance.

The story of the developments in bacteriology which led to a virtual scientific revolution in the second half of the nineteenth century has been told and retold many times. The movement was led by Louis Pasteur (1822–95) in France and Robert Koch (1843–1910) in Germany, who were soon followed by a host of eager disciples, the majority of whom came from Germany and France. As a result bacteriology came quickly into being as a new and exciting science of great significance.

Although Pasteur was responsible in his later years for many practical discoveries in the field of medicine, his early experiments had been concerned with more fundamental problems. These had led to the undermining of that ancient doctrine of "spontaneous generation," a notion based on the idea that all kinds of lower forms of life arose de novo in some mysterious way from materials in which they were usually found. Worms from rotting wood and maggots from putrescent flesh were common examples.

To quote Hans Zinsser, Pasteur's work "marked the ending of biological medievalism."[2]

As for the striking observations affecting practical aspects of medicine, the leap from old entrenched positions to the new concepts which Pasteur and Koch had introduced was almost too great to be managed all at once. Even the great Virchow found himself caught up in a controversy about concepts of disease and, as a result, was almost faced with waning prestige. Previous efforts of clinicians and pathologists, which had centered around an anatomical classification, now gave way to a taxonomic system in which *etiology* was given precedence. This was certainly an advance for those interested in understanding infectious diseases, which occasionally had a variety of different lesions, all of which might be due to the same etiological agent. The concept of an *etiologic* relationship between a specific agent and a given disease provided an infinitely better understanding of the underlying processes and, incidentally, strengthened the arguments of those who believed that diseases were specific entities—not mere figments of man's imagination.

Yet there was a fallacy in this explanation which soon came to light. In the early years of the development of microbiology the popular concept of multiple etiologic factors was rapidly reduced to the idea that diseases were due to a *single* cause, a conviction which the medical profession has been reluctant to relinquish almost ever since. Indeed, a single etiology has great appeal to the average physician. It is simple and particularly satisfying in the present age of antimicrobial drugs and vaccines. Specific therapy often cures infections rapidly; and, from the standpoint of preventive medicine, if the right vaccine is chosen, not only is the individual vaccinee protected, but the spread of infection within the community may be prevented as well. This has been demonstrated in recent times with poliovirus vaccines.

Nevertheless the single cause idea which started in the era of Pasteur has been, and still is being, ridden hard—too hard. It has gradually come to be regarded as an oversimplification. To produce a plant takes more than a seed, just as it takes more than a microbe to produce a disease. Man's *susceptibility*, conditioned by both hereditary and environmental factors, occupies a dominant position in determining his reaction to microbial infection. Acquired resistance is generally gained through *specific immunity*, a state which is either the result of a recognizable attack of the disease in question or an inapparent infection with the causative agent. For an extraordinarily long time the role of immunity (whether transient or permanent) was not fully appreciated. This created a stumbling block for the

---

2. H. Zinsser: *Rats, Lice and History*. Boston, Little, Brown, 1935, p. 51.

students of infectious diseases at the turn of the century and in the early
decades of the twentieth century. A bacterium—or a virus—was supposed
to be *the* cause of a disease, and that ended the matter. The idea that it
made all the difference whether the exposed individual was immune or
susceptible was disregarded. It has been claimed by many that Pasteur
failed to recognize the importance of the immune status of the individual
because he was so preoccupied with the idea that infection had a single
cause, i.e. a pathogenic microbial agent. Rather, it was his immediate followers who overemphasized the role of the microbe. Pasteur himself fully
recognized the role of induced immunity. At the end of his life, he allegedly
said, "Le microbe n'est rien, le terrain est tout."[3]

Few lives have been recorded more completely and are more familiar
than that of Louis Pasteur.[4,5] Understandably, it is in the light of a legendary hero of France, personifying the genius of discovery, that most
of his biographers have portrayed him.

As for Robert Koch, he soon took up the cause of bacteriology for the
Germans. He was typical of the serious and distinguished German professor of his day, and his laboratory was thronged with pupils eager to learn
the new secrets of bacteriology. As a measure of his eminence in science, he
received a Nobel Prize—two years before his death in 1910. Pasteur and
Koch, so different and yet so truly representative of their respective countries, were the luminaries of a movement that transformed speculative
theories of contagion and infection into a soundly based science. Many
other investigators joined them in what eventually became the golden age
of bacteriology, but these two were the pioneers.

How did poliomyelitis fare in this scientific revolution? Although many
new pathogenic bacteria and the diseases for which they were responsible
were identified between 1880 and 1908, and although frequent false claims
were made, this era failed to come up with anything in the way of an etiologic agent for poliomyelitis. Nevertheless, in spite of this failure, the idea
developed that poliomyelitis could indeed be an infectious disease with a
specific cause, and gradually this view took over during the new era.
Around the turn of the century it became almost a certainty, despite the
fact that it was eight years before the virus was actually discovered.

In the nineteenth century, contributions toward a better understanding
of poliomyelitis had come largely through neuropathology. With the aid of
the microscope it was at last possible to tackle the problem of the exact
site of the lesion in the spinal cord. Neuropathologists had practically

3. H. Selye: Stress and disease. *Science, 122*: 625–31, 1955.

4. R. Vallery-Radot: *The Life of Pasteur*, trans. by R. L. Demonshire. New York, Double-
day, Page, 1923.

5. R. J. Dubos: *Louis Pasteur*. Boston, Little, Brown, 1950, pp. 22–23.

started from zero. Not only was nothing known about the nature of the damage in the central nervous system; nothing was known about the nature of the disease which caused it. But after 1860 progress came rapidly. Abercrombie had hinted early in the nineteenth century, and Heine, of course, had already expressed his view, in 1840, that the symptoms "point to an affection of the central nervous system, specifically of the spinal cord." He believed that the congestion associated with the lesions in the cord produced an exudate coupled with edema which caused sudden paralysis; the transitory nature of some attacks of paralysis was explained by the assumption that the fluid exudate was reabsorbed. Heine's main difficulty came in reconciling his hypothesis with the fact that the anterior horns of the cord seemed to be more involved than the posterior ones.

A timely question was whether Heine's inference could be confirmed by employing the new methods of pathologic anatomy. As yet (by 1860), no material evidence existed that there was any lesion either in the brain or spinal cord or in the larger nerves. The answer was to prove difficult, especially since the opportunity to perform autopsies on patients who had succumbed in the acute stages of the disease seldom occurred. In fact, Dr. Mary Jacobi said that "until 1863 only five autopsies had been made upon persons affected with infantile paralysis."[6] In the few cases examined, the cut surface of the cord failed to reveal any gross abnormalities, and attempts to prove that the trouble actually was in the spinal cord must have been a very discouraging business indeed. Several French physicians were not even prepared to accept the central nervous system as the real site of the damage. Thus, the pediatricians Barthez and Rilliet[7] took no stock in Heine's views. Heine, they said, had not had the opportunity of examining a case at autopsy, whereas they had done so in 1843, when a patient who had long since recovered from the acute stage, but who had been left with residual paralysis, came to postmortem. On gross examination they found no changes in the central nervous system—let alone the spinal cord—and immediately came to the conclusion that the unknown cause of the paralysis lay outside of this system. Hence the name which they proposed—*paralysie essentielle chez les enfants.*

Rilliet chose to continue this view, maintaining that he and his coauthor, Barthez, had been the first to draw the attention of the medical profession

6. M. P. Jacobi: "Infantile spinal paralysis," in *A System of Practical Medicine by American Authors,* ed. by Wm. Pepper and L. Starr. Philadelphia, Lea Bros., 1886, vol. 5, pp. 1113–64.

7. F. Rilliet: De la paralysie essentielle chez les enfants. *Gaz. méd. Paris,* 3rd s., *6:* 681–85, 704–07, 1851. Eight years earlier Rilliet had been the coauthor of a textbook on children's diseases which included an article on infantile paralysis. E. Barthez and F. Rilliet: *Traité Clinique et Practique des Maladies des Enfants.* Paris, Baillière, 1843, p. 681. Here they said "L'anatomie revelant une matiere imparfaite de la nature de la maladie. . . ."

to the idea that here was a form of paralysis unaccompanied by any gross lesions. Thus they presented negative evidence based on examination of a single case, which they thought sufficient to prove their point. Since they did not examine the spinal cord microscopically, it is small wonder that they had not been able to see anything abnormal.

Despite the vigor of the opposition to the view that the spinal cord was involved, it could not last long. Soon, evidence pointing to the cord was derived from observations of a neurophysiological, rather than morphological, nature. In France, Duchenne de Boulogne[8] pointed out in 1853 that acute paralysis occurring in childhood—*la paralysie essentielle chez les enfants*—was followed by degeneration of the muscles and loss of electromuscular irritability in much the same way that such changes followed in patients who had suffered from traumatic injuries of the spinal cord. He reasoned by analogy that the primary site of the lesion in the paralysis of infancy must be within the spinal cord. Confirmation of this view came ten years later (1863) from Cornil, who was then working in Charcot's clinic in Paris.[9]

Jean-Martin Charcot (see fig. 9) achieved great distinction as a neurologist, which later resulted in his winning a place in the French Academy. Cornil's report concerned a patient of forty-nine years with residual paralytic poliomyelitis, whose death was due to cancer. She had sustained an attack of paralysis at the age of two, followed by permanent loss of the use of both legs. At autopsy, although it was forty-seven years after the acute episode, examination of the spinal cord revealed atrophy of the anterolateral columns (i.e. the white portion), which contain the nerve fibers. Little was said in this report about the nerve cells in the central gray matter, except that they shared this atrophy to some degree. This led Cornil, who maintained that this demonstration was the first of its kind ever to be published, to consider the gray matter as essentially unaltered. Seven years later (1870), despite the Franco-Prussian War and the fact that the Germans were knocking at the gates of Paris and were soon to lay siege to that city, Charcot was able to correct this observation. From Cornil's own microscopic sections, which had been preserved for some years, he was able to demonstrate a loss of large motor nerve cells in the gray matter of the cord.

In the meantime, also in France, Prevost[10] had already reported in 1866 that he had observed a similar finding. Shortly thereafter another case had

8. Duchenne de Boulogne: *De l'électrisation localisée et de son application à la physiologie et la pathologie et à la therapeutique*. Paris, Baillière, 1855.

9. V. Cornil: Paralysie infantile; cancer les seins; autopsie; altérations de la moelle épinière, des nerfs et des muscles; généralisation du cancer. *C. R. Soc. Biol. (Paris)*, 3rd s., 5: 187, 1863.

10. J. L. Prevost: Observation de paralysie infantile; lésion des muscles et de la moelle. *C. R. Soc. Biol. (Paris)*, 2: 215, 1866.

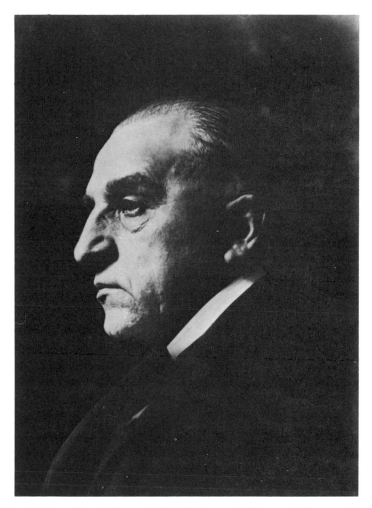

Fig. 9.   Jean-Martin Charcot (1825–93). From the Historical Library of the
Yale University School of Medicine.

come to the attention of Charcot and his colleague Joffroy.[11] Death had
occurred in this instance at the age of thirty-nine. Previously, in childhood,
the girl had suffered an attack of poliomyelitis which had resulted in paralysis of her left leg. At postmortem examination a section of the spinal
cord revealed (under a low-power view of the microscope) that both white
and gray matter appeared shrunken and scarred on the left, with a particular loss of substance in the anterior horn of the gray matter. The original
drawing, included as an illustration in Charcot and Joffroy's paper, shows

11. J. M. Charcot and A. Joffroy: Cas de paralysie infantile spinale avec lésions des cornes
antérieures de la substance grise de la moelle épinière. *Arch. Physiol. norm. Pathol.*, Paris, *3*:
134, 1870.

a microscopic section that indicates the condition of the spinal cord in this case. It appears in figure 10. Credit also must be given to Vulpian in France, who described a similar case almost simultaneously—in the same journal[12] in which Charcot and Joffroy's paper appeared. An appreciation

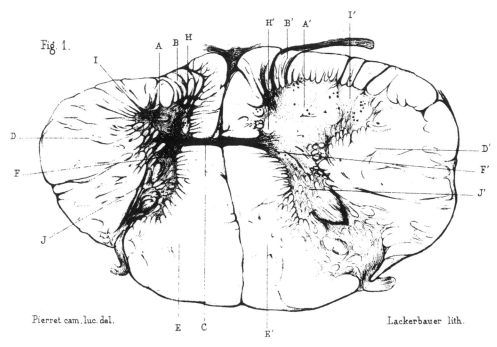

Pierret cam. luc. del.   Lackerbauer lith.

FIG. 10. Camera lucida drawing of a low-power microscopic section of the spinal cord in the case described in note 11. On the left, both gray and white matter appear shrunken with a loss of substance particularly in the anterior horn.

Legends: A, A'—Gray matter—Anterior horns
J, J'—Gray matter—Posterior horns
B, B' and D, D'—White matter

of conditions in the cord had come at last, and moreover, this was due to Charcot. He recognized that it was these particular motor cells which were extremely vulnerable to the "poison," or whatever it was, that was generated in the course of the acute disease. This had reduced the cells almost to nothing. Here was the true seat of the trouble. For within the nerve cells of the gray matter the motor impulses arose and were transmitted. Destruction of these cells meant paralysis. Not only had Heine's original views of thirty years before been correct, but also the lesion had been finally narrowed down to a tiny microscopic area within a circumscribed part of the spinal cord.

12. A. Vulpian: Cas d'atrophie musculaire graisseuse datant de l'enfance; lésions des cornes antérieures de la substance grise de la moelle épinière. *Arch. Physiol. norm. Pathol.*, *3*: 316, 1870.

Later that same year (1870) Charcot's colleagues Parrot and Joffroy[13] were able to confirm the new findings in a striking manner. They described the spinal cord of a child of three who had suffered an acute attack of poliomyelitis with paralysis of the left leg during the previous year. It was the most revealing case yet. Changes included an infiltration of small round cells into the area immediately surrounding the blood vessels—so-called perivascular cuffing (dans la production d'eléments nouveaux autour des vaisseaux et dans le reticulum)—so characteristic of acute and subacute lesions of the central nervous system. This report in essence laid the foundation of all subsequent interpretations of acute microscopic findings in the central nervous system in poliomyelitis.

It might seem that I have gone to undue lengths to emphasize the cord lesions, but any casualness with regard to their exact location would not be tolerated by neuropathologists or neurophysiologists. Because of the discoveries of Charcot and others, the principles and the beginnings of the neuropathology of poliomyelitis had been clearly established. The histological examination of the spinal cord in fatal cases had come into its own —to enable the final word to be given for the differentiation of poliomyelitis from other kinds of acute and chronic diseases in which the central nervous system was involved. Pathological diagnosis became a matter of the utmost significance not only for pathologists but, after 1875, for the medical profession as a whole.

Later, discussions which had begun in the 1870s soon grew into altercations. These were generated over the question whether destruction of the large motor nerve cells in the anterior horns was really the *primary* involvement; or whether this lesion was part of a general inflammatory reaction and edema in which the nerve cells were inevitably caught up. Charcot and his pupils favored the former interpretation, but their views were not by any means universally accepted. One of those scientific wrangles, an occurrence so common in the annals of poliomyelitis research, soon developed. Actually, the controversy was to last for nearly a half century. But with the discovery of the virus some forty years later and the advent of experimental poliomyelitis, neuropathologists were finally able to settle the matter, and Charcot's thesis finally prevailed. If I can skip over a half century, by examining the central nervous system of monkeys sacrificed early in the course of infection, it was possible to document the initial degeneration of the nerve cells in the anterior horns of the cord and the secondary inflammation of the interstitial tissue.[14] One particularly illus-

13. J. Parrot and A. Joffroy: Note sur un cas de paralysie infantile. *Arch. Physiol. norm. Pathol., 3*: 309, 1870.

14. See the excellent review by E. W. Goodpasture: "The pathology and pathogenesis of poliomyelitis," in *Infantile Paralysis*. A symposium delivered at Vanderbilt University April 1941, the National Foundation of Infantile Paralysis, Baltimore, Waverly Press, 1941, pp. 83–

trative set of high-power microphotographs, which was not made until
1941, is reproduced in figure 11. These are from an article by Sabin and
Ward.[15] One can see the progressive destructive changes that motor cells
sustained in the course of a few days or even hours, during an acute attack
of experimental poliomyelitis. Also shown is the manner in which inflammatory cells wander into the gray matter and accumulate for the purpose
of clearing up the detritus left by a dead motor nerve cell. Such infiltrates
collect not only in the sites of actual cellular destruction but also around
blood vessels. They represent a singularly characteristic type of response
which has become so familiar to pathologists in describing the lesions of
acute poliomyelitis.

With this picture of the neural lesions of poliomyelitis thus illustrated
one can perhaps better appreciate the problems that members of Charcot's
Clinic had to surmount in arriving at their interpretations.

However, the *extraneural* lesions of poliomyelitis were yet to be reckoned with. Long before the advent of modern neuropathologists, Rissler,
a Scandinavian, pointed out in 1888 that besides changes in the central
nervous system there were extraneural lesions in acute poliomyelitis. These
were widespread throughout the body but fortunately, unlike the central
nervous system lesions, did no damage as far as the patient was concerned.
Such a development was decidedly a new angle for pathologists. Rissler's
important work[16] marked the beginning of the ascendancy of the Scandi-
navians, who were to dominate advances in the subject of poliomyelitis for
the next twenty years. He had the advantage of having access to pathological material from cases which had occurred during a recent epidemic in
Norway. His observations were based upon the examination of five patients, three of whom had died at the end of the first week of illness. This
gave him a unique opportunity, which had so far been denied to other
pathologists. He was the first to note enlargement of the spleen and of
lymphoid follicles in the intestines and adjacent lymph nodes. These
findings indicated the widespread nature of the infection during the early
phases and led Rissler to suggest that poliomyelitis was primarily an acute
systemic infection with lesions not necessarily limited to the central nervous system, although the latter were obviously the most serious and indeed
the only serious lesions. He was convinced of the correctness of Charcot's
hypothesis that the motor nerve cells were the site of destruction (myelitis)
caused by some injurious agent, on the heels of which neuronal degenera-

125. Also see A. B. Sabin: Pathology and pathogenesis of human poliomyelitis. *J. Amer. med.
Ass., 120*: 506–11, 1942.

15. A. B. Sabin and R. Ward: Nature of nonparalytic and transitory paralytic poliomyelitis in rhesus monkeys inoculated with human virus. *J. exp. Med., 73*: 757–70, 1941.

16. J. Rissler: Zur Kenntniss der Veränderungen des Nervensystems bei Poliomyelitis anterior acuta. *Nord. med. Ark., 20*: 1, 1888.

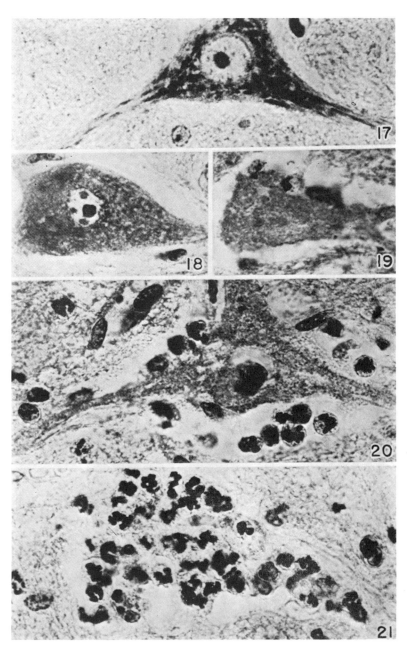

FIG. 11. Fate of the motor cells in the anterior horn (from A. B. Sabin and R. Ward, n. 15).

Legends of individual photomicrophs: 17—essentially normal cell; 18—chromotolysis; 19—complete necrosis; 20—leukocytes invading necrotic cells; 21—complete neuronophagia. Reproduced by permission of the *Journal of the American Medical Assn.*

tion rapidly occurred, leaving atrophy and scarring in its wake. Also, he was the first to describe phagocytosis[17] of the motor nerve cells by leukocytes and macrophages—a process known today as *neuronophagia*.

As for developments in pathology after Rissler, leading to a further revised understanding of the *pathogenesis* of human poliomyelitis, or any interpretations of the mechanisms involved, there was a notable lag. It is altogether surprising that a lapse of about fifty years ensued, during which the majority of pathologists made little progress in dealing with crucial problems of pathogenesis or in determining how the virus entered the human body and spread to invade the central nervous system. But it was too much to expect of the science of pathology to answer all the questions of an overeager world. Eventually came the realization that morphology did not in itself tell enough to allow one to trace the course of what actually happens to an infectious agent in the human or in the experimental disease; it could only represent visible footprints of what had gone before. The medical world would have to turn for help to other sciences such as the newly emerging one of virology. Particularly at first the way was difficult, and some of the answers which were heralded with such enthusiasm in the end proved quite wrong. Hence the long delay.

17. Phagocytosis: the process of the engulfment of dead cells or particles by living cells.

CHAPTER 7

Clinical Ideas in the 1870s and 1880s

Even if the flowering of the new medical sciences failed to touch the bulk of mid-nineteenth-century physicians, particularly in America, we should not be too hard on them. Their background in science was limited, and in medicine it was at a time when a number of empirical and bizarre treatments considered to have distinct curative and restorative powers were in vogue. Physicians were under great pressure to *do* something for their patients, whether such action was scientifically justified or not. They were expected to prescribe the accepted drastic measures, such as dosing with "opening medicines," bleeding, applying leeches, or raising blisters. For example, in the early part of the century Dr. Miner, a worthy Connecticut physician, was so impressed with his own omniscience and skill in handling cases of fever as to make exorbitant claims concerning his therapeutic prowess in using remedies to overcome fevers due to diseases which were in all probability self-limited anyway.[1]

But a certain amount of reform was in the wind, and in the 1830s, after Dr. Miner's extravagant statements were made, Jacob Bigelow of Boston, professor of medicine at Harvard, introduced a seemingly revolutionary idea in an address before the Massachusetts Medical Society:[2] he maintained that some diseases actually were self-limited and might be cured by nature alone. These included fevers, generally the eruptive ones—erysipelas, smallpox, measles, and even mumps. Such an idea was heresy to many physicians, although with the contemporary rise in the Paris school of pathology and the decline in purely empirical medicine, the notion did seem to make sense.

Bigelow did not mention poliomyelitis as a self-limited fever, but in his day acute cases of infantile paralysis had been detected only occasionally. However, in the second half of the century they were recognized with increasing frequency, and in 1867 Charles F. Taylor, a physician of New York City with pronounced orthopedic interests, published a small book on infantile paralysis. As far as I know it was the first book by an American author which dealt solely with this disease and its dire results. In the opening

1. Thomas Miner: Part I, in *Essays on Fevers and Other Medical Subjects* by T. Miner and William Tully. Middletown, Conn., E. & H. Clark, 1823, p. viii.
2. J. Bigelow: On self-limited diseases. *Med. Communications. Mass. Med. Soc.*, pp. 319–58, 1830–36.

pages of the paper-bound volume Taylor says: "There seems to be no doubt that this disease is much more frequent now, and in this country, than formerly, and is rapidly increasing."[3]

In a way it is a mistake to claim that this was the first American book on poliomyelitis, for it actually does not deserve this position. Dr. Taylor makes no pretext of having the slightest idea about the nature of the disease but acknowledges that by his use of the term *infantile paralysis* in the title, he means simply, "to indicate that form of paralysis which occurs only in infancy." He then goes on to describe in the remaining 100 out of 119 pages the deformities which he has seen as the result of paralysis in infancy. In an earlier book, *The Swedish System of Localized Movements,* published in 1861, Taylor seems not to have been especially impressed by teething as a cause; at least he puts it in quotation marks.[4]

Early in the 1870s, professors of medicine and surgery in the United States were already demonstrating cases of paralytic poliomyelitis in their clinics and in some instances were expounding in their lecture halls what seemed to be the latest points of view, especially as to therapy. In spite of these teachings, or perhaps because of them, members of the medical profession in the United States, and no doubt elsewhere, continued mostly in the dark about the nature of the affliction.

An example is a lecture on infantile paralysis delivered in 1872 by that distinguished surgeon, Samuel D. Gross of the Jefferson Medical College of Philadelphia. There is little to indicate whether Gross actually agreed with the majority of contemporary authorities in the United States, or whether his opinions were reported accurately. For Professor Gross was noted for his individuality of thought, and it is only an assumption that he did edit the transcription of his lecture before it was published.

The lecture starts off with a case report of a pale child of thirteen months who had been severely paralyzed shortly after birth; the implication was that the patient was still within the limits of the stage when active treatment of the subacute disease could be expected to be of some benefit. Gross describes infantile paralysis as a nervous affection in which both lower limbs are generally involved and says that it is "met with in young children about 10 months old, occurring during teething or a little before or after. . . ." The lecturer emphasizes the drama of *morning paralysis,* stating:

3. C. F. Taylor: *Infantile Paralysis and its Attendant Deformities.* Philadelphia, Lippincott, 1867.

4. C. F. Taylor: *Theory and Practice of the Movement-Cure;* or *The Treatment by the Swedish System of Localized Movements.* Philadelphia, Lindsay and Blakiston, 1861.

In the late nineteenth century there seems to have been an inclination to compare the Swedish system of movements to the cult of *osteopathy.* This cult was little known in America before 1900. It established its identity in the United States with the founding of the first American School of Osteopathy, in Kirkesville, Missouri in 1892.

The child is put to bed at night apparently well, with a good appetite, and nothing to indicate the onset of the disease. During the night he perhaps wakes up thirsty, and appears restless and feverish. When the mother goes to him in the morning she finds the lower limbs powerless and generally lowered in temperature.[5]

Dr. Gross further reported that "the pathology of the affection is manifestly some lesion of the spinal cord, the brain being unimpaired in the exercise of its functions, and special senses unaffected." He goes on to describe his notions on the nature of the trouble and states his belief that the lesions are in part caused by pressure due to an effusion of serous fluid into the spaces surrounding the spinal cord.

This inflammation extends to the sheaths of the nerves, producing thickening. In this way the nerves are compressed by the effusion and by their investments in the intervertebral canals, thus interrupting the nerve-fluid or current. Paralysis follows in those muscles which obtain their nervous supply from trunks which have their action interfered with at the seat of the disease.

Obviously he disagreed somewhat with views currently being expressed at Charcot's clinic in Paris; or, it is very likely that he did not know of them, for it may be recalled that Charcot and his pupils had announced only recently that the disease was caused by an actual destruction of motor nerve cells within the anterior horns of the gray matter of the cord. Gross, on the other hand, took the older view. In this he was not alone, for he had a following among clinicians, a following which continued for well over half a century. It is not fair to blame Dr. Gross for taking the wrong side in this matter. The only purpose of mentioning his error is that he based his somewhat medieval form of treatment on the assumption that the pathology of the myelitis, or whatever it was, resulted from pressure produced by edematous fluid.

The recorded lecture goes on:

This affection is very obstinate, and does not respond well to treatment; in the majority of cases the paralysis remains, crippling the pa-

5. Notes of Hospital Practice. Jefferson Medical College. Surgical Clinic of Prof. S. D. Gross (reported by Frank Woodbury). Lecture on Infantile Paralysis, August 1, 1872. *Phila. med. Times,* 2: 408–09, 1872–73.

Surgeon Samuel D. Gross should have been in a position to evaluate the spinal cord lesions in infantile paralysis better than most surgeons in this country, having been one of America's earliest pathologists. Not only had he taught pathology in the Medical Department of Cincinnati College but he had been the author of a textbook: *Elements of Pathological Anatomy,* published in 1839. See E. S. Long: Some Early American pathologists. *Trans. Stud. Coll. Phycns. Philad.,* 4th s., *36*: 22–28, 1968.

tient for the rest of his life. After some time, the muscles become soft and atrophied, and their fibres finally undergo fatty degeneration.[6]

However, before this condition of fatty degeneration is complete, the patient may improve by judicious and persistent treatment.

If my opinion regarding the pathology of the affection is correct,— that it is produced by pressure, due to inflammation, on the nerves at their origin,—then counter-irritants and sorbefacients[7] would be useful. Bleeding, either by leeches or cut cups, and blisters, produce good effects if used early and some benefit may be derived from rubefacients and dry cupping immediately over the lesion. To my mind, the best and most efficient means of treating the disease is by establishing with a red-hot iron, a good issue[8] over the affected spot. The eschar (scab) formed comes away in a few days, leaving an ulcer, which should be encouraged to discharge freely. It is a valuable adjunct in the treatment of nervous diseases caused by subacute inflammation, or by a deposit the result of inflammation existing in the spinal cord or its membranes.

Also, no doubt in the cause of physical therapy, he recommended that "during the treatment the muscles must be rubbed and shampooed, and steadily exercised with the battery." He added that mercury ointment should be applied in the following manner:

Put a piece the size of a marrowfat pea twice a day, over the entire spine and along the back of the limbs.

After bathing, wring the end of the towel out of cold water, and with it strike the entire surface of the body, quite smartly, until the skin is reddened. This treatment to be continued for a month; at the end of which time, his mother was directed to bring the child back.

There is no mention made of late convalescent therapy or aftercare, such as splinting of the paralyzed and atrophied limbs, or of orthopedic operations. As this demonstration was of a case in the subacute stage, Dr. Gross seemed to feel that continued heroic efforts were still indicated if all was not to be lost. The aftercare was apparently a different story.

These therapeutic recommendations, made less than 100 years ago to medical students who were destined to have little in the way of further academic training, were not an improvement on those proposed by Michael Underwood or Monteggia. The spectacle of the dignified surgeon brandishing a red-hot iron and applying it to the back of a thirteen-month-

6. *Paralysie atrophique graisseuse de l'enfance* was the name Duchenne de Boulogne had applied to poliomyelitis in 1855 (see chap. 2).
7. Sorbefacient: A substance or preparation causing absorption.
8. An issue: A discharge of blood or other matter from the body generally induced by an ulcerous lesion.

old infant gives us pause for thought. And yet such treatment was recommended by the distinguished Dr. Gross, who had undergone a long training
period on the science of pathology and was easily one of the top surgeons
of the country. In due course his widow was to marry Dr. William Osler.
It is astonishing that Gross's ideas, put forth in 1872, could be so different
from the infinitely more rational ones of the new era that arrived so soon
thereafter and were exemplified in Osler's *Principles and Practice of
Medicine*.[9]

To pursue the story of poliomyelitis through the 1870s and 1880s is to
document a period when the disease, although common enough in many
countries, was still in the stage when a report of a single case was sufficiently
interesting to warrant publication. Innumerable such descriptive reports
found their way into professional journals of the Western world. At least
one, however, contains vestiges of a new idea about the nature of the disease. It describes two cases that occurred simultaneously in the same family,
in a brother aged two and one-half and a sister of one and one-half years.[10]
What makes the report so significant is that the author, Dr. Frederick A.
Packard of Philadelphia, went to some pains to speculate on what this
"family epidemic" might mean. In 1879, although there had been rumors
that poliomyelitis was contagious, such an idea really had hardly been entertained at all. But Dr. Packard (who was soon to become Osler's promising young assistant during Sir William's Philadelphia years [1884–89])
suggested that the events described pointed perhaps to an *infective* character of the disease.

Some fourteen years after Dr. Gross's lecture had been published, notions about poliomyelitis had advanced somewhat. Practically all the
American knowledge about the disease up to 1886, including its neuropathology and neurophysiology, had been summarized in a fifty-page review article in Dr. William Pepper's *System of Medicine*.[11] It was written
by Mary Putnam Jacobi (see fig. 12), at that time professor of therapeutics
in the now defunct Woman's Medical College of New York. This was a
remarkable achievement for a contemporary American woman physician.
Nor does her article lack erudition; almost half of it is taken up by the
subjects of "pathogeny" and pathology, features which must have seemed
relatively abstruse to the average practitioner of pediatrics or medicine
even in the latter part of the nineteenth century. She also took special
pride in being able to give firsthand an exhaustive review of the European

9. W. Osler: *Principles and Practice of Medicine*. Edinburgh, Young & Pentland, 1892.

10. F. A. Packard: Acute anterior poliomyelitis occurring simultaneously in a brother and
sister; with remarks upon its etiology. *J. Nerv. ment. Dis.*, 26: 210, 1879.

11. M. P. Jacobi: "Infantile Spinal Paralysis," in *A System of Medicine by American
Authors*, ed. by Wm. Pepper (assisted by Louis Starr), 5 vols. Philadelphia, Lea Bros., 1886, vol.
5, pp. 1113–64.

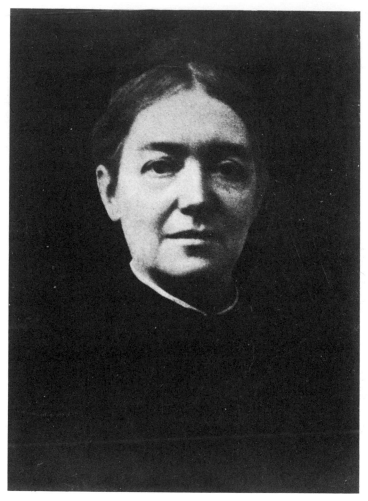

Fɪɢ. 12. Mary Putnam Jacobi, M.D. (1842–1906). Kindness of G. P. Putnam's and Coward McCann.

literature, which, to say the least, was an unusual accomplishment for a young American physician. The reason Dr. Jacobi could write such a scholarly and up-to-date account of poliomyelitis was that this remarkable woman had a background of training that peculiarly qualified her for the task.[12]

As a member of the well-known New York publishing family, Mary Corinna Putnam's special heroine had been Elizabeth Blackwell, the first woman ever to become a graduate M.D. in the United States and who, despite enormous opposition, had maintained a medical practice in New York for several years. Mary Putnam, at the age of nineteen, had faint hope

12. R. Putnam: *Life and Letters of Mary Putnam Jacobi.* New York, Putnam, 1925.

of becoming a full-fledged physician; as a substitute she chose to study pharmacy and received her degree in 1863. To become a druggist fell short of her ambition, and she decided to enter the Woman's Medical School of Philadelphia, where, after a singularly abbreviated training, she received her medical degree in the spring of 1864. Difficulties and uncertainties beset her during the next two Civil War years, and she came to realize that her training in medicine had been inadequate. Since she was ill equipped to accomplish what she had set out to do, she decided to seek another medical degree, this time in Paris, and enrolled in what must have been premedical courses at the Sorbonne in 1866. Here, for the first time, her interest in two basic medical sciences, pathology and physiology, was aroused. A year before she was admitted to the medical school she was attending surgical lectures, doing autopsies, and studying histology. Quite by accident she fell under the spell of Ranvier, Cornil, and later Vulpian, whose exciting work on the neuropathology of poliomyelitis was in full swing and about which we have heard in relation to contemporary studies in Charcot's clinic.

Mary Putnam's intimate knowledge of the French language enabled her to make the most of this experience, and she soon brought her newly acquired knowledge to the United States. After her return in 1873, she entered upon the practice of internal medicine in New York City and in the same year married Dr. Abraham Jacobi, who had emigrated from Germany in 1848 and was destined to become the virtual father and founder of American pediatrics. The following year she published in a journal which her husband had started, a definitive report describing the pathogeny of infantile paralysis.[13] She laid stress on the latest French discoveries and on the idea that the spectacular paralysis and deformity were due to tiny microscopic destructive lesions within the gray matter of the spinal cord. This was a completely new concept which supplanted the inadequate descriptions of the pathology and the long-winded emphasis on treatment of the subacute disease which had gone before. Dr. William Pepper, professor of medicine at the University of Pennsylvania in Philadelphia and the acknowledged dean of American physicians,[14] was quick to detect Dr. Jacobi's ability and her superior knowledge of the subject. Dr. Pepper must have had a wide range of authors to choose from when it came to selecting physicians most competent to contribute to his *American System of Medicine.*

13. M. P. Jacobi: Pathogeny of infantile paralysis. *Amer. J. Obstet.,* 7: 1, 1874–75.

14. F. N. Thorpe: *William Pepper, M.D., L.L.D. (1843–1898)*. Philadelphia, Lippincott, 1904.

In the early days of his professional career, Dr. William Pepper had also been a pathologist. When barely twenty-five years old, he spent much time in recataloging the huge collection of pathological specimens that had been amassed at the Pennsylvania Hospital in Philadelphia. See W. Pepper: *Descriptive Catalogue of the Pathological Museum of the Pennsylvania Hospital.* Privately printed, 1869.

For the chapter on poliomyelitis he did not choose a well-known name or a man established in the practice of medicine; instead he chose Dr. Mary Jacobi, who had had less than a dozen years of clinical experience, but who in his opinion possessed the most up-to-date knowledge about the neuropathology and neurophysiology of infantile paralysis and was capable of writing an article on the subject in which useless recommendations about treatment did not take up at least 50 percent of the text.

Nevertheless in Dr. Mary Jacobi's article she says with more humbleness than her predecessors had displayed that there is little definite knowledge of the nature of poliomyelitis. Her views of etiology are given in a few short paragraphs in which the probability is mentioned that "traumatisms have a more decided influence than is generally assigned to them."[15] A second cause she ascribed to "almost certainly the presence of some poison circulating in the blood." The article goes on:

> The evidence . . . has led, not unnaturally, to the theory that all cases of acute infantile paralysis are due to a specific infecting agent, some as yet unknown member of the great class of pathogenic bacteria.

Apparently she was hinting that the disease was infectious but was rightly unwilling to commit herself on this score.

Another cause mentioned is "the influence of exposure to cold." However, to Dr. Jacobi's credit, the time-honored causes of teething or foul bowels had, as far as she was concerned, at last faded out of the picture.

As was natural for an era in which the emphasis in scientific medicine was largely on pathology, the epidemiology of poliomyelitis received short shrift; indeed, it was hardly mentioned except for the terse statement that children are usually affected between the ages of eighteen months and four years, and attacks are more likely to occur in the summer.[16]

Dr. Jacobi goes into meticulous detail in describing the sequential events in the clinical disease: its apparent brief prodromal symptoms, the duration of fever, and the usual anatomical distribution of the paralyses. When it comes to neuropathology, naturally she leans heavily on the views of vari-

---

15. See n. 11, pp. 1151–52.

Even today *trauma* is recognized as a *precipitating* cause. Arguments have been put forward pro and con but very largely pro, in which the claim has been made that if an individual is in the late incubation period of poliomyelitis and experiences a severe injury or indulges in physical activity, this will influence the course of the disease unfavorably. See W. R. Russell: Poliomyelitis; the preparalytic stage and the effect of physical activity on the severity of paralysis. *Brit. med. J.*, 2: 1023, 1947; and D. M. Horstmann: Acute poliomyelitis; Relation of physical activity at the time of onset to the course of the disease. *J. Amer. med. Ass., 142:* 236–41, 1950.

16. On the latter point Dr. Jacobi quotes Dr. Wharton Sinkler of Philadelphia who had noted the summer incidence in an unusually large series of sporadic cases which he had collected over the short period of four years. W. Sinkler: On the palsies of children. *Amer. J. med. Sci.,* n.s., *69:* 348–65, 1875.

ous European physicians, particularly her former professors in Paris who, it will be remembered, maintained that the main lesion was "the deformation, atrophy and final disappearance of the large ganglionic cells of the anterior cornua [of the spinal cord] . . . which explains admirably, as will be seen, the permanent symptoms of the disease." In summary, she repeats that old aphorism of Rilliet and Barthez which had held the stage so long but was soon to be disproved by Rissler, Medin, and his followers: "la paralysie est toute la maladie."

As to treatment, Dr. Jacobi was not quite ready to give up the time-honored remedies. She says that almost all modern authorities advise that ice be applied to the spine and that ergot be administered either internally or subcutaneously in an effort to divert the circulation of blood to the surface. She recommends, as Dr. Gross had before her, that mercury ointment be rubbed in along the spine, followed by blisters, and that treatment with iodides be started. Electrical treatment should begin at the end of the first week after paralysis; but as for massage and passive exercise, here she was less vocal. Her views seem to indicate a certain lack of experience with these forms of physical therapy.

Mary Jacobi was the first to bring to physicians in America the idea and the evidence that meticulous studies of the neuropathology of poliomyelitis could be rewarding and that the real seat of the trouble lay in destructive lesions in motor nerve cells in the spinal cord. She was also the first to write a really scholarly and exhaustive textbook article on the disease, indicating that there was much more to the concept of infantile paralysis than could be covered by a clinical description of its resulting paralysis and detailed methods of treatment of the acute disease. True, she acted only as a messenger, but she was a dedicated messenger on a particular errand, somewhat in the fashion of Dr. William H. Welch, who brought the sciences of pathology and bacteriology to America.

Six short years later a fresh wind started to blow from another direction in the matter of therapy. This was inherent in the views expressed by Dr. Osler in a short article on infantile paralysis in the first of many editions of his *Principles and Practice of Medicine*. Osler castigated, with his customary courage, the irrationality of medieval treatments then in vogue. He recognized that, as the major pathological lesion had been demonstrated clearly as a destructive myelitis, there was little to be accomplished in the way of therapy until the day should come that new methods could be shown to be effective. He said:

> No drugs have the slightest influence upon an acute myelitis, and even in subjects with well-marked syphilis neither mercury or iodide of potassium, is curative.
> Electricity should not be used in the early stage of myelitis.

The child should be in bed and the affected limb or limbs wrapped in cotton. . . .

The application of blisters and other forms of counter-irritation to the back is irrational and only cruel to the child.[17]

It is clear that Dr. Osler considered that contemporary physicians, in their efforts to *do* something, had allowed themselves to drift into the posture of trying to treat the acute disease in a mood of desperation, not of wisdom; let alone one based on scientific principles. It had taken a long time to reach this stage and was still to require a painfully long time before more effective approaches were devised.

17. See n. 9, p. 834.

CHAPTER 8

Epidemics in Sweden
Medin and His Clinical Contributions

Between 1890 and 1905, clinical medicine had decidedly come of age, even on this side of the Atlantic. It was a period characterized by great clinicians, many of whom profited from an association with a university clinic while carrying on large private practices: Dr. William Pepper at the University of Pennsylvania in Philadelphia, Weir Mitchell in the same city, the elder Janeway in New York, and Osler, who is claimed by several North American cities including Montreal, Philadelphia, and Baltimore. It was an exuberant period for medicine, a time when clinical knowledge was being accumulated with remarkable volume and rapidity. In a heroic effort to keep pace with this progress, ponderous multivolume systems of medicine appeared on the scene, such as those edited by William Pepper[1] in the United States and Clifford Allbutt[2] in England. The authors apparently attempted to document almost everything that was known about a given disease in terms of its physiology, pathology, immunology, clinical course and treatment—obviously an impossible task in view of the ever-increasing number of new facts that were being garnered each year. Many of the articles about familiar individual diseases in these voluminous systems ran to 100 pages or more!

Poliomyelitis was swept along in this vigorous movement of the late nineteenth century, with new clinical features being detected almost every year. I shall not attempt to document each one in the long list of firsts, but perhaps a few deserve special mention. One had to do with the recognition of the disease in older age groups. As early as 1858, Vogt[3] in Switzerland had described what was thought to be the first case in an adult. This was the beginning of a new trend. Until the last quarter of the century poliomyelitis had always been considered a disease solely of infants and young children. It then began to be recognized in adolescents and, particularly when the disease appeared in epidemic form, even in a fair quota of young adults.

1. W. Pepper: *A System of Medicine by American Authors,* 5 vols. Philadelphia, Lea Bros., 1886.

2. T. C. Allbutt: *A System of Medicine by Many Writers,* 8 vols. London, MacMillan, 1899.

3. W. Vogt: *Die essentielle Lähmung der Kinder.* Bern, Haller, 1858.

Seeligmüller,[4] in 1880, had the unusual opportunity of collecting a series of seventy-five sporadic cases seen in various stages of the illness and was able to make detailed studies of the early symptoms and of the distribution of the paralyses. He was among those who deserve credit for first suggesting an infectious element in poliomyelitis, although, as I have mentioned, this idea had been cautiously advanced in 1879 by Dr. F. A. Packard of Philadelphia.[5]

In 1884 the first accurate account of the cerebral type (i.e. the encephalitic form) was given by Strümpell[6] in Vienna. He suggested that the causative agent, whatever it was, could occasionally localize in the brain as well as in the spinal cord, as was to be abundantly proven in the years to come (see fig. 1). The following year this observation was corroborated in Paris by Pierre Marie,[7] who has been described as Charcot's ablest pupil. The cerebral type thus came to be referred to as the Strümpell-Marie form of poliomyelitis. Both authors also had some inkling that the disease was of an infectious nature, an idea then unacceptable to the medical profession but soon to have added support by the appearance of epidemics of infantile paralysis.

Who reported the first epidemic of poliomyelitis in Scandinavia has never ceased to be a controversial matter, but, I may say, one which is not of great importance. According to Wickman and his teacher Medin, both Swedes, Bergenholtz deserves the credit for observing a small outbreak of thirteen cases occurring in Umeo, in northern Sweden, in 1881. Apparently his report was made verbally before the Swedish Medicinal-Collegium. It was never published in medical literature but was recorded in the Swedish Public Health Reports.[8]

Lavinder, Freeman, and Frost et al. give credit to Bull for describing an even earlier epidemic in Scandinavia. This occurred in 1868 in the Modums district of Norway, not far from Oslo. Bull treated fourteen patients, of whom five died from what he thought was spinal meningitis; but on careful examination of his account there seems to be little doubt that he was dealing with an epidemic of poliomyelitis, in spite of the unusually high fatality rate. To support this opinion Lavinder and his colleagues[9]

4. A. Seeligmüller: "Spinale Kinderlähmung," in *Handbuch d. Kinderkrankh.* (Gerhardt) Abt. 1, Heft 2. 1: Tübingen, Laupp., 1880.

5. F. A. Packard: Acute anterior poliomyelitis occurring simultaneously in a brother and sister; with remarks upon its etiology. *J. nerv. ment. Dis., 26*: 210, 1879.

6. A. Strümpell: Ueber die acute Encephalitis der Kinder (Polioencephalitis acuta, cerebrale Kinderlähmung). *Allg. Wien med. Ztg., 29*: 612, 1884.

7. P. Marie: Hémiplégie cérébrale infantile et maladies infectieuses. *Progrès méd., 13*: 167, 1885.

8. The acceptance of Bergenholtz' claim to priority can only be based upon Medin's and Wickman's authority, which seems reliable enough.

9. C. H. Lavinder, A. W. Freeman, and W. H. Frost: Epidemiologic studies of poliomyelitis in New York City and the northeastern United States during the year 1916. *Publ. Hlth Bull.* (*Wash.*), no. 91, 1918.

quote Leegaard's article on the history of poliomyelitis in Norway, in which a full account of the epidemic reported by Bull is given.[10] As to the contagious nature of this malady Bull is said to have written:

> It does not seem apparent in this small epidemic that contagion played any role, because the disease occurred here and there in different places of the district without the possibility of establishing any relation between various cases or the families of the same. Yet I will state that in one court two children were taken sick at the same time. Moreover, in two places where cases occurred the brother or sister in the same house sickened, but not with an evident spinal meningitis—rather with light and unimportant form, so that the patient, after the course of a couple of days, was entirely well.

In the foregoing account we must admit that Bull was observant, though not quite perceptive enough. At least he made a natural mistake that was to be repeated by many an astute clinician and public health worker who followed him. Clinical epidemiologists continued to wrangle for the next fifty years over questions of contagion and indeed over the way the infection traveled from one person or place to the next. The fact that Bull's series included cases of "a light and unimportant form," which were in all probability the characteristic "minor illnesses" of poliomyelitis, might have alerted him as to what was happening. And yet, understandably enough, he did not realize that minor illnesses, or abortive cases as they eventually came to be called, play a major role in transmitting the infection. It remained for Wickman, who in due time came after him, to make this important observation. Certainly Bull was not aware that during epidemics these "light and unimportant" forms occur at a rate at least several times that of the overt cases. In fact, for at least a half a century frustrated epidemiologists were to make the same mistake, a mistake which led to the hiring of untold numbers of nurses and fieldworkers who trudged throughout affected cities during poliomyelitis epidemics attempting to trace relationships between multiple overt or paralytic cases.[11] Countless forms and questionnaires were filled out with the aid of families of patients. Such forms were eventually subjected to statistical analyses aimed at tracing the manner in which the infection spread between frank cases—truly an impossible task. So it seems that Bull was not alone in his estimate of the difficulty of establishing a relationship between paralytic cases.

Outside of Scandinavia, epidemics of poliomyelitis were also just begin-

10. C. Leegaard: Die akute Poliomyelitis in Norwegen. *Dtsch. Z. Nervenheilk.*, *53*: 145–262, 1914. Leegaard himself described two epidemics in Norway.

11. A fundamental fallacy in this type of surveillance has been that the usual fieldworker has generally lacked the clinical judgment to decide what should be called "minor illnesses of poliomyelitis" and what should not, a question which generally requires the knowledge of an astute clinical investigator.

ning to be reported. In 1888, Cordier in France described in retrospect thirteen cases in the small village of Sainte-Foy-l'Argentière, which is near Lyon.[12] The outbreak had occurred in June and July of 1885. Yet the first case did not come to Cordier's attention until October 1886, fully fifteen months later. Only then was he able to visit this village, "pour juger par mes propres yeux," in order to find out what actually had happened. On this visit he uncovered twelve additional cases, but obviously he must have missed others since the outbreak was investigated at such a late date. Although the total compilation of cases and their exact ages were almost surely inaccurate, one thing is clear—the representative patients were very young. Of twelve patients, five were under the age of seven months; three were between seven and twelve months; two were one year old; and only two were between two and three years. This little village must have received a particularly heavy exposure to poliovirus in June 1885, as more than a third of the cases were in infants less than seven months old, suggesting that the dosage of virus had apparently been great enough to overcome the maternal passive immunity of infants of such a tender age. Furthermore, the age incidence was an indication that the village population over the age of three or four years was solidly immune. Thus Cordier's epidemic was almost comparable to Colmer's Louisiana outbreak twenty-five years earlier. Obviously it did not at all resemble the epidemics in Scandinavia which were to come a very few years later.

Cordier was scornful of the theoretical causes of poliomyelitis which had been consistently mentioned by previous writers, such as teething, stomach upsets, and trauma, events which he claimed are common enough in early infancy and therefore incidental—not causative. He maintained that since infantile paralysis occurred in epidemics, this was proof that it was "a specific infectious disease—one might say a microbial disease."

In this period, it is to Sweden that we should turn for contemporary advances in poliomyelitis, advances which were to continue for the following twenty-four years, i.e. from 1890 to 1914. Besides Rissler, early progress was largely due to the contributions of the Stockholm pediatrician Oskar Medin (see fig. 13), who deserves the credit for detecting and assembling various clinical features of the disease in a more concise yet comprehensive way than had ever been accomplished. His observations received worldwide attention after Medin's convincing presentation of them before the Tenth International Medical Congress held in Berlin in 1890.[13] It was the first time that physicians of Europe and elsewhere had heard about the epidemic disease which had beset Scandinavia from a thoroughly reliable,

12. S. Cordier: Relation d'une épidémie de paralysie atrophique de l'enfance. *Lyon méd.,* 57: 5–12, 48, 1888.

13. O. Medin: Ueber eine Epidemie von spinaler Kinkerlähmung. *Verh. X Internat. med. Kongr., 1890.* 2: Abt. 6: 37–47, 1891.

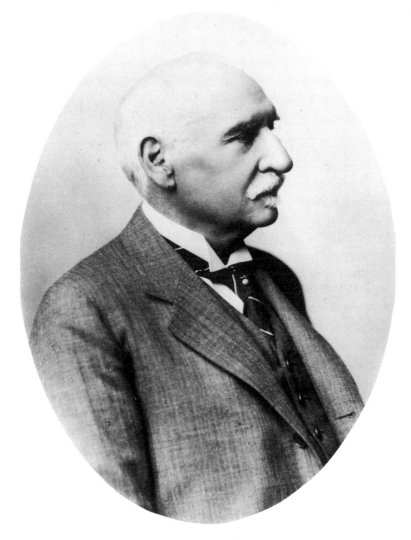

Fig. 13. Karl Oskar Medin, M.D. (1847–1927). Photograph obtained through the kindness of Dr. W. Koch, Museum of the History of Medicine, Stockholm.

articulate, and experienced pediatrician. No wonder they felt justified in naming the disease after him. Besides clarifying the picture of poliomyelitis, he succeeded in gaining for Sweden the unenviable reputation as the country where the worst epidemics occurred. Little did the medical profession realize that the rest of the world would soon catch up.

In 1887 Medin had investigated an epidemic of forty-four cases. Before that year, poliomyelitis, he said, had been infrequent not only in Stockholm but also in all of Sweden. An experience of fifteen years at the Polyclinic Hospital in Stockholm testified to this, since only about one or two cases had been admitted annually.

The opportunity of dealing with so many acutely ill or even mildly ill school-age children, gave Medin a decided advantage. He brought to it all the talents of a keenly perceptive clinician. However tragic the consequences of a sizable epidemic may be, at least the physician gains some benefit in terms of greater insight than is possible from sporadic observations made over a period of years. He is able to concentrate his attention on features which often come sharply into focus and may have escaped him at other times. Moreover, during an outbreak the physician is likely to be on the lookout for illnesses both typical and atypical.

Medin divided his forty-four cases into two groups: those of the spinal type, consisting of twenty-seven more or less typical paralytic cases; and those remaining, which presented less common signs owing to unusual localizations of the lesions. But his most important contribution was his comprehension of the clinical course of the disease. That the site of the usual pathological lesion was the spinal cord had been well established, but it was Medin who expressed the view that in the beginning there is a systemic phase. It was his claim that early, minor symptoms and signs such as slight fever and malaise signified a generalized process, which coincidentally and later was occasionally followed by serious damage to the central nervous system. As such, the involvement of the central nervous system almost amounted to a complication. In this astute conclusion Medin scored a triumph. Here his views were in line with those expressed earlier by the pathologist Rissler. Medin followed his patients closely and was thus able to document the early clinical features by observing that the course of the acute disease was sometimes interrupted by a brief afebrile period, resulting in a biphasic pattern with a first and second bout of fever. This was the forerunner of Draper's biphasic "dromedary form" (so named in 1917) in which the *minor illness* of poliomyelitis represented the first phase. Particularly were Medin's ideas taken up by his pupil Wickman and by the remarkable team of clinical virologists, Kling, Pettersson, and Wernstedt, about whom we shall hear much more in subsequent chapters. Yet, although Medin's views were in advance of his time, the period of Swedish ascendancy was comparatively short lived. It lasted only twenty or so years and was eclipsed during the 1920s and 1930s by rising interests in the study of *experimental* poliomyelitis. Eventually the clinical concept held by these early Swedish investigators of what was actually going on in the human disease in contradistinction to the disease in the monkey was vindicated, but this took a long time.

Karl Oskar Medin, who became in his later years the "grand old man of Swedish pediatrics," had many interests besides poliomyelitis.[14] Born in

14. Through the kindness of Dr. Sven Gard of Stockholm I have obtained an obituary note of Dr. Medin prepared by A. Lichtenstein and published in *Svenska lakartidningen* in 1927, pp. 1530–34. I am indebted to Mrs. Frank H. Stowell for a translation.

1847 in a small town near Stockholm, he prepared for his medical studies at Uppsala and obtained his medical licentiate at Stockholm in 1875. He became the leading pediatrician of Sweden and, during his long career, held many hospital positions of prominence; among them, professor of pediatrics at the Karolinska Institute, to which he was appointed in 1880, and head physician at the General Orphan Asylum in Stockholm. This latter institution, of which he was in charge for thirty years, was a model in terms of child care from both the pediatric and social points of view.

Medin must have been superb as a clinical teacher, in addition to his other commanding and attractive qualities. He was concerned about the *community* care of children and was chairman of the Stockholm Board of Health from 1906 to 1915. In his later career, in the same way and at about the same time as Dr. Osler in England, he turned his attention to the prevention of tuberculosis and to medical history.

Medin died in his eightieth year. Obviously he had touched the minds and hearts of his pupils as well as his patients. He was the symbol of the best in pediatrics in the late nineteenth century. This was an age when any prominent pediatrician or physician could have a fling at poliomyelitis provided he had the opportunity to see cases, possessed intelligence and clinical ability, and was willing to carry out the hard work entailed in clinical investigation. It was before the day when specialists of one kind or another, some expert and some not so expert, began to "take over" and restrict investigation of the disease to a particular aspect or form of treatment.

Reasons why Scandinavia should have been virtually the first place to feel the brunt of the extensive epidemic form of poliomyelitis in the late nineteenth century (Medin's time) are not clear, except for the suggestion that it was because the area was sparsely settled and lay far to the north. This might account for its people having had less immunity to poliomyelitis compared to most of the contemporary populations of Europe. Similarly the first sizable epidemic in the Western Hemisphere occurred in the state of Vermont. But quite apart from the fact that these outbreaks added materially to existing knowledge about the disease, it was natural that Europe and North America should look upon Scandinavia with a certain amount of alarm as a breeder of epidemics. That geography and climate had some bearing on this is probable, because even in modern times the greater the distance in either direction from the equator the less chance has this disease of remaining endemic. Whether in the years after 1880 travel to rural areas in Sweden in the summertime was increased, resulting in more frequent introduction of the virus by visitors, is not known; but at least in the sparsely settled Scandinavian countryside, the juvenile population, then as now, was more vulnerable to poliomyelitis than was the population in most cities, Scandinavian or otherwise. Indeed, as Medin's pupil Wickman was soon to point out, in the Swedish epidemic of 1904 the disease appeared in places far from large centers and seemed to avoid the more densely populated sections. This phenomenon points to a higher degree of immunity in urban residents and less immunity in rural populations, particularly in more remote areas.

Medin possessed that intangible quality that makes a great clinician, and when the suggestion was made that he deserved a place in the history of infantile paralysis, there was a quick response—hence the name *Heine-Medin* disease. But although it may have been satisfying nomenclature-wise, a disease as common as poliomyelitis could not remain designated by proper names for long. Physicians and pediatricians from far and wide were surprised that they should have had to put to use so promptly the information about epidemic poliomyelitis that Medin had supplied, when they faced epidemics themselves. The world did not have long to wait for another epidemic—just three or four years. This time it came to North America.

CHAPTER 9

The Earliest Sizable Epidemic in the United States

In 1893, two Boston physicians, John J. Putnam and E. W. Taylor, published a paper with the provocative title: "Is Acute Poliomyelitis Unusually Prevalent This Season?" They reported twenty-six cases in the summer of 1893 in and around the city of Boston and compared this with past summers when only a few cases had been seen: six in 1892, six in 1888, and three in 1889. The authors seemed concerned but were ultracautious in their claims that this was anything more than a modest increase in incidence. Nonetheless, they were aware that the disease had recently occurred in distinct epidemics and quoted Cordier, Medin, Sinkler, and others on this point. Regarding the local distribution of cases they went on to say:

> It is noteworthy, as against any strongly marked epidemic influence, that the patients did not come to any extent, from any one locality, but from different parts of the large area of the suburbs of Boston. The Charlestown and Chelsea district, however, furnished several cases. Very few of the patients came from Boston proper; and, as further evidence of the immunity of the city, it may be said that the records of the City Hospital yield but one case for this summer and autumn (onset in October), and none for last year.[1]

This recalls an observation made 100 years earlier by Underwood in the first clinical description of debility of the lower extremities in infants—that the disease occurred "seldomer in London than elsewhere." Putnam and Taylor, however, were the first to suggest a reason for this. They surmised that the city population may be more *immune* than its suburban counterpart. This bit of intuition, to say the least, was far in advance of the times.

A year later than the Boston article, in 1894, America suffered its first substantial epidemic of poliomyelitis. This occurred in Vermont and was reported in detail by Dr. Charles S. Caverly (see fig. 14), physician and public health officer of that state. His first and preliminary account of the outbreak begins as follows:

> Early in the summer just passed, (1894) physicians in certain parts of

1. J. J. Putnam and E. W. Taylor: Is acute poliomyelitis unusually prevalent this season? *Boston med. surg. J., 129*: 509–10, 1893.

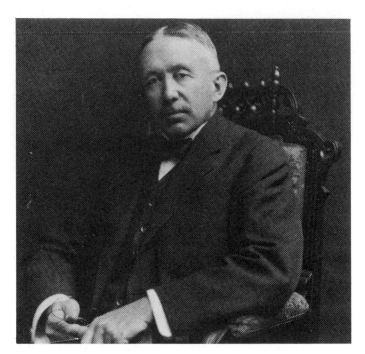

FIG. 14.   Charles S. Caverly, M.D., Sc.D. (1856–1918). Kindness of Vermont State Dept. of Health.

Rutland County, Vermont, noticed that an acute nervous disease, which was almost invariably attended with some paralysis, was epidemic. The first cases observed occurred in the city of Rutland and the town of Wallingford, appearing about mid-June. The disease prevailed locally up to about the middle of July when other towns about this city began to report cases.

From my own observation and conversation with other physicians, and the general feeling of uneasiness that was perceptible among the people in regard to the "new disease" that was affecting the children, I determined during the last of July to undertake a systematic investigation of the outbreak, in my capacity as a member of the State Board of Health.[2]

The Vermont epidemic turned out to be by far the largest one (132 cases on the final count) that had ever been reported in one year anywhere in the world. And, as far as can be ascertained, it was the first epidemic to be studied by a full-time local public health official. As was to become more apparent later, any local (or national) health officer who is in an authori-

2.   C. S. Caverly: Preliminary report of an epidemic of paralytic disease, occurring in Vermont, in the summer of 1894. *Yale med. J., 1*: 1, 1894.

tative position during epidemic times has certain advantages. This is evident in matters concerning an overall view of the community, in conducting sickness or follow-up surveys and in encouraging and organizing meetings of physicians and pediatricians in order to exchange individual clinical experiences.

Caverly's meticulous search for patients probably accounted for the unusually large number of reported cases in the 1894 epidemic, but if the outbreak had been only half its actual size it would have still been the largest to date.

In retrospect, it seems likely that the Vermont epidemic could have been anticipated by the increase in cases in the Boston area during the previous summer, for Rutland, in the neighboring state of Vermont, is only 125 miles from Boston. This interrupted progression of an epidemic is by no means rare. Certainly it has been a common experience for an epidemic to terminate in a given area with the coming of cold weather and then start up again the following spring or summer in an adjacent city, county, or rural district. The appearance and character of *epidemic* poliomyelitis in the northern lands of Scandinavia and in the sparsely settled parts of America's New England were part of the same general epidemiological phenomenon. This was to become manifest by the shift in age incidence which occurred in these two areas. Between 1890 and 1905, increasingly older children were attacked during epidemics, in contrast to the situation in other, middle European countries and in most of the United States, where the disease retained its endemic character and sporadic cases were still confined to infants and very young children.

As late as 1886, Dr. Mary Jacobi, whose exhaustive article on poliomyelitis has already been mentioned, maintained that the disease occurred mainly between the ages of eighteen months and four years. A more liberal opinion was expressed by no less an authority than Dr. Allen M. Starr, professor of diseases of the mind and nervous system at Columbia University, New York, whose chapter on poliomyelitis appeared in Albutt's *System of Medicine,* published in Britain in 1899.[3] Starr prepared a compilation of five series of endemic cases from European and American sources, all of them reported between 1880 and 1900. Each series had presumably been derived from as large a collection of *sporadic* cases as could be assembled. As shown in table 1, Starr came up with estimates which indicated that the cases of poliomyelitis had strayed but little from the infantile age group. Less than 1.0 percent of a total of 609 drawn from several sources were older than ten years! How different this was from the ages of *epidemic* cases, occurring between 1895 and 1905 in Scandinavia and Vermont (see table 2). In the 1905 outbreak in Sweden reported by Wickman, 45 percent

3. A. M. Starr: "Poliomyelitis anterior acuta," in *A system of Medicine by Many Writers,* ed. by Thomas Clifford Albutt, 8 vols. London, Macmillan, 1899, vol. 7, pp. 186–206.

TABLE 1. Age distribution of sporadic cases reported during the period 1880–1900 from Europe and the United States

Author	Year	Place	Total in Series	Number in Each Age Group (years)					Percent in Each Age Group (years)			
				0–3	4–6	7–9	10–14	≥15	<6	6–10	10–14	≥15
Seeligmuller	1880	Germany	77	73	4	0	0	0	100	0	0	0
Galbraith	1894	U.S.A.	75	70	5	0	0	0	100	0	0	0
Sinkler	1880+	Phila.	243	191	40	9	3	0	94.0	4.9	1.4	0
Gowers	1890+	England	109	67	30	12	0	0	88.9	11.1	0	0
Starr	1899	New York	115	81	23	8	3	0	90.4	9.0	2.6	0
Total			619	482	102	29	6	0	94.4	4.8	0.9	0

Data quoted from Starr (see n. 3).

TABLE 2. Age distribution of cases occurring in epidemics, largely in Scandinavia, during the period 1894–1905*

Author	Year	Place	Total in Series	Number in Each Age Group						Percent in Each Age Group	
				0–3	3–6	6–9	9–12	12–15	≥15	Over 6	≥15
Medin	1895	Stockholm	65	50	13	1	0	0	1	3.1	1.5
Wickman	1899	Stockholm	53	34	12	1	1	0	5	13.2	9.4
Wickman	1903	Göteborg	20	11	5	2	0	0	2	20.0	10.0
Wickman	1905	Sweden	1025	183	214	179	123	106	220	61.4	21.4
Caverly	1894	Vermont	122	90			20		12	26.2	9.1
				0–4	5–9	10–14			≥15	≥5	≥15
Leegaard	1899	Norway	54	12	5	7			30	77.7	55.5
Leegaard	1905	Norway	734	208	207	140			179	71.0	24.4

*Scandinavian data quoted by Wickman (see n. 6).

of the patients were over the age of ten, and 21 percent were over fifteen years!

The striking shift in age incidence marked the beginning of a pattern that the behavior of poliomyelitis was to follow from then on. In subsequent years it became apparent that, in a given population, once the disease began to involve sizable numbers of children older than four or five years, the trend toward periodic epidemicity and higher and higher attack rates in older individuals was relentless. Dr. Starr of New York, whom Dr. Caverly called in for consultation about the Rutland epidemic, said, in speaking of the 132 Vermont cases, that although they "chiefly appeared in infants and children, adults were not exempt." This statement runs counter to Dr. Starr's previous writings about the age incidence of the disease, whose meaning he was apparently unaware of. Clearly he had witnessed a new phenomenon in the epidemiology of "infantile" paralysis, although its significance escaped him completely. Thus poliomyelitis assumed an entirely different role in certain highly developed countries where repeated epidemics of increasing severity, affecting older and older individuals, began to appear. The changing age incidence was a crucial event in the history of the disease, and the secret of the shift from *endemic* to periodic *epidemic* poliomyelitis was partially contained in it. A dozen years later Wickman detected this relationship and was the first to appreciate what was going on. The subject is also discussed at length in a subsequent chapter.

In the second of several papers published on the 1894 Vermont epidemic,[4] Caverly did much more than point out that older children had become involved. He also was responsible for a number of original observations which, along with Medin's findings, soon made some of the statements in the erstwhile authoritative textbook articles of Jacobi and Starr seem out of date. He analyzed clinical manifestations in detail with a view toward classifying cases according to sites of paralysis. It is presumed that the majority of these patients eventually recovered from their disability. At least 56 of them are stated to have recovered completely. The remainder, 30 of whom were followed by Caverly for eighteen months, all suffered permanent paralysis. The death rate in the epidemic was high, 13.5 percent. This is not surprising, considering that the ages of the patients were greater by far than had been recorded in any previous epidemic, for it is a fundamental rule that the older the poliomyelitic patient, the higher the death rate.

However, a more fundamental and original observation than any of those mentioned above was the one upon which Caverly's fame was to

---

4. C. S. Caverly: Notes of an epidemic of acute anterior poliomyelitis. *J. Amer. med. Ass.,* *26*: 1, 1896.

rest. Of the 132 cases, *6 were stated to have no paralysis,* but "all had distinct nervous symptoms explainable only on the supposition that they belonged to this epidemic." Dr. Lovett of Boston, an ardent student of poliomyelitis himself, said, "He [Caverly] recognized the abortive cases, which were not so named and recognized until a great many years later."[5] A few years later, in 1907, Wickman had occasion to follow up Caverly's observation on this point with many examples of his own, and it was he who established the frequency of the abortive or nonparalytic form. Nevertheless, Caverly deserves priority at least for noticing these cases, infrequent as their presence seemed to him.

During the Vermont epidemic Dr. Caverly reported another curious finding, which has not been confirmed. It was that there was in the same geographical area an acute nervous disease, paralytic in nature, which affected domestic animals. Horses, dogs, and fowls died with various paralyses. One of the fowls, with paralysis of its legs, was subjected to a pathological examination by the distinguished neuropathologist Dr. Charles L. Dana, professor of nervous diseases at Cornell University Medical College, New York, who found "an acute poliomyelitis of the lower portion of the cord." Nevertheless a common etiologic connection between paralysis in animals and human poliomyelitis has never been established. In retrospect, Dr. Dana may have been led astray by the myelitis or inflammation of the spinal cord that is quite common in chickens with paralysis due to a variety of causes, none of which is ascribable to poliovirus.

And finally it is interesting to learn what Caverly thought about the cause, or causes, of poliomyelitis and of the idea that contagion played no role (see n.4).

The immediate apparent cause is stated in 37 instances. Of these overheating is mentioned 24 times, chilling of the body 4 times, trauma 4 times, while fatigue, typhoid fever, pneumonia and whooping cough are mentioned. There was a general absence of infectious disease as an etiologic factor in the epidemic. The element of contagium does not enter into the etiology either. I find but a single instance in which more than one member of a family had the disease, and as it usually occurred in families of more than one child, and as no efforts were made at isolation, it is very certain that it was noncontagious.

In this statement it must be admitted that Caverly went too far in attempting to negate Cordier's earlier and more correct claim concerning contagion, made six years before, in 1888. However, Caverly's place in the history of poliomyelitis is assured in spite of his denial of contagion. It rests

5. *Infantile Paralysis in Vermont, 1894–1922; A Memorial to Charles S. Caverly, M.D.* State Dept. of Public Health, Burlington, Vt., 1924, pp. 13–14. R. W. Lovett wrote a foreword to the collection of papers in this volume.

on his two major contributions: he was the first American physician and health officer to make a systematic study of a large epidemic, and he was among the first to recognize the occurrence of a few nonparalytic cases. His description of six patients without paralysis was the initial indication, outside of observations mentioned by Bull of Scandinavia, that lesions in the spinal cord might be so minimal that they were not reflected by any clinical signs, or that the central nervous system might escape neuronal lesions altogether. Yet Caverly's concept of the relationship of paralytic to nonparalytic poliomyelitis, soon to be supported by more extensive Swedish data,[6] was temporarily forgotten in the rush of experimental work which took place immediately after the discovery of the virus a few years later.

But what of Dr. Caverly himself? Fortunately there is available an account by Dr. Robert W. Lovett, who wrote the biographical note on Caverly in *Infantile Paralysis in Vermont, 1894–1922*, published in 1924 (see n.5). Charles S. Caverly was born in Troy, New Hampshire in 1856. He was educated in New Hampshire schools and graduated from Dartmouth College in 1878, where, it is stated, he was a member of Phi Beta Kappa. He then attended the University of Vermont, receiving the M.D. degree in 1881, and subsequently went on to the College of Physicians and Surgeons in New York City where he did postgraduate work for eighteen months before engaging in medical practice in Rutland, Vermont.

According to Dr. Lovett, Caverly was "always successful in private practice," but his major interest in public health soon came to the fore, superseding his interest in the practice of medicine. He became a member of the Vermont State Board of Health in 1890, and its president and animating spirit in 1891. He held this office until the time of his death. Caverly was also professor of hygiene and preventive medicine at the University of Vermont, from which he received the honorary degree of Sc.D. in recognition of his distinguished service in the field of public health. He died in 1918 at the age of sixty-two.

Obviously Dr. Lovett, who knew Caverly well both professionally and personally, had a high regard for "this quiet cultivated man" who had a singleness of purpose and a lack of pretense, and kept himself in touch with the progress of medicine in all departments. As a practitioner and experienced public health officer, he knew his community, and indeed, the entire state of Vermont. He had already been president of the state board of health for three years before the epidemic broke, and he also knew the proper consultants to bring up from New York City.

In judging his contribution to poliomyelitis, it would seem that Dr. Caverly was the right man in the right place at the right time. While he

6. I. Wickman: *Beiträge zur Kenntnis der Heine-Medinschen Krankheit (Poliomyelitis acuta und verwandter Erkrankungen)*. Berlin, Karger, 1907.

did not pursue most of his original observations on poliomyelitis further, he was so impressed with the tragic quota of paralyzed patients left in the wake of the 1894 outbreak that, as health officer of his state, he felt it his own special responsibility to provide facilities for the rehabilitation of patients with residual deformities. Moreover, he had the feeling that he should do something about a disease which had singled out his state and cruelly invaded it; thus he was instrumental in establishing a privately endowed poliomyelitis research laboratory under the auspices of his department of health. In the 1920s, the Harvard Infantile Paralysis Commission contributed in no small degree to the development of this laboratory —and to poliomyelitis in general—but that is anticipating our story.

CHAPTER 10

Ivar Wickman

Considering the importance of the contributions of Ivar Wickman, I do not believe that his work is fully appreciated today. Wickman was a pupil and ardent admirer of Medin and had been thoroughly indoctrinated by him in the then current knowledge of poliomyelitis. Subsequently, as an assistant in the Medical Clinic in Stockholm he also had the benefit of witnessing on his own two epidemics of the disease in Sweden, one in Stockholm in 1899 and one in Göteborg in 1903. His ambition to be recognized as an authority on poliomyelitis had become manifest early, for as a young man of thirty-three he had already brought out an ambitious 300-page monograph,[1] which was a thorough textbook review of the disease. This dealt with the development of knowledge to date, but for the most part concentrated on his own interpretations of the pathology and to a lesser extent his views on the pathogenesis of the infection. He remained skeptical of claims which various workers had made, that bacteria had been isolated from the spinal fluid and other sources, and unwilling to commit himself as to their significance. He was otherwise concerned with numerous unanswered questions: how the agent (whatever it was) traveled through the community, how it entered the human host, how it spread throughout the body, and how it was eliminated; did it travel to the central nervous system by way of the nerves, or by lymph channels, or through the blood stream? His views at this point in his career regarding the contagious nature of the disease were cautious and conservative, and he really dodged this particular issue, but not for long.

Wickman's background and experience logically placed him in the role of a trained investigator who was ready and anxious when the devastating Scandinavian epidemic of 1905 (more than 1,000 cases!) broke. He came to the epidemic with a mind already made up, confident that he knew what were the important studies to be done—and he was avid in the pursuit of them. The pathological picture had by this time already been described —almost as far as current histological methods would allow, and this aspect could rest for a while.[2] Wickman was after bigger game. To him the real

1. I. Wickman: Studien über Poliomyelitis acuta; zugleich ein Beitrag zur Kenntnis der Myelitis acuta. *Arb. path. Inst. Univ. Helsingfors, 1*:109, Berlin, Karger, 1905.

2. Obviously new details and descriptions of the pathology of poliomyelitis have inevitably continued to appear. Indeed Wickman himself made a histological study some years after the

questions were: What was the nature of the disease? Was it actually contagious? If contagious, how did it spread? Was it spread by direct contact with infected sick persons, even by "healthy" carriers of the virus? Was it waterborne or food-borne in the fashion in which typhoid fever was disseminated? Seldom has such an opportunity been presented to a young man who had prepared himself for just such a challenge and was at the height of his powers.

The Scandinavian epidemic of 1905 is described in Wickman's second monograph.[3] He proposed for the first time the name "Heine-Medin disease." Admiration for his teacher did not stop there but is further expressed by his dedication of the volume to Medin, on the "occasion of his 60th birthday." The epidemic of 1905 reached the staggering figure of 1,031 cases. It was by far the largest one that had occurred up to that time anywhere in the world. No doubt the total number was enhanced by Wickman's practice of including abortive and nonparalytic cases as well as those with paralysis. He went far beyond Caverly's view that such cases were uncommon, for Wickman pointed to their frequency, even emphasized that they were instrumental in the spread of the disease. Whether to accept all nonparalytic cases as examples of poliomyelitis has been a constant problem to this day, especially for statisticians. But by including them, Wickman went far to emphasize their importance, which was exactly what he wished to do. To a parent, the difference between a child who is ill and is left with paralysis and one who has escaped with no muscle weakness whatever is like comparing the difference between black and white. Yet to Wickman, the epidemiologist, who was attempting to trace the spread of poliomyelitis, the two had equal significance, as both varieties seemed equally infectious.

A graphic picture of the precipitous character and the magnitude of this Swedish epidemic of 1905 appears in figure 15. It was inevitable that in such a large outbreak the geographical distribution of cases should be widespread throughout Sweden and equally inevitable that the disease should spread to Norway. Among Wickman's early observations was that infected foci were not influenced by the density of the population in the manner in which an infection such as tuberculosis might have behaved. In contrast, the rural districts were ravaged, while cities were spared. This tendency to attack villages, especially remote villages, in Sweden's sparsely settled countryside was a fundamental principle of the epidemiology of the

1905 epidemic (in 1910). I. Wickman: Weitere Studien über Poliomyelitis acuta; ein Beitrag zur Kenntnis der Neurophagen und Körnchenzellen. *Dtsche Z. Nervenheilk.*, *38*: 396–437, 1909–1910.

3. I. Wickman: *Beiträge zur Kenntnis der Heine-Medinschen Krankheit (Poliomyelitis acuta und verwandter Erkrankungen)*. Berlin, Karger, 1907. Unfortunately this work was not translated into English until four years later.

disease and a fortunate break for Wickman. It enabled him to trace the comings and goings of Heine-Medin disease more readily and more accurately than ever. This success was due in some measure to the small size and circumscribed nature of many of these communities, the consequent

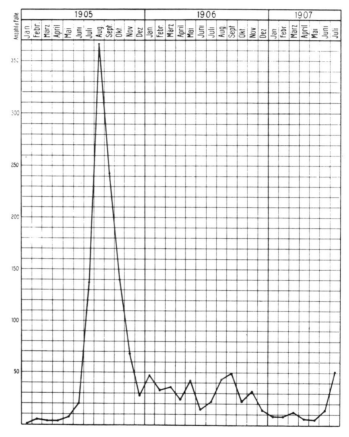

FIG. 15.   Graph indicating the number of cases of poliomyelitis recorded in Sweden from January 1905–July 1907 (from Wickman, n. 3).

intimacy with which he was able to carry out his studies, and to the simple fact that the incidence of poliomyelitis in rural areas happened to be exceedingly high in the 1905 epidemic. Total attack rates were 5 or 6 per 1,000 in some villages; and 3.0 to 3.7 per 1,000 if only the paralytic cases were counted—considerably above the usual rates. The high incidence could have meant one or both of two things: either the strain of poliovirus responsible had an unusual degree of virulence; or, what is more likely, the children were particularly susceptible because of the remoteness of the villages and the infrequent contact with people from the outside world. This had the inevitable result of a lack of immunity in the infantile and even the juvenile population. The pattern is a familiar one today, as illustrated by the extreme vulnerability of Eskimos and other isolated populations when exposed to visitors who harbor infectious agents; only in this case the susceptibles were Swedish children living in remote rural communities.

Almost at the onset of the epidemic Wickman began to appreciate that in some instances the infection might miss the central nervous system altogether, obviously not a new observation. But Wickman was definitely the first to grasp the implications of these observations. He was also the first to realize that abortive cases might equal or even outnumber the paralytic ones and, what was more important, that they had a profound significance in the spread of human poliomyelitis! Thus the emphasis was shifted away from the view that the lesions of the disease were entirely confined to the central nervous system. Even though paralysis was the more spectacular aspect of poliomyelitis, Wickman appreciated that it was a mistake to concentrate his attention entirely upon it. He grasped the idea early in the epidemic that the (infected) patient who was lucky enough to have escaped paralysis or who developed only minor symptoms was not any the less dangerous to the community from the standpoint of contagion. Wickman estimated that in one village more than 50 percent of the cases were of this nonparalytic type. The findings strongly suggested that the infection must be spread in large part through the intermediary of such cases —a concept which required reevaluation of the whole clinical and epidemiologic picture of poliomyelitis.[4]

Wickman certainly did not arrive at such a conclusion all at once. For a time he was in a quandary as to how to deal with the problem. Should he include *all* of the abortive illnesses, however mild, in the *total* number of cases? Among the forty-nine examples which he described, the range was from an illness in which a stiff neck and pain and stiffness in the back were evident to one in which the only manifestation was fever lasting from one to five days. His descriptions went from what we would today call clear-cut nonparalytic cases to those which would be considered as the mildest of "minor illnesses" of poliomyelitis. In recent times both paralytic and nonparalytic types are included and so specified in any official report giving the total number of cases occurring in any particular epidemic in a given city or state, while minor illnesses are omitted because of their entirely nonspecific clinical features. But what Wickman faced was the question

4. Today abortive and nonparalytic forms of the disease make up a considerable proportion of all cases seen in epidemics in unvaccinated communities. The exact ratio of *reported* paralytic to nonparalytic cases is inconstant, shifting with each outbreak, depending on many variables including the alertness of local physicians. Wickman's overall estimate of the nonparalytic cases in the entire Swedish epidemic of 1905 was about 15 percent. This is approximate, for he stated that precise enumeration was possible in limited districts only; so the total number of such cases in this epidemic was therefore underestimated.

whether all suspicious nonparalytic illnesses, however slight the symptoms, should be called poliomyelitis. This might be theoretically sound, but practically impossible. Such a practice deviated sharply from accepted medical custom of his day, and it was unlikely that elder clinicians would go along with so radical a shift in point of view about the disease. To diagnose infantile paralysis in the absence of paralysis must have seemed ridiculous to the rank and file of the medical profession, and so it remained until more than a generation later.

But over and above the classification of the different forms of the disease, Wickman reached a fundamental decision: that poliomyelitis must be regarded as a highly contagious disease, and the mild cases should be considered along with the severe because they too were infectious. He ascribed the tardiness of recognition of this concept partly to the small size of former epidemics and partly to the fact that the possibility of the spread of infection by slightly ill persons or even healthy carriers (inapparent cases) had not even been considered. This last point he made with singular perspicacity—through, I suspect, a process of what I may call epidemiologic instinct—for evidence of the transmission via the agency of inapparent cases did not receive laboratory confirmation until two years later.

As to the routes of spread of the 1905 Swedish epidemic, the relation to main roads and railways was striking. A study of local conditions showed that dissemination was associated with the busy traffic centers, which permitted more frequent communication between rural and urban people. In all of these investigations one gets the picture of Wickman going up and down throughout the Swedish countryside in the disastrous summer of 1905, tirelessly following up cases and examining local conditions. This was the manner in which W. H. Frost, one of America's leading epidemiologists who came after Wickman by some six or eight years, investigated epidemics in the midwestern states of the United States. It was a method of tireless and careful clinical study which was not to last long.

Among the many focal outbreaks that Wickman investigated the summer of 1905 were at least four in which he was able to designate the local school as the primary site from whence the infection was disseminated. One such small town (Tingsryd) some 200 miles southwest of Stockholm had at the time a population of "more than 3,000 inhabitants." This community yielded eighteen cases during the period from mid-August to mid-October 1905, a high incidence even if the population had totaled 4,000. A diagram of the manner in which the infection was thought to have spread has been reproduced from Wickman's monograph and is shown in figure 16. It will be seen that twelve of the eighteen patients attended the local school, and three of the twelve (case nos. 328–30) dwelt in the schoolhouse. By tracing the spread of the disease through abortive as well as paralytic cases Wickman was left with only six children, occupying four houses, for

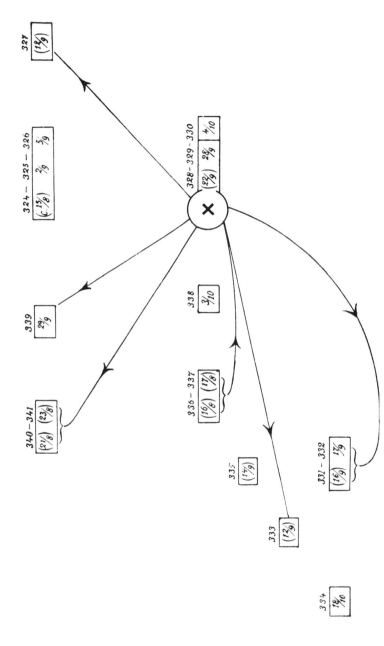

FIG. 16. A school outbreak near the small town of Tingsryd, Sweden. The X (within the circle) designates the location of the school. Arrows indicate the radial spread of the infection. Individual numbers (324–41) of the 18 cases appear above the oblong boxes. Within these boxes the dates of onset of the cases are given. Eleven such dates, enclosed in parentheses, indicate abortive cases (from I. Wickman, n. 3).

whom no contact with the other fifty-two children who attended school could be traced.

Besides recognizing the frequency of abortive cases and establishing the contagious nature of the disease, Wickman described a number of other features. With more than 1,000 cases which he had painstakingly collected, he certainly did not lack material. In fact his series included the largest array of clinical forms that had ever been assembled. His classification and description of these cases reads like a modern textbook.

There is one other point that I should stress among the many important clinical observations which Wickman made. This has to do with the length of the incubation period in poliomyelitis, an important matter if one is attempting to trace the comings and goings of disease and to follow contact spread. Wickman was correct when he maintained that this period averages 3 to 4 days. Before his time, and for many years afterward, the question was disputed whether the incubation period should be measured from the time of exposure to the beginning of the minor illness (3 to 4 days), or to the onset of fever associated with the paralytic phase (the major illness), which was often 8 to 10 days. Anyway, for nigh on to half a century authors of textbook articles on the clinical features of poliomyelitis (the writer among them) were to state that the incubation period averages 8 to 10 days with a minimum of 5 and a maximum of 35.[5] It was not until the live attenuated poliovirus vaccine came into use that it was possible to establish the length of the incubation period of the *human infection* on a large scale, and it turned out to be 3 to 4 days, just as Wickman had maintained all along.

Only a year or two after Wickman's second monograph had appeared, the discovery of poliovirus was announced in 1908, in Vienna, by Landsteiner and Popper. Actually this discovery, monumental as it was, probably had only minor significance as far as Wickman's epidemiological interpretations were concerned. Personally he must have been technically interested in this discovery, but he was not profoundly stirred by it for the simple reason that he had anticipated that an infectious agent would be discovered sooner or later. Yet he had neither the desire nor the experience to go on to a career in clinical virology; nor to pursue the paths which the discovery of the virus opened up, for he was fundamentally a clinical epidemiologist and pediatrician, and he had already made other plans for his future. Once he had made the decision that the disease was contagious, perhaps highly contagious, it mattered little to him whether the infectious agent was a bacterium, a virus, or indeed any other kind of a microbial

5. The longer estimate was based in part on analogies drawn from the experimental disease in rhesus monkeys. Such evidence had the advantage that the exact time of inoculation of the animal was known, but the decided disadvantage that the infection was produced in a highly artificial manner, by a different route from the natural one in many, and furthermore in a totally different species of primate from *homo sapiens*.

agent. To others, it made all the difference in the world, for with the discovery of the etiological agent came the possibility of isolating the virus
for diagnostic purposes, of measuring immune reactions resulting from infection, and the hope of immunization as well. But unfortunately this was
not Ivar Wickman's dish. Although he perhaps did not realize it, Landsteiner's discovery was to turn the main direction of poliomyelitis research
into new channels for all time. Because of this, Wickman probably sensed
that poliomyelitis was not to be his major interest in the future. He did
not become a member of Sweden's famous team of clinical virologists that
followed close upon the heels of Landsteiner's discovery (by less than five
years) and capitalized on his work in a remarkable fashion.[6]

As a matter of fact, at about the time of the discovery of the virus Wickman had decided that he needed broader training in clinical medicine and
pediatrics if he was to achieve the professorship for which he had ambitions. He had hoped to secure the chair of pediatrics which his former
teacher and idol Medin had occupied, and he set out on an intensive course
of training on the Continent to prepare himself in the best possible manner.

To start from the beginning, Ivar Wickman (see fig. 17) was born in
Lund in 1872; he studied in Lund and Stockholm, passed the state medical examinations in 1895, and promptly became Medin's assistant in the
Stockholm Pediatric Clinic. In 1906 he was granted the advanced degree
of doctor of medicine, and a year later he occupied the position of docent
for neurology. A year later, his finest work (his second monograph, which
dealt with the 1905 epidemic) had appeared. It was a publication which
brought universal acclaim from his colleagues. Then, after some five years
in which he added to his medical experience in Sweden, there followed two
years of training in neurology and pediatrics abroad. This took him to
Berlin and Paris and ended with assistantships in pediatrics in Breslau and
in Strasbourg.

With such a promising candidate, who had trained so assiduously, it
would seem that the Stockholm Faculty of Medicine should have appointed
him as the professor of children's diseases and successor to Medin. But tragically enough, it was not to be—Wickman was turned down. The blow was
evidently more than he could bear, and shortly thereafter, in 1914, he took
his own life. He was only forty-two years old.

What were the reasons? No doubt disappointment over the loss of the
professorship was paramount. However, what may have hung in the background was a feeling that whereas his greatest contribution had been made
in the field of poliomyelitis, his efforts had perhaps suffered an eclipse by

6. C. Kling, A. Pettersson, and W. Wernstedt: The presence of the microbe of infantile
paralysis in human beings. *Communications Inst. méd. État, Stockholm, 3*: 5, 1912; and other
papers by individual members of this remarkable team.

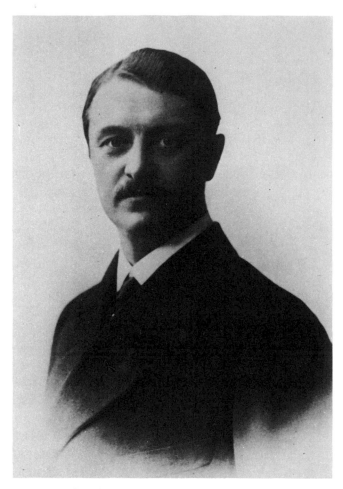

FIG. 17. Ivar Wickman, M.D. (1872–1914).

the discovery of the virus. In addition was the tragedy that he himself had turned away from this, his first love, to prepare through a long and arduous training period for Medin's chair—all to no avail. He probably thought that in the meantime the field of poliomyelitis had gone far beyond him and into different channels, of which he had little knowledge.

Ivar Wickman has been described as an attractive, intelligent, even brilliant young man, though one who was outspoken and had no use for Philistines and fools. He was also one who never made concessions. Perhaps it was this last quality, combined with a psychasthenic temperament, which led to his untimely death.

But there was another tragedy, which concerned the disease itself. Wickman had established the concept that human poliomyelitis was highly contagious and was not entirely, or even chiefly, a disease of the central nervous system. In fact his observations indicated that it was spread primarily through the medium of subclinical infections. Yet before he died he must have had grave doubts that his views would hold. For with the discovery of the virus and the rush of enthusiasm for experimental work, the mainstream had soon been diverted away from Wickman's correct concepts of the human disease gained from clinical epidemiological work carried out so painstakingly in the field. His ideas were about to be supplanted. Particularly in the United States the new era centered rapidly in the laboratory; it was dominated by investigations on experimental pathology in the monkey, with most of the interest focused again on the neurotropic aspects of the virus and the central nervous system lesions it could produce. Indeed the human disease was not shaken free from this one-sided approach for many years. The course of events was typical of the way knowledge in poliomyelitis seems to have progressed—always by fits and starts, often punctuated by long periods of frustrating inactivity followed by spurts of sometimes misdirected effort. One does not have to look far for the cause of this. It soon became easier to work at the laboratory bench than in the field, or to do both. For it has been said of this particular time that everything one discovered through the use of the microscope must be true. Also, the stakes were so high and certain authorities were so eager to have their own pet theories accepted that they ignored any inconvenient facts which had been established previously about the human disease. But in the end, no amount of experimentation on the monkey could upset the fundamental clinical epidemiological truths that Wickman had discovered.

CHAPTER 11

Landsteiner and the Discovery of the Virus

Within a year after the appearance of Wickman's second monograph, came a discovery which was to change the direction of poliomyelitis research for all time—the discovery of the virus of poliomyelitis. For nearly a generation a fruitless search had been going on to find such a microbial agent. Numerous false hopes had been raised by claimants who championed this or that particular species of bacteria.[1] A search for so-called filterable viruses probably had been made less often, for this presented many more difficulties than did tests for bacteria. Indeed, at the turn of the century techniques for dealing with viruses were in their early infancy—not to say an embryonic state.

By 1908 only a few filterable viruses as agents of human and animal diseases had been detected. These included the viruses of smallpox and vaccinia, rabies, and foot-and-mouth disease. The use of tissue cultures for the growth of viruses was unknown. If any laboratory animals out of the ordinary were to be inoculated, no one knew which ones were likely to be susceptible, and no one knew how such inoculations ought to be done. Furthermore, if one were lucky enough to produce a hopeful result with presumably infectious material from cases of poliomyelitis, there was the added difficulty of proving it by histological means. This meant reproducing in experimental animals spinal cord lesions comparable to those seen in the human disease—not to speak of the task of maintaining the agent alive by transferring it serially in continuous passage.

Nevertheless, at a medical meeting in Vienna on December 18, 1908, the immunologist Landsteiner (see fig. 18) and his assistant Popper[2] were able to demonstrate microscopic slides of one human and two monkey spinal cords, all showing the familiar histological picture of acute poliomyelitis. Sections from the human infection came from a boy of nine years who had died after an illness of three days. Bacterial cultures of the spinal cord had

1. For an account of the negative and false positive results of this period the reader is referred to E. F. Hutchins: "Historical summary," chap. 1, in *Poliomyelitis*. International Committee for the Study of Infantile Paralysis, Baltimore, Williams & Wilkins, 1932, pp. 24–26.

2. K. Landsteiner and E. Popper: Mikroscopische Präparate von einem menschlichen und zwei Affenrückenmarken. *Wien. klin. Wschr., 21*: 1830, 1908. A further report by these same authors appeared in May 1909 amplifying these findings: I. Übertragung der Poliomyelitis acuta auf Affen. Z. *Immun.-Forsch.* (Orig.), *2*: 377, 1909.

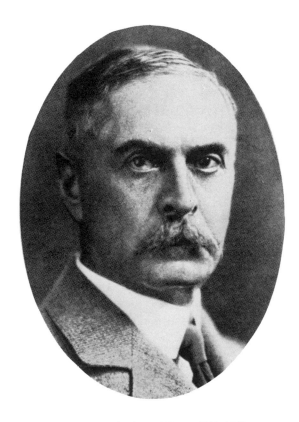

Fig. 18. Karl Landsteiner, M.D. (1868–1943). From the Historical Library of the Yale University School of Medicine.

been sterile, and injection of a suspension of the ground-up cord into rabbits, guinea pigs, and mice also had given negative results. But the team went further than this in their choice of experimental animals. They selected the right ones in the form of two monkeys, animals which probably represented an expensive luxury for these young scientists. Nevertheless, they were willing to risk what might have been considered a useless expense for an experiment which did not have any particular promise of success. The monkeys were of different species, one being a *Cynocephalus hamadryas* and the other a *Macaca rhesus* (*Macaca mulatta*). The choice turned out to be fortunate. Both of these species of primates are known today to be highly susceptible to experimental poliomyelitis, although to somewhat different degrees. The selection of Old World monkeys rather than the relatively insusceptible New World ones was just as fortunate.

The bacteriologically sterile material obtained from the spinal cord of the fatal human case was injected into the two animals intraperitoneally.

The *Cynocephalus* monkey succumbed eight days later, following a short illness of two days; although no paralysis was noted, this could have escaped observation. The real test came when histological sections of the spinal cord revealed typical and extensive lesions which had a remarkably close resemblance to the lesions of human poliomyelitis. Similar, though not such widespread, changes were found in the sections of the cord from the second monkey, which developed complete flaccid paralysis of both legs after a long incubation period—seventeen days. The authors must have been amazed, and not a little pleased, at the nature of the experimental disease produced in this animal, which resembled so closely the paralytic disease in man. They made the modest suggestion that poliomyelitis might be caused by an invisible virus, an opinion soon confirmed by other experiments.

Landsteiner and Popper were well aware of the immense amount of work that remained to be done before they had proved their case. They were working at a time when it was necessary to follow the rules strictly to achieve acceptance of a claim that a particular microorganism had been shown to cause a given disease. These rules, formulated by Robert Koch in 1884,[3] stipulated that the following points should be demonstrated: (1) the presence of the organism in all cases of the disease in such distribution as to explain the lesions; (2) the isolation of the organism in pure culture; and (3) the reproduction of the disease in animals by inoculation of the specific organism.

Landsteiner and his teammate had succeeded only in partially fulfilling two of these postulates—the first not at all. It was apparently going to take several years to collect enough cases to prove the correctness of the conclusions based on their first experiment. Nevertheless they had succeeded in reproducing the disease so exactly in the monkey and the record was so genuine that not only were the investigators themselves impressed, but the evidence was enough to convince the rest of the scientific world almost immediately. Seldom has the record spoken louder or in a more convincing manner than it did when one of these monkeys "came down" with paralysis, and louder still when they were shown to have lesions within the spinal cord exactly like those seen in human poliomyelitis. Landsteiner and Popper had not attempted to pass the "virus" from monkey to monkey, but they soon carried out this step successfully, as did several others. By late 1909 almost the whole microbiological world had accepted the viral etiology of poliomyelitis.

It is a truism in science that discovery of some new fact, or even of a

3. Koch's postulates were modified time and again, but they represented the rules that dominated the science of microbiology for half a century, until in 1937 Rivers led a movement for their modification which has been going on ever since (T. M. Rivers: Viruses and Koch's postulates. *J. Bact., 33*: 1, 1937).

method that is really new, is bound to lead the investigator further along the uncertain path he has begun to explore. There were innumerable questions to be answered about poliomyelitis, which obviously could not be tackled all at once. Landsteiner was therefore left with the difficult decision of having to choose the most important of these. Could the virus be recovered elsewhere in the human body besides the spinal cord? Was it present in the blood, or in the spinal fluid? What was the ideal method of inoculating monkeys so as to ensure the maximum number of "takes"? Could experimental poliomyelitis turn out to be a model for demonstrating how the human disease might evolve in its natural host—in other words, its pathogenesis in man? Did a single attack of the experimental infection confer immunity? And, more hopefully, could the discovery of the virus lead quickly to a method of immunization against this terrible disease?

Available means for pursuing investigations of experimental poliomyelitis were not open to everyone. A well-equipped laboratory with an accessible department of pathology was necessary. Monkeys were not only expensive, but also they required special animal quarters—quite different from the usual cages or bins for mice, guinea pigs, and rabbits. Besides, monkeys needed an entirely different kind of care from that required by smaller animals. This included the services of a full-time keeper who was skillful in catching and handling them. In addition to cleaning the cages and preparing special food, his duties were to observe and exercise the animals daily, to assist in inoculations, and to perform sundry other duties. In fact, if work was to go forward as it should, the facilities needed amounted to those offered by a well-staffed, well-equipped, and well-endowed pathological institute.[4] Within some university settings, or at the Pasteur Institute in Paris or the Rockefeller Institute for Medical Research in New York, there were suitable facilities for investigating poliomyelitis, but these were not available to Landsteiner at the time of his discovery, for his position was only that of pathologist to a general hospital.

However, so quickly was the value of Landsteiner and Popper's discovery recognized, and their results confirmed in a number of laboratories, that it was inevitable that scientists in many countries should rush to take advantage of the new leads. Overnight, investigation of the pathogenesis of poliomyelitis became a popular cause, and, as such, it was soon taken over. It was equally inevitable that Landsteiner himself, with all his other interests in immunology, should have felt crowded out—to a certain degree. But this did not occur until he had answered certain fundamental questions he probably considered as the ones deserving first priority. It was in the course of these studies that he teamed up with Levaditi (a member of the Pasteur Institute of whom we will hear later), a prolific and tireless worker in the

4. In 1909, many university departments of pathology included bacteriology and immunology and were often dignified by the name, *Institute of Pathology.*

field of poliomyelitis and in infectious diseases in general. Together they published at least a dozen papers on experimental poliomyelitis within the incredibly short time between 1909 and 1911. Their first and most immediate quest was to determine whether the virus existed and perhaps traveled through the human body outside the central nervous system, i.e. extraneurally. This was in spite of the known fact that the agent apparently produced no lesions, or only lesions of an insignificant nature, in these other anatomical regions.

The team of Landsteiner, Levaditi, and Pastia was soon able to detect poliovirus in nonnervous tissues from fatal human cases. They recovered the agent from tonsils and from the lining membranes of the throat.[5] In a remarkably few months they were also able to demonstrate its presence in nasal secretions, in parotid and submaxillary salivary glands, and in intestinal (mesenteric) lymph nodes. Obviously the idea they had in mind was to determine the portal of entrance, the route along which the virus progressed on its way to the central nervous system, and perhaps the mode of exit.[6]

Both neural and extraneural sites of predilection of the virus occupied the attention of workers in several other laboratories at the same time: Dr. Simon Flexner at the Rockefeller Institute in New York, Leiner and von Wiesner in Vienna, and Römer in Marburg, Germany, to mention but a few of the more prominent ones. These workers soon focused their main attention on the infection in monkeys, believing this to be an excellent model for elucidating problems of the human disease—as it surely was, before interpretations based on the image of the experimental infection were carried too far. For a short time, however, poliovirus research was kept within the channels Landsteiner and Levaditi had begun to explore.

Factors which were eventually to lead Landsteiner away from further studies of the etiology and pathogenesis of poliomyelitis must have been his appraisal of the trend toward leaning heavily upon observations on the monkey instead of on the disease in man; and that several of the successful and eager workers who crowded in to exploit his discovery worked in well-equipped laboratories or institutes, with many facilities at hand, whereas, as previously noted, Landsteiner had only a minor position as pathologist at the Wilhelminspital in Vienna. I have been reliably informed[7] that he

5. K. Landsteiner, C. Levaditi, and C. Pastia: Étude expérimentale de la poliomyélite aiguë (maladie de Heine-Médin). *Ann. Inst. Pasteur, 25*: 805, 1911.

6. See chap 13 for further investigations along these lines.

7. In correspondence with Landsteiner's son, Dr. E. K. Landsteiner of Providence, Rhode Island, on this point, he stated: "According to what he (my father) told me in later years, he recognized that any advancement beyond the point to which he had carried the work would come only after many years of arduous and costly effort. Thus he quite voluntarily turned to other projects which gave promise of shorter-term results." How right the elder Landsteiner was to prove.

sensed the manner in which powerful figures in the field of experimental medicine had begun to take over and decided, like the true and unselfish scientist he was, that if others were in a position to carry out the work better and more easily than he was, then let them do it. Perhaps they would move faster than had been possible for him. It was in consideration of all these points, plus the fact that he must have been eager to get on with his earlier researches in the budding science of immunology, that Landsteiner relinquished opportunities in a field in which he had already blazed a trail, but the full potential of which he had barely begun to explore. Landsteiner may be ranked with the great pioneers in the burgeoning field of immunology. Subsequently for nearly half a century he was to witness the steady development of this science to which he himself contributed so much new knowledge.

Of his biography, we happily know a number of important details. Karl Landsteiner was born in Vienna in 1868 and graduated there in medicine at the age of twenty-three. Six years later he became an assistant in the Vienna Institute of Hygiene, starting his work with the director, Max von Gruber, in 1897. It was at this time that he began his immunological investigations, which were continued later when he moved to the Pathological Anatomical Institute of the University to pursue studies under Weichselbaum.

The problem Landsteiner had set for himself was to determine if immunological differences might exist among the various types of human blood. At that time few had any idea of the eventual importance of this. Before the turn of the century, if one transfused a patient with blood obtained from another individual, the outcome was often disastrous, resulting in the immediate death of the patient. Such tragedies were due to incompatibility between the blood types of the donor and of the recipient. To make a long story short, Dr. Landsteiner's studies in the early 1900s on such practical immunological problems were to pave the way for the identification of the four major blood groups, thus laying the groundwork for the science and techniques of blood transfusion as they are practiced today. To quote from an obituary note in the *Lancet:*

> It is to Landsteiner's credit that order was brought out of chaos. In 1901 he described three types of blood which he believed were not developed through a pathological change but were manifestations of a constitutional difference. Shortly afterwards a fourth type of blood was described by Decastello and Stürli. These findings were soon confirmed and extended by other workers until the exact relation of the different blood-group factors to their corresponding iso-antibodies[8]

8. Isoantibodies are antibodies present in the blood of some individuals of a given species; they react against cells of certain other members of the same species.

became clear, and a practical result of immense importance emerged —the successful transfusion of whole blood.[9]

Landsteiner's discovery at the turn of the century remained almost unnoticed for some years, although he specifically pointed out its possible application both in the practice of blood transfusion and in the determination of paternity. However, within about ten or fifteen years the use of transfusions began to increase tremendously, particularly in connection with the casualties during World War I. The correctness of Landsteiner's predictions was proved, not only in terms of therapy but also with respect to the hereditary transmission of blood groups.

In 1908 Landsteiner had been appointed pathologist to the Wilhelminspital in Vienna, and it was there that he succeeded in isolating poliovirus. Yet this discovery and all the vistas which it opened held his interest for only two or three short years. It was the field of immunology that attracted him more, and to it he soon returned. Intricate details of his work on specific and nonspecific antibodies[10] need not concern us here. Suffice it to say that he had a long and most distinguished career and it was for his work in this field that he was eventually rewarded with the Nobel Prize.

Soon after his return to immunological research, Europe became engulfed in World War I, and he was forced to remain in Vienna under the trying circumstances which existed in that city during the war and postwar years. Because of difficult living conditions in Austria, after the war he decided to leave his native city and seek a livelihood elsewhere. First he went to Holland (in 1919), where he was appointed pathologist at the R. K. Ziekenhuis at the Hague, but a few years later he accepted an invitation to become a member of the Rockefeller Institute for Medical Research in New York. There he was able to continue his immunological studies on human blood groups, investigations begun so brilliantly nearly a quarter of a century earlier. He became a member emeritus of the institute in 1939 but continued working at the same pace until his death in 1943.

It is rare for a scientist to live to see the fruits of his work ripen as did Landsteiner; almost as rare as it is for an inventor to witness the success of his invention before the patent rights have run out. For Landsteiner, his long career was a real triumph. By nature he was a stern man, though modest, simple, and sincere. It was natural that these qualities impressed everyone who met him, including the author, who will always remember his remarkable dignity and the sense of genius that his person evoked. Seldom have I felt that I was in the presence of such a great scientist.

9. Karl Landsteiner (1868–1943): *Lancet, 2*: 110–11, July 24, 1943.

10. Some of these details are set forth in a small book that has been described as a classic on the subject: K. Landsteiner: *The Specificity of Serological Reactions.* Springfield, Ill., C. C. Thomas, 1936; 2nd ed. Cambridge, Harvard Univ. Press, 1945.

At the time of the award of the Nobel Prize to him in 1930, Sinclair Lewis, who received the prize for literature that same year, minimized his own importance as compared with the contributions made by Landsteiner. "As for myself," said Mr. Lewis,

I might be able to write another book which would suit your tastes or would not. May I say that I shall be happy on that day I can write a book the hero of which should personify the ethical and material value to humanity of Dr. Landsteiner. What more could I say?[11]

The humbleness and modesty of this remarkable man of genius had little in common with the character of an ambitious and self-seeking scientist.

By 1912 the state of knowledge about poliomyelitis had reached at long last, after one hundred or more years, the stage where a correct concept of the nature of the disease could begin to take shape. The etiological agent had been established as a virus, and from then on it was generally agreed that infantile paralysis was an infectious, contagious disease with epidemic potentialities. Yet almost forty years were to elapse before the three distinct immunologic types of poliovirus, all members of one and the same family, were definitely separated, and their relationship to one another clarified. In view of the quick success of Landsteiner's earlier work on the immunology of blood groups, it is conceivable that had he worked on the family of polioviruses in the same manner, he might also have achieved comparable headway in this field, and the world would not have had to wait so many years for progress in the understanding and control of the disease.

But Landsteiner's discovery and his work with Levaditi, which followed within three years, certainly opened doors sufficiently wide for the investigation of all kinds of problems whose solution had up to that time seemed hopelessly obscure. It was unfortunate that many who followed him became so entangled in the intricacies of research on the experimental infection that they were never able to shake themselves sufficiently loose to explore the human disease. At the moment there were so many leads to be followed and so many eager investigators ready to pursue them, it is not surprising that in the rush of activity some wrong turns were taken. It was typical of the crablike method in which poliomyelitis research was to proceed. But nonetheless the heightened activity had the aura of great progress. In the period between 1912 and 1930 it was as if some of the main investigators, particularly in the United States, had become so transfixed with the importance of laboratory work on experimental poliomyelitis that they had, for the time being, arrived at the assumption that it was the only type of poliomyelitis research worth doing. It was a premature assumption but highly understandable.

11. Obituary notes, *New York Times*, June 27, 1943.

On the other hand, all this sudden upsurge of interest beginning in 1910, and the subsequent extensive laboratory work on the experimental disease, were of immense and timely value. My criticism is that it was carried on far too long, to the exclusion of other forms of endeavor. But in the years immediately after the discovery of the virus (1909–14), to say that advances were made and hopes were bright would be understatements. The windfall which had brought important new knowledge to the field of poliomyelitis was full of promise. It was even anticipated that a quick and ready laboratory solution of many crucial problems lay just around the corner. Little did the eager scientists of the day realize that it would be almost another half century before such major questions were resolved.

CHAPTER 12

Simon Flexner and Experimental Poliomyelitis

As soon as the news reached this side of the Atlantic that Landsteiner had discovered an agent thought to be responsible for poliomyelitis, Simon Flexner, the recently appointed director of the Rockefeller Institute for Medical Research, was quick to grasp its significance and to act upon it. Here was news that he had long been awaiting. Flexner seemed to be the ideal man to take advantage of the new discovery and to implement the necessary experimental work promptly. His institution had just completed a highly successful attack on meningococcal meningitis, and it was thought that poliomyelitis would go the same way. The Rockefeller Institute was well endowed, well equipped to work with viruses, and had adequate facilities to handle monkeys; it also had a staff of enthusiastic and willing young assistants. The omens were indeed favorable, and the stage was set for a major scientific advance.

Actually, poliomyelitis was just the kind of disease to interest Flexner, and, in fact, he had followed its progress for a number of years. New York City had been visited by an outbreak of some 750 cases (1,200 according to one report) in 1907. Recognizing the importance of the disease, the New York Neurological Society, under the chairmanship of Dr. Bernard Sachs, had appointed (in October 1907) a committee of twelve, including Dr. Flexner, to study this epidemic. The membership consisted of the foremost authorities in the country, although admittedly in 1907 such authorities were few. Incidentally it was almost the last time that neurologists as a professional body were to assume a position of dominance with respect to poliomyelitis, at least in the United States. Subsequently the disease was gradually taken over by virologists, internists, pediatricians, orthopedists, specialists in physical medicine, and public health officials, with neurologists only serving as consultants. The field was crowded with quite enough specialists.

Although the epidemic had occurred in 1907, the New York committee did not get around to publishing its formal report until 1910.[1] In the interim, the electrifying news had come across the Atlantic that the micro-

---

1. *Epidemic Poliomyelitis in New York, 1907.* Report of the Collective Investigation Committee on the New York Epidemic of 1907, Nervous and Mental Disease Monograph Series, no. 6, New York, Journal of Nervous and Mental Diseases Publishing Co., 1910.

bial cause of poliomyelitis had been discovered. As a result, a whole section of the committee's report dealing with the pathology of poliomyelitis[2] was quickly revised by Flexner to include an extra section on the pathology in the monkey. Here he described his own (and his colleagues') experiences with the experimental disease in animals inoculated with central nervous system tissue—from two fatal cases that had occurred in New Jersey and New York in 1909. These American viruses had all the characteristics of the agent which Landsteiner and Popper had succeeded in isolating in Vienna in 1908. Flexner, with the help of Dr. Martha Wollstein, had, however, gone a little further than the Viennese workers in that he had successfully passed the two virus strains from monkey to monkey, reproducing the disease serially, thus fulfilling the second of Koch's postulates. Others were soon to achieve successful passage of the virus also, or had already done so.

Recovery of the agent by the Rockefeller scientists represented the first time that poliovirus had ever been isolated in this country. The new observations appeared in the committee's report under the authorship of Flexner and Strauss,[3] with the interesting title of "The Pathology and Pathological Anatomy of Epidemic Poliomyelitis." There was a noticeable omission here of the word *experimental* in describing this work which was concerned only with poliomyelitis induced artificially in the monkey. Indeed this was a major mistake that was to dog Flexner's footsteps throughout his entire professional life—his failure to distinguish between certain aspects of experimental poliomyelitis in the monkey and the disease in man. This led him to misinterpretations, not so much in terms of pathology but of pathogenesis. It was an error with unfortunate implications that were to influence thought at the Rockefeller Institute for a generation. Eventually Flexner recognized well enough that in different species of monkeys (chimpanzees had not yet come into the picture) poliovirus behaved somewhat differently, but by this time it was too late. In 1910, and for years thereafter, his mind was set in the belief that the experimental infection simulated so exactly the disease in man that conclusions about pathogenesis could be drawn equally well from observations on either species—and he chose the monkey.

This attitude was probably a natural one for Flexner in view of his background. He had received his early training in both general and experimental pathology at the newly created and highly modern Johns Hopkins Medical School in Baltimore under Dr. William H. Welch, in the authorship

2. The section, entitled: "The Pathology of Acute Poliomyelitis," had been written by I. Strauss (pathologist to the Mt. Sinai Hospital, New York, and of the Cornell Medical School). See n. 1, pp. 68–104.

3. See n. 1. Subcommittee No. IV. S. Flexner and I. Strauss: The pathology and pathological anatomy of epidemic poliomyelitis. Submitted December, 1909, pp. 57–67.

of whose biography, he was eventually to share.[4] He had been greatly influenced by his experience at Johns Hopkins and by his frequent contracts
with German universities, associations which had given direction to his
ideas about experimental pathology in the unscientific age that characterized American medicine of the time. As a result he became a militant early
leader in the fields of experimental pathology and microbiology.

Simon Flexner was born in Louisville, Kentucky in 1863.[5] He was educated at local schools and received his medical degree from the University
of Louisville in 1889 at the age of twenty-six. He then became a postgraduate student at the newly established medical school of Johns Hopkins
University, where he was soon appointed a fellow in pathology in Welch's
department, and, in short order, resident pathologist of the Johns Hopkins
Hospital.

During this period of apprenticeship Flexner had been delegated by the
Maryland State Board of Health to investigate an epidemic of cerebro-
spinal meningitis in Lonacoming, Maryland, a town of some 5,000 inhabitants in a mining region in the Allegheny Mountains. This early epidemiological tour was to serve him in good stead. It sensitized him to the
community aspects of the sudden tragedy of an acute outbreak of disease
and specifically to problems of meningococcal meningitis, which led eventually to his significant contributions in the understanding of this infection
some fifteen years later. But more than that, it fired his enthusiasm for
pioneering in the investigation of other infectious diseases of potential
epidemic character.

Also, during his early years in Baltimore, Flexner made the first of several trips to Europe, visiting clinics in Strasbourg and Prague. Welch had
immediately recognized Flexner's ability, and in 1895, five or six years
after his arrival at Johns Hopkins, he appointed him associate professor of
pathology. Three years later he was promoted to a full professorship.

It would seem that at the turn of the century Flexner's enthusiasm for
studying the pathology, the epidemiology, and the pathogenesis of all kinds
of infections was endless. As if the diseases of Baltimore were not enough,
he launched an adventurous scheme to study tropical diseases in the Philippines. To this end, in 1899, he and his good friend and colleague at the
Johns Hopkins Hospital, Lewellys F. Barker, applied to President Gilman
of the Johns Hopkins University for permission to go to the Philippines,

4. S. Flexner and J. T. Flexner: *William Henry Welch and the Heroic Age of American
Medicine*. New York, Viking, 1941.
   5. Several members of his immediate family were to win distinction in their respective
fields. His brother Abraham achieved eminence in education and eventually became the first
director of the Institute for Advanced Study at Princeton, New Jersey. Another brother,
Bernard, was a noted lawyer.

which had just been taken over as a result of the Spanish-American War. Their request was granted, and the two young physicians set off for Manila, "with the hope not only of making contributions to the Science of Medicine, but also of being of service to the American forces in those islands, to the natives of the country, and to humanity at large."[6] It was just at the time of the Philippine insurrection.

Suffice it to say that, between them, they were unable to cover the whole broad field of tropical medicine, but Flexner did manage to see many diseases that plagued that part of the world, and he made at least one important discovery. This was the isolation of an organism which eventually became known as the Flexner bacillus, an agent responsible for many cases of bacillary dysentery.

The expedition to the Philippines took place in 1899. In the meantime Flexner had succeeded to the chair of pathology at the University of Pennsylvania, and along with other academic duties he took on the directorship of the Ayer Clinical Laboratory at the Pennsylvania Hospital. This was in 1900, when a professor of pathology, and especially a director of a clinical laboratory in a general hospital, was supposed to "know everything about scientific medicine," at least everything that might be of value to clinicians, and a great deal more besides. He was expected to be both a general and surgical pathologist, a bacteriologist, an immunologist, and a clinical chemist. Although clinicians on the whole were apt to be a trifle scornful, they were none the less tolerant of the idea that something might be learned from the laboratory which could sometimes be of direct assistance to them in their diagnostic and other practical problems. It was a period when the director of the hospital laboratory was affectionately referred to by fellow members of the clinical staff as "Bugs."

But Flexner was not yet through with investigations of an epidemiologic nature. Early in 1901, the surgeon general of the Marine Hospital Service, Dr. Walter Wyman, had been disturbed over conflicting reports of the existence of cases of bubonic plague in San Francisco. To investigate this problem, men with the necessary experience to recognize plague were needed, and Dr. Wyman, recalling the success which Flexner and Barker had had with diseases endemic in the Philippine Islands, appointed the three-man Federal Plague Commission, with Flexner as chairman, and Barker and Professor F. G. Novy of the University of Michigan as members (see fig. 19). The commission was charged with the duty "of ascertaining the existence or non-existence of bubonic plague in the City of San Fran-

6. Other members of this group included Frederick Gay, Joseph Flint, and John W. Garrett. Accounts of the expedition were later published: see S. Flexner and L. F. Barker: Report upon an expedition sent by Johns Hopkins University to investigate the prevalent diseases in the Philippines. *Johns Hopk. Hosp. Bull., 11*: 37, 1900; and L. F. Barker: *Time and the Physician.* New York, Putnam, 1942, pp. 62–72.

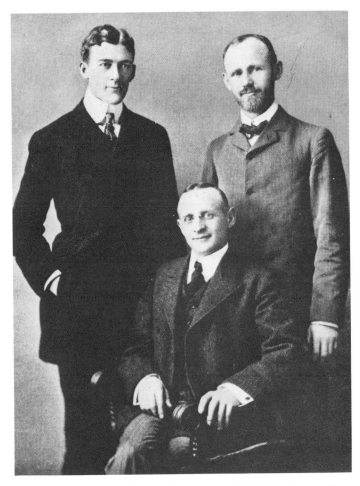

Fig. 19. The Federal Plague Commission (1901). Standing, left to right: L. F. Barker and F. G. Novy; seated, S. Flexner, chairman (see n. 6). Reproduced by permission, G. P. Putnam's & Coward McCann.

cisco, California." In an age when academic advice was sought far less frequently by government agencies than it is today, it must have been gratifying to the young, newly appointed professor of pathology at the University of Pennsylvania to think that he had been the one singled out to lead a group with such an important assignment.

The upshot was that within a few days of the commission's going into action in February 1901, a few cases of plague were discovered in San Francisco's Chinatown, and it was the opinion of Flexner and the others that similar cases probably had occurred there for more than a year. The California authorities had done little about the problem because of the obvious fear of stirring up needless alarm; for it was indeed a delicate situation, fraught with dangers of a medical, economic, and political nature. In subsequent years Flexner faced similar situations many times in connection with poliomyelitis epidemics, when even health officers or, more often, civic authorities were guilty of suppressing the ugly information that cases of poliomyelitis were beginning to appear in their city. Such actions were guided by a fear of prematurely spreading news of an incipient epidemic, thus causing visitors to shun the whole area—a result which might spell disaster not only for business but for the community at large.

What the origin of cases of plague in San Francisco's Chinatown was, i.e. whether the infections were acquired from rodents which had strayed in from the hinterland or whether infected rats coming off the ships in the harbor were the source, was not a problem to concern the Plague Commission in 1901.[7] The delicate question as to whether local health authorities were justified in admitting the existence of a potential threat to the community was one requiring a swift but accurate decision by the commission. The answer, made according to the knowledge available at the time, was the only one possible, namely, to announce that a potential epidemic situation existed. This judgment was accepted. It scored another triumph for the young Dr. Flexner.

Flexner did not remain in Philadelphia for long. In 1903 the board of the newly established Rockefeller Institute for Medical Research, after a careful search, chose him as the first director of its already well-planned and well-financed institute. He was recommended and selected as one of the ablest young pathologists in the country—a man who, besides having received superior training, had witnessed the scientific achievements of the European universities, had enjoyed success on his various academic missions concerned with epidemiologic investigations, and had already successfully administered a university department.

Almost immediately after Flexner had assumed his new position, he became an active champion of the experimental pathological laboratory as a virtual shrine. His view was that a well-equipped laboratory provided infinite opportunities for solving any number of fundamental questions which currently faced the medical profession in America, particularly in the field of infectious disease. In an address delivered in 1907 before the American Association for the Advancement of Science, he left no doubt as to where his interests lay and what he meant to do. He spoke with confidence and authority:

7. I am greatly indebted to Dr. Karl F. Meyer of the University of California, San Francisco, for further detailed information about this episode and the incidence of bubonic plague during the years of 1900–04 in San Francisco. See K. F. Meyer: Ecology of Plague. *Medicine,* *21*: 144–55, 1942. He has described these years as one of the darkest periods of public health in San Francisco.

The resultant of the discoveries in the newer fields of pathological knowledge constitutes the period of etiological pathology which, dating its beginnings from the middle of the last century, is today the dominant influence affecting medical thought.[8]

Also during this period, Simon Flexner had a distinguished and successful ally in the form of his brother Abraham,[9] who was to come into prominence as a result of his report on the extraordinarily poor quality of the bulk of the country's medical schools. This 1910 report, which was not published in detail until 1925, was a milestone in the history of American medical education. Its conclusions were very different from those of reports today, which call frantically for an increase in the number of medical schools in the United States. On the contrary, Abraham Flexner stated that 120 of the 155 existing schools in the United States and Canada were of such poor quality that they should either be closed or affiliated with other institutions. This was good news only to those physicians who had been struggling desperately to establish medicine on a sound scientific basis. To others it was a bombshell, but it had the desired effect.

Thus, in the early decades of the twentieth century there was much stirring of the waters in the matters of reform of medical education and of clinical practice; there was also a determination to make medicine in the United States more of a science. Physicians were encouraged, even admonished, to make greater use of the laboratory in an effort to bring timely and exact measurements into clinical medicine, something which had been long neglected. Simon Flexner occupied a position in the middle of the reform movement. He had come to his position as the first director of the Rockefeller Institute for Medical Research as a resolute and quiet champion of scientific medicine. He was determined to do all in his power to make his institute far more than a laboratory dedicated to experimental investigation and the advancement of those fields nearest his heart—pathology, bacteriology, and immunology. He visualized it as a beacon—as a haven of scientific medical thought in America.

Landsteiner's discovery of poliovirus, coming just five years after Flexner's appointment at the institute, had proved a windfall. The position that he then occupied on the American medical scene and his ardent desire

8. S. Flexner: Tendencies in pathology. *Science*, 27: 128–36, 1908.

9. In 1908, Abraham Flexner was asked by Henry S. Pritchett, president of the Carnegie Foundation, to undertake a study of American medical schools. He had had no training in medicine but had studied the principles and practice of American education extensively. For his report, see A. Flexner: *Medical Education in the United States and Canada.* Bull. no. 4. New York, Carnegie Foundation for the Advancement of Teaching, 1910. It was subsequently published in book form. See A. Flexner: *Medical Education—A Comparative Study.* New York, Macmillan, 1925.

to further the cause of scientific medicine in this country made the timing absolutely propitious. Infantile paralysis was the ideal disease on which he could set his sights. Isolation of the etiologic agent held out the promise of a better appreciation of the pathogenesis of poliomyelitis and better diagnostic facilities for the clinician—perhaps even a diagnostic test. Conceivably, these features might lead to the next prodigious steps: a means of prevention, possibly of cure. All sorts of interesting possibilities presented themselves, and the dream that scientific medicine would conquer the disease seemed near realization. It was obvious that Flexner was *the* man in the United States to accomplish this task.

In the meantime, during the years 1908–12, poliomyelitis in the United States had been sharply on the increase. Cases were being detected and reported from almost every section of the country, although records of the actual national incidence during this period are inaccurate since statistics from different states were not collected in a uniform manner. But the disease was quickly becoming a national problem, and there were few, if any, experts who knew how to cope with it.

Although in 1910–11, Flexner's was perhaps the most authoritative voice in the land on matters concerning poliomyelitis, his position as "a laboratory doctor" militated against his being able to handle the practical questions addressed to him by general practitioners from all parts of the country. In his Philadelphia days he had been a director of the laboratory of a general hospital, which had brought him into constant contact with clinicians, but as head of a great research institute he had now withdrawn from clinical medicine. He made few attempts to be even a clinical investigator, such as the members of the contemporary Swedish team headed by Carl Kling had proceeded to do (see chap. 13). Flexner considered the gap between experimental pathologist and clinician to be almost too great. True, he was the outstanding and most publicized expert in the field of experimental poliomyelitis, and so physicians inevitably turned to him for advice; but in 1911, neither he nor, for that matter, anyone else had the knowledge to answer the questions that clinicians were constantly asking. How long was a child with poliomyelitis to be considered infectious? How could one explain the apparent lack of contagiousness of the disease? What was the best form of treatment?

Flexner was hardly the man to deal with such practical inquiries.[10] For instance, when he countered a physician's question concerning therapy by exhorting him to send autopsy material from fatal cases, his response could hardly have satisfied the doctor charged with the responsibility of caring for acutely ill patients. Flexner had gone beyond that earlier phase of his

10. I am indebted to Dr. Saul Benison, historian of the National Foundation for Infantile Paralysis in New York, for many data and correspondence dealing with the anxious inquiries which came from physicians throughout the entire nation during the period of 1909–12.

career when he had been ready to drop other duties and visit epidemic areas, and to travel up and down the countryside, as Wickman had done in Sweden and Frost was soon to do in the United States, talking to doctors and discussing the innumerable practical problems which inevitably arose. That was clinical epidemiology—which he had abandoned. In his present position at the Rockefeller Institute he preferred to work at his base laboratory with its many facilities, instead of in the field. He had set his sights on two fundamental objectives—a cure and a means of prevention.

But the nation's physicians, during the years 1908–12, were anxiously seeking knowledge which might better equip them to handle the day-to-day *clinical* problems of the new disease that had suddenly sprung up to plague them every few summers. So in this period of waiting they became increasingly frustrated. The notion that the disease was caused by a virus did not help the general practitioner at all, for prior to 1920 viruses were ultramysterious and their actions unpredictable. There was a crying need for more descriptions of infantile paralysis written in English by top-notch clinicians with a practical knowledge of the disease. Publication of such material in prominent United States medical journals and textbooks would provide the up-to-date information which physicians were seeking, but who was there to write such articles? Flexner, having recognized a certain amount of urgency in this matter, tried to arrange for good translations of the works of Römer,[11] Leiner and von Wiesner,[12] and Wickman, but these valuable monographs appeared in English somewhat belatedly, in 1913.

Following closely on Flexner's first publication (see n.3) on the pathology of experimental poliomyelitis, he and his colleagues Paul Lewis and Paul Clark were tireless in their efforts to cover the fields of pathology, pathogenesis, and the distribution of the virus in the organs and tissues of infected monkeys. A great many experiments were performed and reported in the short time between 1909 and 1913. Flexner's team was able to publish promptly during this period a series of some fifteen notes in sequential issues of the *Journal of the American Medical Association*. These were put out in the manner of news bulletins, reporting the "latest thing on poliomyelitis." The papers even attracted attention abroad and were widely quoted by foreign workers, which was unusual at that time. American medical science was supposed to be way behind that of Europe. Flexner may not have been of much help in solving the immediate clinical problems the disease presented, but he made such progress in the experimental laboratory, and there was no doubt in the minds of American physicians

11. P. H. Römer: *Epidemic Infantile Paralysis; Heine-Medin Disease,* trans. by H. R. Prentice. New York, Wm. Wood, 1913.

12. C. Leiner and R. Wiesner: "Zur Ätiologie und experimentellen Pathologie der Poliomyelitis acuta," in *Studien über die Heine-Medinsche Krankheit (Poliomyelitis acuta).* Leipzig and Vienna, Franz Deuticke, 1911.

that he had become the leading authority on poliomyelitis in this country, if not in the world. All of this made for confidence, and Flexner was apparently so satisfied and so sure of the way his experimental work was going in 1911 that he was quoted as follows in a press release:

New York. March 9.—The Rockefeller Institute in this city believes that its search for a cure for infantile paralysis is about to be rewarded. Within six months, according to Dr. Simon Flexner, definite announcement of a specific remedy may be expected.

"We have already discovered how to prevent the disease," says Dr. Flexner in a statement published here today, "and the achievement of a cure, I may conservatively say, is not now far distant. We have been working on this problem for a year and a half. The germ has been known only that long, and, advancing from that point, we have learned where it resides, how the disease is spread, how the germ enters the body, the main sources of infection and the means of combating the disease.

The germ is so excessively minute that the most powerful microscope fails to reveal it, yet there are accurate methods by which its nature and presence have been determined."[13]

Whether or not this news report actually reflects Flexner's views is not apparent; it at least reflects some of his early confidence.

It is difficult to follow events of this period (1909–12), to determine who actually deserves priority for this or that discovery in Europe or in the United States, or who devised one or another of the new techniques. Discoveries were being made at an altogether astonishing rate. Besides the investigations of Landsteiner and Levaditi, significant contributions were emanating from laboratories in Germany and Austria as well as the United States. A few attempts, painfully few it would seem, were made to determine in what tissues and organs the virus could be found during different stages of the human infection. Substantial progress was made when immune mechanisms were explored by testing the resistance of monkeys to reinfection; and tremendous efforts were made to develop methods of active and passive immunization. In line with the latter, Flexner and collaborators had embarked on a program which demonstrated in 1910 that the serum of monkeys convalescent from experimental poliomyelitis contained antibodies, spoken of as "germicidal substances"[14]—a finding that was made almost simultaneously by Landsteiner and others. These inves-

13. "Cure for Infantile Paralysis near." *New York Times*, Mar. 9, 1911. This news item was obtained, many years after its first publication, through the kindness of the late Dr. C. H. Bunting, emeritus professor of pathology at the University of Wisconsin, Madison, Wis.

14. S. Flexner and P. A. Lewis: Experimental poliomyelitis in monkeys; active immunization and passive serum protection. *J. Amer. med. Ass., 54*: 1780, 1910.

tigators all showed that when such serum was mixed with a small amount of active poliovirus, the antibodies in the serum, which had been formed as a result of experimental infection, actually could inactivate (neutralize) the virus and render it inert. Shortly after this, Netter and Levaditi[15] and others also found these neutralizing substances in the blood of humans recovering from poliomyelitis. This demonstration of antibodies in convalescent patients was to prove another landmark in the therapeutic history of the disease. Its significance ranked almost on a par with the discovery of the virus, a fact unappreciated until some years later.

Although Flexner's pioneer contributions to experimental poliomyelitis, particularly his discovery of poliovirus antibodies, were landmarks, his early confidence that he and his colleagues could quickly conquer poliomyelitis subsided gradually. The hopes that had seemed so promising at first proved to be decidedly premature. By 1913, to most poliomyelitis workers, it was painfully apparent that such questions as how to prevent the disease by immunization, or how to cure it, posed innumerable difficulties. In any event, Landsteiner, Leiner and von Wiesner, and Römer, after surveying the field, did not pursue the subject further; at least they did not publish further on matters concerning poliomyelitis, either experimental or human. Also world events interfered. World War I caused an interruption of work in most of the laboratories in Europe and probably had a dampening influence on investigations elsewhere. Nevertheless, Levaditi continued his researches at the Pasteur Institute relentlessly, and Flexner was in no mood to give up. Perhaps it might have been better had he called a scientific holiday for a few years, but it was a long time before he recognized that the objectives he had set for himself could not be achieved—at once. Painfully enough, he would not even live to see the intricacies of the family of polioviruses unraveled; nor the various aspects of the pathogenesis of the human disease straightened out, which, paradoxically, he himself had entangled.

Flexner retired as director of the Rockefeller Institute in 1935, and his death occurred some eleven years later. That was almost a decade before the final "conquest" of poliomyelitis. The experimental path he had elected to follow in later years only led him further and further away from the human disease and deeper into the woods. He had convinced himself and his colleagues that the virus was a strictly neurotropic one that entered the body by the nasal route and proceeded directly to the central nervous system. He developed with Noguchi a strange enthusiasm for "globoid bodies," which together they considered, but only for a while, as a substitute for poliovirus. He once even intimated that these bodies might be found

15. A. Netter and C. Levaditi: Action microbicide exercée sur la virus de la poliomyélite aiguë par le sérum des sujets antérieurement atteints de paralysie infantile; Sa constatation dans le sérum d'un sujet qui a présenté une forme abortive. *C. R. Soc. Biol. (Paris)*, *68*: 855, 1910.

in the human buccal and nasal mucosa. He steadfastly held out against the alimentary tract as the portal of entry. Remarkably enough, he was resistant to the idea that polioviruses are actually a family composed of several types with different antigenicity. But more than that, he held out doggedly against methods of clinical investigation which included clinical virology—approaches that eventually made possible the unraveling of the whole story.

A belief in the desirability of separate and distinct spheres of activity for clinicians (i.e. doctors) versus laboratory medical scientists unfortunately colored Flexner's thinking and his decisions in the early years of his directorship of the institute. The integration of these two functions was proceeding rapidly, right at his very doorstep, under the able direction of the founders of the American Society for Clinical Investigation.[16] But Flexner stubbornly held out for his own point of view. He was not without allies, for many European medical schools continued to be resistant to this movement, claiming that doctors should be doctors and not pose as scientists.

An immediate result of this attitude was the limitation imposed on the team of investigators at the Rockefeller Hospital who undertook a study of clinical poliomyelitis during the large epidemic of 1911. Flexner seized the opportunty presented by this epidemic to initiate a project in his institute's hospital which would lead to the publication in America of a much needed comprehensive review of the clinical disease, worthy of the best European clinics. The result was a substantial monograph, published in 1912 by the remarkable team of Peabody, Draper, and Dochez.[17] This report, based on the investigation of almost 200 cases, added some new clinical data, but there was little that was new in their approach, and none of the attempts to elucidate the clinical virology of the disease such as characterized the work in Sweden during an epidemic in the same year. I believe the reason for this lay in Flexner's rigid separation of the character of the work to be carried out in the Rockefeller Hospital as opposed to his own research laboratory in the institute. He supported clinicians to the limit of

16. Clinical investigation had become a contemporary American development which went along with the increasing number of *full-time* medical schools being established in this country. Since this development was to contribute much to the flowering of American medicine it deserves a word of definition here.

The American Society of Clinical Investigation, founded in 1909, was dedicated to the ideal that academic physicians should possess the appropriate clinical knowledge of how to deal with patients properly and intelligently, but besides that, they should have more than a passing knowledge of the preclinical sciences as well. It was a movement reflecting the fact that medicine had suddenly graduated from being an applied science.

See F. G. Blake: Clinical investigation. *Science, 74*: 27–29, 1931; and A. E. Cohn: "Medicine and Science," chap. 4, in *Medicine, Science and Art.* University of Chicago Press, 1931, pp. 138–63. It was with these principles that Flexner felt reluctant to go along.

17. F. W. Peabody, G. Draper, and A. R. Dochez: *A Clinical Study of Acute Poliomyelitis.* Monograph of the Rockefeller Inst. Med. Research, no. 4, New York, 1912, pp. 1–187.

his own beliefs, but he clung to the idea that physicians were supposed to practice their craft at the bedside—not in the experimental laboratory. They were not even allowed access to monkeys to perform clinical virological tests.

The scope of the Rockefeller Hospital's study was the source of considerable contention between Dr. Rufus Cole, the director of the hospital, and Dr. Flexner. Nowhere is the case for the laboratory aspect of clinical investigation more succinctly expressed than in the correspondence between these two men, carried on in 1911. I shall quote directly from Corner's book:

> When in 1911 Cole's attitude was questioned in the Board of Scientific Directors, he gave Flexner a forthright statement of his position. "Men who were studying disease clinically," he wrote, "had the right to go as deeply into its fundamental nature as their training allowed, and in The Rockefeller Institute's hospital every man who was caring for patients should also be engaged in more fundamental study. It had required some energy and effort," he continued, "to get the men to adopt this view, but they were all now convinced of its soundness, and he hoped that some of them, at least, might share in the revolution, or evolution, of clinical medicine that was bound to come. Of course," wrote Cole, "collaborative studies by the hospital and Institute laboratories might be extremely valuable, but unless the hospital first accomplished something independently, the other laboratories would never respect its work. Co-operation might develop spontaneously.[18]

Unfortunately Flexner got the best of the argument.

And yet the Rockefeller Hospital study, although it suffered mightily by comparison with the Swedish work of the same period, was to start a new trend in clinical investigation. As such, it represents a definite landmark. What Peabody, Draper, and Dochez did accomplish for American medicine was to point the way to a new style of teamwork in which a group of clinical investigators worked enthusiastically for a common cause in an academic atmosphere, in a well-equipped and well-run institution. It was a kind of investigation peculiarly appropriate to the new organization of house-staff physicians then being introduced into the best of American

18. Correspondence between Rufus I. Cole and Simon Flexner, Oct. 30, 1911, Flexner Papers. See also G. W. Corner: *A History of the Rockefeller Institute, 1901–1953; Origins and Growth.* New York, Rockefeller Institute Press, 1962, p. 107.

Dr. George Corner gives an account of this reform as it affected the Rockefeller Institute in above mentioned history of the institute. The relation of the institute's ideals and activities was tied closely to medical educational practices in this country; so much so that sixty years after it was founded, the Rockefeller Institute became Rockefeller University.

I am indebted to Dr. George Corner for further information about this 1911 letter from Rufus Cole to Dr. Flexner.

teaching hospitals. In this case the objective was to examine the acute febrile and subacute stages of poliomyelitis in a more meticulous manner than had ever been done before. To accomplish this the investigators organized their interns and residents for round-the-clock clinical observations and for the performance of simple laboratory tests. Since crucial events frequently happen with surprising rapidity in the severely ill, paralyzed patient, this exacting standard was set by Cole's team. Thus the tradition of clinical investigation was established. The years of 1911 to 1940 represented its golden age in America, and gradually, as a result, leadership in medicine shifted from Europe to the United States.

To return to the study by the team of investigators at the Hospital of Rockefeller Institute: although it was focused almost entirely on the course of the acute clinical disease, the report began with a recognition of Wickman's fundamental contribution.

> An entirely new light was thrown on the obscure question of dissemination by Wickman's recognition of the so-called abortive and meningitic forms or types of the affection. Until then, attention had been riveted on the paralysis, and the possibility of cases of epidemic poliomyelitis occurring in which paralysis is entirely absent seems not to have been entertained. It is at once clear that the existence of such cases would throw an entirely new light upon the mode of transmission of the infection.[19]

One curious item contained in the Rockefeller Hospital monograph was also concerned with the epidemiology of the disease. It consisted of a paragraph or two in which the three authors apparently had little part. Indications are that it had been contributed by Dr. Flexner, and it is completely out of keeping with the rest of the clinical account. The idea expressed is that during epidemic times domestic animals as well as man are apt to be afflicted with paralysis, a view which had been mentioned by Caverly in describing the Vermont epidemic some twenty years previously. Flexner admitted, and even stressed, that the presence of poliovirus had never been demonstrated in such animals, yet he felt that it was a point of sufficient importance to be inserted in a clinical study of the disease! He had gone on record at an earlier date in at least two publications indicating that he already possessed evidence that certain lower animals, among them poultry, dogs, and possibly horses, were subject to poliomyelitis, due in each instance to a cause peculiar to the species affected. Unfortunately he did not mention mice, for by so doing he would have uncovered one grain of truth. Actually, from none of the above species mentioned by Flexner

19. See n. 17, p. 117.

have polio or polio-like viruses ever been recovered. Perhaps Flexner thought that the possible involvement of animals emphasized the universality of the infection. In any event this digression into speculative epidemiology did little good as an adjunct to an otherwise factual bedside study. Shortly after 1912 Flexner reversed himself, and the idea that domestic animals were involved met the same fate as many another ill-founded theory regarding poliomyelitis.

The bulk of the 1912 monograph is taken up with a detailed description of thirty-four patients; fifty pages are devoted to symptoms and physical signs in the acute disease; and thirty-five pages to results of orthodox laboratory examinations of blood and cerebrospinal fluid at different stages of the illness. In the typical Oslerian manner of the day, methods of treatment received short shrift. Only seven pages (less than 4 percent of the report) were spent on this subject, which is not surprising since there was no effective therapy for the acute infection. For the uncomplicated paralytic case, the authors recommend absolute bed rest, mild sedatives, and medication for the control of pain.

Practical points mentioned in connection with the handling of patients on a hospital ward reflect the thinking then current in America concerning the nature of the disease. In line with Wickman's ideas, the authors concluded that poliomyelitis should be treated like any other contagious disease. Cases should be notified, and quarantine and terminal disinfection carried out; this was required by law in some places. At the Rockefeller Hospital,

> All doctors and nurses wore caps and long gowns when working with the patients. When leaving the ward, the hands were thoroughly scrubbed with soap and a nail brush, and soaked in corrosive sublimate. The occasional use of a hydrogen peroxide spray (1 per cent.) was recommended. . . . All visitors were compelled to wear gowns while in the ward, . . . and use a hydrogen peroxide mouth wash on leaving the ward. . . . All urine and feces were sterilized by heat. . . . After being used, the rooms were disinfected with formaldehyde gas, and the walls and floors were thoroughly scrubbed with soap and water.

Some of these precautions seem unnecessarily stringent. Few are in use today. They were the forerunners of the rather inexpedient rules upon which the New York City Health Department shaped its sanitary code four years later when the severe epidemic of 1916 broke out.

Nowhere in the report are attempts to isolate the virus from patients mentioned. The late Dr. A. R. Dochez has on numerous occasions recounted to me his vain efforts to persuade Dr. Flexner that by 1912, a proper clinical investigative study did call for such efforts. The denial of

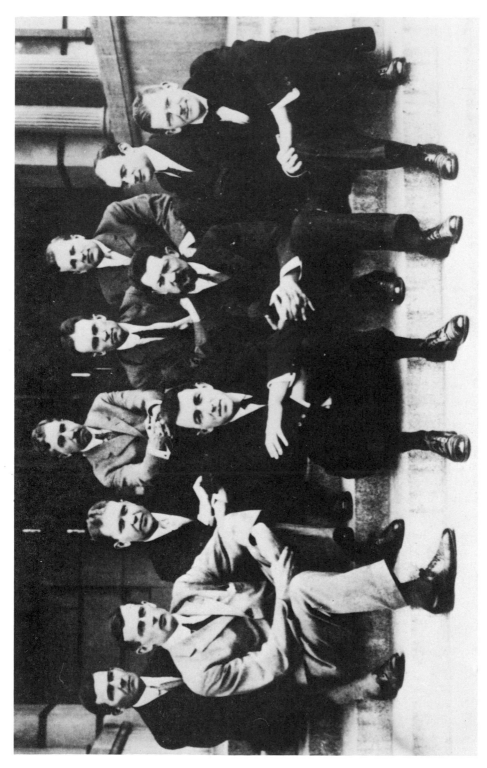

Fig. 20. The staff of the Hospital of the Rockefeller Institute (1911). FRONT ROW: Drs. A. Ellis (later Sir Arthur Ellis), F. Fraser (later Sir Francis Fraser), unidentified physician from Rumania, another unidentified physician. MIDDLE ROW: Drs. A. R. Dochez, F. W. Peabody, G. Draper, and H. F. Swift. BACK ROW: Drs. R. I. Cole (director) and G. C. Robinson. Kindness of Dr. Maclyn McCarty of the Hospital of the Rockefeller University.

this request was understandable, considering Flexner's insistence that his own special department in the institute would take care of the experimental aspects of poliovirus work. Furthermore, he upheld the rule that projects, no matter who initiated them, were not to overlap in their scope, for fear of jealousies arising when it turned out that several staff members were working on the same subject.

Thus the study by staff members of the Hospital of the Rockefeller Institute (see fig. 20) was not so novel or so important that it deserves a particularly high place in the history of poliomyelitis. But one should recall that it was undertaken at a time when there was great urgency to produce a good American study, even though conservative and clinical in nature. The result was indeed a pioneer effort as far as this country was concerned. The earlier authoritative European monographs had appeared in the German language only and had not yet been translated. The trio of young medical scientists were all gripped with a certain amount of excitement that they were going to make medical history. Indeed they did make their mark subsequently. Of Draper we shall hear more in a later chapter, for he continued his interest in poliomyelitis.

Francis W. Peabody, born in Boston and educated at Harvard, became in this era one of the best-known and best-beloved professors of medicine at the Harvard Medical School within a few years after he had left his apprenticeship at the Rockefeller Hospital. From his initial interest in poliomyelitis he went on to develop as wide an interest in medicine as a respected professor of medicine is suppposed to have—and more too. In 1923, he became the first medical director of the Thorndike Memorial Laboratory of the Boston City Hospital. Overnight this laboratory achieved an almost fabulous reputation for training and clinical investigation, and from it a host of disciples emerged. Dr. Peabody's students and house officers and colleagues idolized him. It was indeed a nationwide tragedy when his life was prematurely cut off at the age of forty-six, by death from cancer.

Of Francis Peabody, Dr. Hans Zinsser subsequently wrote: "A rare blending of learning and humanity, incisiveness of intellect and sensitiveness of the spirit, which occasionally come together in an individual who chooses the calling of Medicine; and then we have the great physician."[20]

The third of the three members of the team was Alphonse Raymond Dochez, or "Dō," as he was familiarly and affectionately known to his intimates. Dr. Dochez was educated at Johns Hopkins University, both at its college and medical school. Within a year of graduation (1907) he received a fellowship at the Rockefeller Institute and later served as senior house officer at the affiliated hospital. During his five-year residency at this insti-

20. Hans Zinsser: "Introduction to collected papers of Francis W. Peabody," in *F. W. Peabody: Doctor and Patient*. New York, Macmillan, 1930.

tution, he developed an interest in microbiology and infectious disease which was to last throughout his career.

He joined the faculty of the College of Physicians and Surgeons of Columbia University in New York in the early 1920s and became chairman of its Department of Bacteriology in 1940. His consuming interests were in the field of acute infections—pneumonia, scarlet fever, and the common cold. Yet he was always ready to talk about poliomyelitis and its problems, and it was in these practical and theoretical discussions on the subject of acute bacterial or viral infections that he excelled. His name will always rank among the greats in the field of infectious diseases.

But what of Flexner's subsequent career? To leave him on the disappointing note of his failures with poliomyelitis would be grossly unfair. Flexner achieved singular distinction as an administrator of one of the finest institutes devoted to medical research that the world had ever seen. It was indeed a pity that success in poliomyelitis research eluded him, particularly since he had started out with such enthusiasm and with high hopes that the riddle of the disease could be promptly solved. The mistakes he made can be attributed to a certain rigidity in clinging to ideas he considered sacrosanct—a characteristic which in some ways was a source of strength. But at least he had given his best efforts in the poliomyelitis fight. Legions of other workers were to go down in the same struggle.

This unsuccessful attempt to solve the poliomyelitis problem was but an episode—a skirmish—viewed in the light of his long and rewarding life. The account given in this chapter would be woefully inadequate in representing Flexner's spirit and ideals and accomplishments unless that point is made abundantly clear. Dr. Peyton Rous, writing a few years after Flexner's death in 1946, said:

> Simon Flexner responded when young to a deep need of what was then the future, and when the future became the here and now he was the appointed man equipped and ready. . . . During the fifty years of his personal effort medicine emerged in the sharp light of science. He helped this happen, and he did vastly more.[21]

Although Flexner did not achieve hoped-for objectives in poliomyelitis, he excelled in many different forms of endeavor. Throughout his productive life he exhibited a devotion to the science of pathology and to its enrichment by all that could be brought to it from physics and chemistry, by intellectual and incidentally by financial means. And he was strong in the conviction that as these sciences grew, freedom from disease would be brought nearer.

Most who knew Dr. Flexner (see fig. 21), and I include myself in this category, were struck by his simplicity, dignity, honesty, and industry. Not

21. Peyton Rous: Simon Flexner (1863–1946). *Royal Soc. Obituary Notices,* 6: 430, 1958–59.

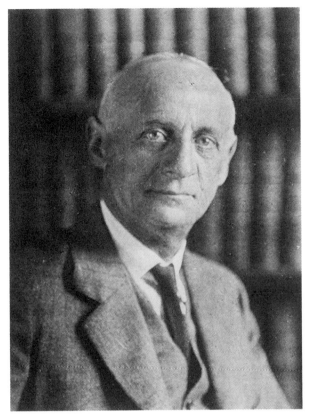

FIG. 21. Simon Flexner, M.D., Sc.D. (1863–1946). From the
Historical Library of the Yale University School of Medicine.

the least of his qualities was his generous and sincere interest in the young
men working in various departments of his institute—and elsewhere. Even
when defending what he strongly thought was right, his approach was
humble and carried the recognition that he might be wrong. He can be
forgiven for making mistakes about poliomyelitis.

CHAPTER 13

Clinical Virology in Sweden

If the Landsteiner discovery had proved a lucky break for Dr. Flexner in 1909, it was no less of a windfall for other investigators in the laboratories of Europe, including Scandinavia. An unforeseen event, however, soon confronted the microbiologists of Sweden, for no sooner had they begun to familiarize themselves with the properties of the virus than they were confronted, in 1911, with the largest epidemic of poliomyelitis that Sweden had ever experienced or indeed the world had ever seen. Within this small country alone there were 3,840 cases by official count! The outbreak went far to strengthen the unsavory and, I may say, unjust reputation that Scandinavia had already acquired, of being not only the original source of the disease but a continuing breeding place for large epidemics. This reputation was to endure from the 1880s on—for almost forty years.

In many ways, though the 1911 outbreak was full of tragic overtones, it provided an opportunity to conduct more thorough clinical virological studies than had ever been possible. By a fortunate circumstance a team headed by the then young Carl Kling, at the State Bacteriological Institute in Stockholm, was quick to respond to the emergency and put the new methods to good use. Kling and his colleagues proceeded at once to carry out tests on tissues from fatal human cases and were successful in recovering poliovirus from various anatomical sites. Of even greater importance was their success in isolating the agent from living patients—not only from those who were in the acute and convalescent stages of typical paralytic poliomyelitis, but also from children with the abortive form of the disease —even from individuals who were considered "healthy carriers."[1] Their study was no pedestrian review of already familiar events and orthodox clinical laboratory tests made in the course of the acute disease, such as the study by the Rockefeller Hospital group that had been conducted in the same year. Rather, they were breaking new ground, undertaking new clinical virologic investigations on a scale never before attempted and, incidentally, not to be tried again for a long time. The Swedish team seemed tireless during the summer of 1911. One of its major accomplishments was

---

1. The term "healthy carriers" was a misnomer. It carried the implication that the individuals were not actually (although inapparently) infected. This in turn tended to downgrade the idea that these individuals had gained immunity from this experience.

the confirmation of Wickman's theories about the clinical epidemiology of poliomyelitis. By isolating the virus from patients with mild or inapparent infections, they proved the importance of such persons in the spread of the disease.

A prompt report of the findings was presented at the Fifteenth International Congress of Hygiene and Demography held in Washington, D.C. in 1912,[2] but unfortunately the work received an indifferent response from those present. However, that is another story—a sad one, to say the least.

During two previous years members of the Swedish team—Kling, Pettersson and Wernstedt—had been aware of the flood of advances on both sides of the Atlantic that had been in the making after Landsteiner's discovery. There was abundant evidence that the etiologic agent was a filterable virus, amenable to laboratory experimentation, and that it caused lesions which were found in the spinal cord and brain of experimentally infected monkeys. The Swedish investigators were also aware that Flexner and Lewis had demonstrated poliovirus in the mucous membranes of the throat and nasal passages of infected monkeys. These same authors had even isolated the virus from lymph nodes adjacent to the small intestines (i.e. mesenteric lymph nodes) in a fatal human case. Various European workers, including Landsteiner and Levaditi, had also found the agent in the tonsils, pharyngeal mucous membranes, and salivary glands of children who had died of poliomyelitis. The Swedish team therefore started with the premise that:

> The microbe had thus been found to exist in the central nervous system, in the mucous membranes of the nose of monkeys, in the tonsils and pharyngeal mucous membranes of human beings, in some of the lymphatic glands of man and monkeys, in the salivary glands of monkeys and, exceptionally, in the blood.[3]

As a preliminary to their work with living patients, Kling and his coworkers decided to do a series of autopsy studies and to attempt a more thorough search than had been made previously to locate the virus in several anatomical sites in material from patients succumbing at various stages of the acute or subacute disease. The Swedish team must have had a remarkable and enviable supply of monkeys at its disposal in order to undertake such an ambitious program at so early a date. Tissues from 14 fatal cases of poliomyelitis that occurred in the epidemic of 1911 were stud-

2. C. Kling, A. Pettersson, and W. Wernstedt: Experimental and Pathological Investigation. I. The presence of the microbe of infantile paralysis in human beings, trans. by A. V. Rosen (report from the State Medical Institute of Sweden to the 15th International Congress on Hygiene and Demography, Washington, 1912). *Communications Inst. méd. État, Stockholm, 3*: 5, 1912.

3. Ibid., p. 12.

ied[4]—the largest single series of fatal cases in which virological studies had
ever been tried. The virus was found to be present in most of the patients
in the oropharynx and trachea, which was expected; but what was not expected was its recovery from the contents and the wall of the small intestine
as well. These significant results, recorded in table 3, were all the more impressive when it is remembered that they were obtained by a group of
young amateurs, less than three years after the virus was discovered. The
findings in fatal human cases left little doubt in the minds of the investigators as to where to look for the virus in living patients.

The next step was to examine specimens from acutely ill individuals.
In these clinical studies the procedures of collection and preparation of
materials for inoculation were in general the same as those used in investigations of the fatal cases.[5] Eleven patients with acute poliomyelitis provided specimens. From materials collected within two weeks of onset of
the disease, virus was recovered by and large from the same sites, and approximately with the same frequency, as from the fatal cases. Success was
achieved both with oral and nasopharyngeal washings (7 positive of 12 so
tested, or 58 percent) and with intestinal washings (9 out of 10, 90 percent).

For the Swedish team these results provided abundant food for thought;
the members pondered long and hard as to what the correct interpretations
were, what theories of the pathogenesis of human poliomyelitis would fit
their findings best. How did the agent get into the body initially? How was
it eventually transported to the brain and spinal cord? Previous experimental work in monkeys had shown that when the virus was introduced
directly into the peritoneal cavity and into a nerve, it somehow traveled
either by the bloodstream or along nerves until it reached the central nervous system. This problem of the pathogenesis of the infection was to em-
broil workers in the poliomyelitis field for at least another generation, and
it has not been entirely settled to this day. So naturally Kling and his colleagues were puzzled. But one thing seemed fairly certain: "that the microbe

4. Techniques for collecting and testing tissues from fatal cases were as follows: small
samples of saline washings from the various sites listed in table 3 were inoculated into monkeys,
three or four animals being used for every fatal case tested. The solutions were filtered to rid
them of bacteria. Monkey inoculations were done by a combination of two routes—intraperitoneal and intraneural (i.e. an injection into the sciatic nerve). Some of the animals succumbed to illnesses other than experimental poliomyelitis; in others paralyses were manifest;
in still others although paralyses were not noted, these animals were sacrificed at an appropriate
time. The spinal cords of all monkeys were examined microscopically for the lesions characteristic of poliomyelitis. On the basis of the presence or absence of these neuronal lesions the
results were recorded in table 3 as: positive (+), negative (—), or indeterminate (±).

5. Washings were collected from the nasopharynx and intestinal tract. Nasopharyngeal
specimens were obtained by instilling a small quantity of saline solution through a flexible
tube placed within the nose, and having the patients gargle the same fluid when it entered
the throat. For intestinal washings, the colon was first cleared by an enema, and then irrigated
with a small amount of saline solution. The returned fluid was then used as the inoculum.

TABLE 3. List of the anatomical sites in 14 fatal cases from which Kling et al. recovered poliovirus

Case No.	Age of Patient	Duration of Acute Disease in Days	Poliovirus Recovered from:			
			Oropharynx	Trachea	Intestine	Spinal Cord
1	18	6	0	+	+	−
2	14	5	+	0	+	+
3	6	3	±	+	±	−
4	2	5	+	+	+	+
5	11	4	−	−	+	−
6	4	9	+	+	−	+
7	8	6	−	+	+	+
8	13	3	+	−	−	+
9	35	4	+	0	+	+
10	14	3	+	+	+	+
11	2	8	+	+	−	−
12	13	8	0	−	0	+
13	6	5	−	−	+	−
14	4	8	0	+	±	+
No. of cases virus positive			7	8	8	9
No. of cases in which trials were made			11	12	13	14
Per cent of positive results			63.6	66.6	61.5	64.3

Legend: (+) = poliovirus recovered; (−) = virus not recovered; (0) = recovery not attempted; (±) = result indeterminate. Only those cases with definitely positive virus recovery have been counted in the percentages. See n. 4.

has been carried to the mucous membrane from outside, has multiplied in the secretions and finally perhaps penetrated the mucous membrane and caused the infection." As regards the oropharynx and the lining of the intestinal tract, it seemed that the oropharynx represented either a portal of entry or of exit of the virus; but the presence of the agent in the intestinal wall was thought to indicate more strongly that it was eliminated by that route.

Besides recording the sites of predilection of the virus in fatal human cases and in living patients with acute poliomyelitis, the Swedish report contained a wealth of other information. The authors, being mindful of the way that Wickman had drawn attention to atypical cases, i.e. "abortive" infection, set out to prove whether such patients were important as carriers of the virus. For this study they divided their patients into two groups: those with slight illnesses or no symptoms at all who gave a history of intimate contact with frank cases of paralytic poliomyelitis; and those in which no such contact, familial or otherwise, could be traced.

Having investigated six families, some of which fulfilled the qualifications of the first group and some the other, they succeeded in demonstrating to their satisfaction the existence of poliovirus in the throats and intestinal excreta of individuals from both groups. Such persons they regarded as "carriers." Kling and his colleagues concluded that "one is therefore no doubt justified in assuming that virus carriers are very common and often exceed the clinically positive cases."

Perhaps the clinical investigators were not aware of the great significance of these findings, which constituted laboratory proof of what several keen students of the epidemiology of poliomyelitis had suspected all along. It is certain that the bulk of the medical profession did not realize the importance of the new discoveries. In time, basic observations on the frequency with which the virus could be detected in the intestinal excreta and the frequency of inapparent infections with poliovirus was to transcend nearly all of the other remarkable discoveries that were made by Kling, Wernstedt, and Pettersson during the summer of 1911. But it was to take many years.

The problem of the *persistence* of virus in the throat and intestinal tract, which the Swedish investigators also tackled, was one of no mean practical importance. Questions concerning this, it may be remembered, had been addressed to Dr. Flexner in New York earlier, and he had been unable to provide answers. The results of tests on patients in the Stockholm series performed on specimens collected within the first two weeks from the onset of the disease revealed that throat and intestinal washings continued to yield virus in the majority of instances during this period. Positive results declined after that. In a single instance the virus is recorded as having persisted in the throat for some seven months (beyond 200 days!); also, it was recovered from intestinal washings after six months (beyond 180 days!). The report goes on:

> The experiment also shows that the microbe rather quickly—already after 8–14 days—loses its power of causing inflammatory exudations in the inoculated animals. This fact is of very great importance from a practical point of view since it perhaps gives us right to assume that the virus, possibly rather soon after the termination of the acute stage, gets weaker.

Regardless of the questionable accuracy of this last statement, the important practical conclusion was that it would obviously be impossible to quarantine convalescent patients long enough after an acute attack of poliomyelitis that they all could be considered free from contagion. But the point that the virus becomes weaker as convalescence lengthens has not been confirmed. It was to prove a fatal mistake for the Swedish team. Eventually it led to a temporary undermining of confidence in their entire series of experiments among poliomyelitis experts on both sides of the Atlantic.

Additional discussions of a number of other theoretical questions occupy many pages in their voluminous report which was given in abbreviated fashion in Washington in 1912.[6] The series of papers concluded with significant epidemiological observation contributed by one member, W. Wernstedt.[7] It would be interesting to know whether other members of the team shared his views, either wholly or in part. Wernstedt noted that some investigators had speculated as early as 1908 that a given district, if visited by poliomyelitis during a certain year, was apt to be spared during the next few years. This sounded reasonable, but he had gone further and had observed that in none of the principal centers of the 1905 epidemic did the disease appear in epidemic form during 1911. He went on to say that although it hardly seemed possible that the natural immunization of thousands of persons could have taken place in a district where only 50 to 100 frank cases were reported, he believed that this was indeed the case. He concluded further that such *general immunization,* naturally acquired, was the explanation of the resistance of large segments of the population during the current disquieting era of periodic epidemics. Wernstedt's opinion had been confirmed by the new evidence accumulated during the 1911 epidemic, that both mild abortive cases and healthy carriers were indeed infected and, as a result, presumably were immunized.

6. Among these reports were: "The isolation of the microbe of infantile paralysis from inanimate objects and flies," by A. Josefson. See n. 2, pp. 169–86. The upshot of this study was that one positive isolation of poliovirus was obtained from a piece of cloth. No isolations were made from flies.

7. W. Wernstedt: (B) Some epidemiologic experiences from the great epidemic of Infantile Paralysis which occurred in Sweden in 1911. See n. 2, pp. 235–267.

Thus Wernstedt was among the first, if not *the* first, to expound the theory that immunity acquired from inapparent infection during epidemic times was the basis of the age incidence of poliomyelitis. He certainly was the first to be able to back up his argument with proof. To him, this explained why the majority of overt cases of the disease occurred in infants and young children. The simple reason was that they were the only ones who were susceptible, i.e. they had not yet been exposed and infected. Older children and adults, on the other hand, were resistant by virtue of having experienced the infection previously, rarely in a form which was diagnosable, but nonetheless in a form adequate to immunize. The new theory soon received confirmation in the United States from Dr. W. H. Frost, one of the U.S. Public Health Service's epidemiologists, about whom we shall hear more subsequently.

A few medical scientists, but painfully few, accepted Wernstedt's interpretation. To the skeptics the idea was incredible. They had other theories to propose. One of these, put forth by Draper, held that susceptibility was largely a matter of constitutional makeup manifested by physical traits, and not necessarily related to acquired immunity. Another and somewhat similar view, championed by Aycock in the 1920s and 1930s, was that immunization was taking place among young children all the time as a result of infections occurring in both winter and summer, not necessarily mainly during epidemic periods. He also believed that immunity was partially gained as a process of physiological growth. In the face of these conflicting ideas, it was not until a quarter of a century had elapsed that Wernstedt's theory was finally recognized as the correct one. This came about in America in the late 1930s, through the demonstration by several clinical virologists that during epidemic times the number of infants who were inapparently infected and had become transient carriers of the virus far outnumbered the paralytic cases.

But to retrace our steps, it is said that when the Swedish team presented their work at the Fifteenth International Congress on Hygiene and Demography in Washington in 1912, their report was somewhat overshadowed by a spectacular announcement which stole the show. The rival presentation was by two Harvard professors who had carried out experiments that were supposed to prove that poliomyelitis was an insect-borne disease transmitted by the common stable fly! This news was apparently greeted at the convention with a tremendous ovation. More will be said about it in the next chapter.

So the findings of the Swedish team seem to have been lightly brushed aside, at least by some of the leading investigators in America. What were the actual reasons? One was that the accuracy of the work of the Stockholm laboratory was questioned. When others tried to repeat it, positive results were meager, which is not surprising since in the absence of a large epidemic the number of individual attempts that could be made was necessarily limited. The failure to isolate poliovirus from intestinal washings was particularly disappointing. In only a single instance was a subsequent positive result reported; W. A. Sawyer, working in the California Health Department, was able to recover the virus from rectal washings from one patient 14 days after onset of illness.[8] Dr. Sawyer often recounted to me in subsequent years how this modest finding of his was disregarded as the work of an amateur and a public health physician at that. Thus, little enthusiasm was generated for the idea that the intestinal tract had anything to do with the pathogenesis of poliomyelitis.

The Swedish work also was challenged by those who raised serious questions concerning the notion that poliovirus underwent a process of weakening or attenuation during convalescence. This was unsupported by the observations of others. Such doubts, though they perhaps discredited only part of the work, nevertheless tended to put the whole project under a cloud. Gradually this cloud became a curtain that was not to be raised, in this country at least, until the late 1930s. The whole cause of poliomyelitis was to suffer accordingly for almost three decades.

But what kind of men made up this Swedish team of investigators who were able to confound all the poliovirus laboratories of the world with their discoveries? Dr. Carl Kling was the only one of the three that I was privileged to know. For a generation he was considered the dean of poliomyelitis workers in Europe and for most of his career went by the title of "Old Papa Kling." Born in a small town in central Sweden in 1887, he decided early to study medicine and earned his doctorate from the Caroline Institute in 1910. The next year found him as an assistant at both the Stockholm Epidemic Hospital and the State Bacteriological Institute.

Both these institutions must have felt the terrific impact of the severe epidemic of 1911, which furnished such a large number of patients. It was the primary feature that allowed Kling, Pettersson, and Wernstedt to carry out their remarkable investigations. Kling was only twenty-four years old at the time and just out of medical school. Yet he had the imagination, leadership, and industry which carried his team of amateurs along a path of brilliant discovery. Within one year of the 1911 epidemic a prodigious amount of work had been completed, analyzed, presented in Washington, and published!

After the epidemic of 1911, Kling spent some time at the Pasteur Institute in Paris, then described as a mecca for young microbiologists. His friendship and collaboration with Levaditi began at this time. Here it was that Kling, regardless of his repudiation in America, soon came to occupy

---

8. W. A. Sawyer: An epidemiological study of poliomyelitis. *Amer. J. trop. Dis., 3*: 164, 1915. Dr. Sawyer eventually headed the International Health Division of the Rockefeller Foundation which was to direct work in many fields of medical study, including that of yellow fever.

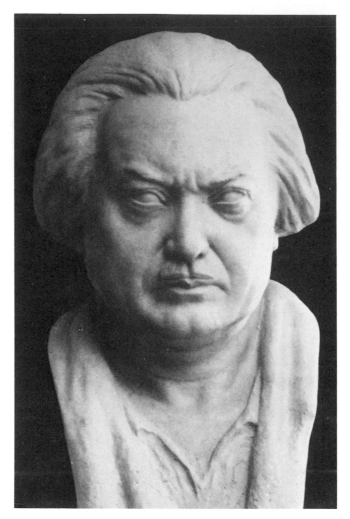

Fig. 22. Bust of Carl Kling, M.D. now in the State Bacteriological
Laboratory at Stockholm. Kindness of Dr. Sven Gard.

the position of an international authority on poliomyelitis. This collaborative association with the Pasteur Institute was to last for at least twenty
years.

Kling succeeded to the directorship of the State Bacteriological Institute
in 1919, a position which he held for twenty-six years. His leadership and
talents were thus recognized and appreciated by his fellow countrymen.[9]
He never lost an abiding interest in poliomyelitis, particularly in matters
concerning its spread. There was one curious idea which he did not relinquish as long as he lived; he considered that poliomyelitis was a water-

9. I am indebted to Dr. Sven Gard of the State Bacteriological and Caroline Institutes,
Stockholm, for many details of Kling's career.

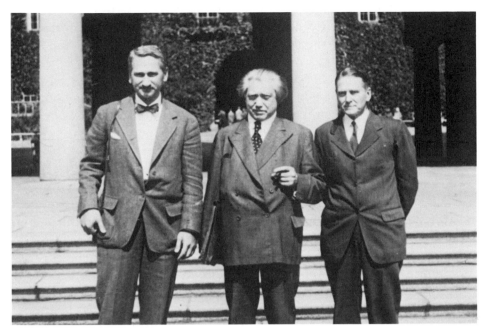

Fig. 23. Stockholm, July 1947. Left to right: Drs. A. B. Sabin, C. Kling, and the author. From the author's collection.

borne disease—at least sometimes.[10] Indeed his ideas about the epidemiology of poliomyelitis were inseparable from his so-called *theorie hydrique*.

In 1961, sixteen years after his retirement from the Bacteriological Institute, Kling gave a radio broadcast entitled "Glimpses of 100 years of Polio Research." He himself had experienced almost fifty of these years; no one else in the history of poliomyelitis research can claim such a record. He died in 1967, at the age of eighty.

Carl Kling was a bachelor, and, like other bachelors in academic medicine in the first half of the twentieth century, such as William H. Welch of Johns Hopkins, his semimonastic existence enabled him to throw all his energies, all his enthusiasm into his work. In some ways Welch and Kling resembled each other. Certainly both men lived in a welter of unanswered letters, manuscripts, and reports of all kinds that scarcely left room for a visitor to sit down.

There are innumerable stories about Kling, most of them concerning his quixotic behavior, illustrated by his habit of telephoning his assistant Sven Gard at five o'clock in the morning with a request to come over right away as he had suddenly thought of something which he would like to dis-

10. In one of the last letters that I received from Kling (Nov. 7, 1955) he took me to task for not recognizing and not giving credit to this theory "hydrique" in an article I had written on the "Epidemiology of Poliomyelitis" which had been published in the *World Health Organization Monograph Series,* no. 26, Geneva, 1955, pp. 9–29.

cuss. His sculptured image (see fig. 22) makes him appear as a more sinister figure than he actually was; another side of him is shown in figure 23 which portrays him in the role I came to know best—as a bluff and kindly man.

The other two members of Kling's original team both went on to distinguished careers, but neither kept up a special interest in poliomyelitis as Kling did. Alfred Pettersson, born in 1867 (and described by one of his students as having the appearance "of an old viking"), became professor of general hygiene at Uppsala University. His chosen subject, urban sanitation, had more than enough ramifications to engage his entire professional attention.

Wilhelm Wernstedt eventually became a professor of pediatrics at the Caroline Institute. It will be remembered that he was the one who had first proposed the correct, but oft to be temporarily forgotten theory that the great majority of children gained their immunity to poliomyelitis during epidemic times from inapparent infections. Wernstedt himself became too busy as a Stockholm pediatrician and professor of pediatrics to be concerned about the pros and cons of his interpretation, but it is heartening to know that before his death his views were universally accepted. America was to learn its lesson the hard and emotional way and not until it had experienced the extensive epidemic of 1916. Even then only a few souls were converted.

CHAPTER 14

W. H. Frost and the Beginnings of Statistical Epidemiology

In the years from 1910 to 1930—during a period of multifarious theories of how the disease was disseminated and what to do about it—a dominant American figure was to preempt the field of the epidemiology of poliomyelitis. Wade Hampton Frost (see fig. 24) was a man of extraordinary gifts who was among the first Americans to comprehend the infinite importance of the manner in which poliomyelitis spreads and the first to put epidemiology on a firm statistical basis in the United States. His approach was different from that of Flexner, and he appreciated the work of the Swedes.

Frost's earliest investigation was concerned with the theory put forth by Rosenau and Brues in 1912, that the biting stable fly (*Stomoxys calcitrans*) was the answer to the epidemiology of poliomyelitis. This idea was quickly hailed with enthusiasm but almost as quickly discarded. Anderson and Frost performed two experiments within a year in attempts to confirm or disprove it; the first partially confirmatory, and the second—not at all.[1] Shortly afterward the theory collapsed. Frost was to learn the hard way, early in his career, that laboratory experiments attempting to elucidate the means of spread of poliomyelitis often went awry.

Despite the failure of his first venture in experimental work, or because of it, Frost went on to become a discerning student of poliomyelitis and, in the 1920s and 1930s, America's leading epidemiologist. Between 1910 and 1913 he proved as energetic as Wickman had been, traveling about the countryside during epidemics, conducting meticulous investigations in the towns which had been hardest hit, searching for clues to explain the puzzling epidemiologic behavior of the disease in rural and urban areas alike. Moreover, he went further than Wickman in that he gathered serum specimens for laboratory tests and data which lent itself to statistical analysis. The new "statistical epidemiology" had already been used successfully in England and was shortly to attain a certain degree of maturity in this country, and Frost deserves no little credit for contributing to the advances that were made between 1910 and 1930. Eventually he was to bring up a whole

---

1. J. F. Anderson and W. H. Frost: Transmission of poliomyelitis by means of the stable fly (*Stomoxys calcitrans*). *Publ. Hlth Rep.* (*Wash.*), 27: 1733, 1912; Ibid., Poliomyelitis. Further attempts to transmit the disease through the agency of the stable fly (*Stomoxys calcitrans*). *Publ. Hlth Rep.* (*Wash.*), 28: 833, 1913.

generation of public health students in the tradition of statistical epidemiology. This would seem to have been an easy task, yet the contrary was true. Many of these public health students were physicians, members of a profession notoriously skeptical and wary of the new science of biostatistics.

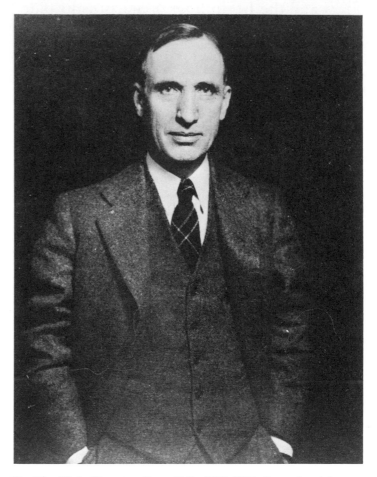

Fig. 24. Wade Hampton Frost, M.D. (1880–1938). Reproduced by permission of the Oxford University Press and the Commonwealth Fund of New York.

Their attitude was that statisticians were not to be trusted as far as either the medical traditions of that era or the current practice of medicine was concerned.

As to concepts about the spread of poliomyelitis which were held in the first decade of the century, we have already heard Wickman's. But his influence had not penetrated to the United States, and at the time Frost entered the scene, in 1910, the epidemiology of poliomyelitis was decidedly not one of American medicine's strong points. For example, in 1909, according to the opinion of H. W. Hill, epidemiologist of the Minnesota State Board of Health, a "conception of this disease may be briefly stated." His notion of clarity and of brevity was a singular one, as illustrated by the following description:

A peculiar gastro-intestinal condition possibly the result of a specific infection, perhaps like summer diarrhea, due to a non-specific, miscellaneous, bacterial interrelation with poor nutritional conditions under abnormal climatic surroundings, resulting in the formation and absorption of poisonous substances which attack the central nervous system diffusely, the exact clinical results depending upon the concentration and the effects of the poison at various points.[2]

This "conception" of the epidemiology and pathogenesis of poliomyelitis, if so it can be called, was obviously in dire need of repair. Fortunately American views were not limited to the above, for a somewhat more sophisticated article published in 1910, in which the New York City outbreak of 1907 was described, contains a statement ending up with the prevailing, yet relatively uninformative conclusion, that the disease is "moderately communicable."[3] On this basis, an eloquent plea had been made in 1910, that infantile paralysis be considered a reportable quarantinable disease. All of this was of little help to Frost as he began his investigations at the very onset of his career.

Details of his life deserve attention. He was born in 1880 in a village near the Blue Ridge Mountains of Virginia, the seventh of eight children.[4] His father was a country physician from Charleston, South Carolina, who had moved to Virginia just after the close of the Civil War. It is said that Frost's early education was entirely informal. Actually he was taught at home by his mother, who must have been a remarkable woman to have undertaken the primary education of such a large family.

Preparation for college demanded more formal teaching, so at the age of fifteen Frost entered a military school at Danville, Virginia, and subsequently attended another preparatory school before he went on to matriculate at the University of Virginia in 1898. Here, after three years, he was successful in gaining admission to the medical school. He was granted the M.D. degree in 1903 and, after a summer as a substitute house officer at Bellevue Hospital in New York, served a year's internship at St.

2. H. W. Hill: The epidemiology of anterior poliomyelitis. *J. Minnesota med. Ass.,* 29: 369–74, 1909.

3. C. F. Boldman, L. C. Ager, and J. F. Terriberry: Epidemiology of poliomyelitis. Report of Subcommittee No. I, in *Epidemic Poliomyelitis; Report on the New York Epidemic of 1907.* New York, J. Nervous and Mental Disease Publishing Co., 1910, pp. 13–28.

4. For these and other details I have drawn heavily on the introduction to: *Papers of Wade Hampton Frost; A Contribution to Epidemiological Method,* ed. by Kenneth F. Maxcy. New York, the Commonwealth Fund, Oxford University Press, 1941.

Vincent's Hospital in Norfolk, Virginia. So far, Frost had gone along with family medical traditions, which, if followed to their logical conclusions, would sooner or later have led to the practice of medicine, for both his father and grandfather had been country doctors. But the idea of becoming a commissioned officer in the Public Health and Marine Service was apparently more appealing than country practice to the young medical graduate. As soon as his internship was completed he decided to apply for a berth in this service and, after passing the necessary examinations, was assigned to duty in 1904 as an assistant surgeon at the Marine Hospital in Baltimore. His first epidemiological assignment was to serve on a team whose task it was to combat a yellow fever outbreak in New Orleans. The experience must have been an exciting one, and not without risk, for it proved to be a large and serious epidemic. All told, there were about 3400 cases with 443 deaths. The role of the mosquito (*Aëdes aegypti*) in the transmission of yellow fever had been well established by 1905, and the effectiveness of measures to eliminate the breeding places of the vector had already been demonstrated by Major Gorgas and others; thus, Frost's team could proceed with a proper and effective plan as to how to combat the disease.

Next came a tour of duty as surgeon on a U.S. Revenue cutter in which, during two summers, cruises were made along the New England coast, to a number of European and North African ports, the islands off the west coast of Africa, and to the West Indies. This varied experience, coming early in Frost's career, sensitized him to the value of observing diseases in a number of different geographical and equally different sociological environments. After this apprenticeship he took advantage of a new opportunity to find out what could be learned from the laboratory in connection with studies carried out in the field. By a fortunate turn of events, in 1908 Frost was assigned to the Hygienic Laboratory of the U.S. Public Health Service, then in the heart of Washington and under the direction of M. J. Rosenau. Rosenau soon left to enter upon his new duties at Harvard and was succeeded in the directorship by J. F. Anderson. Frost's colleagues at the Hygienic Laboratory included a number of busy and distinguished men; Anderson and Goldberger were studying Mexican typhus; Rosenau, Lumsden, and others were conducting an investigation of the prevalence of typhoid fever in the District of Columbia. Other studies in progress in the Hygienic Laboratory were on pellagra, tetanus, and a subject that has been a constant plague to industrial and other civilizations down through the years—water pollution.

Two years after he had joined the laboratory staff, Frost embarked on his first field investigation of poliomyelitis epidemics. It must have been a truly major experience for it gave him the confidence to produce, in the following year, a critique on poliomyelitis, a précis as he called it. This was a general description of the disease—as he had come to know it.[5] In some ways this description simulated Wickman's earliest effort, six years before. Both young men had set out to investigate this disease without knowing much about it, but both had had their interest so aroused that they had turned their hands to writing a monograph on poliomyelitis. Frost's description was only 50 pages long—whereas Wickman's had run to 300 pages. Anyway it was an abbreviated American forerunner of the Peabody, Draper, and Dochez monograph, if only by a year. Though this account has been largely overlooked in poliomyelitis literature, it contained features not in the Rockefeller Hospital monograph, such as the recorded age incidence of cases in various epidemics under different environmental conditions. By this time, Wickman's second monograph had been published, although it had not yet been translated from the original German. This was the article which gave special emphasis to the frequency of abortive cases and made the point that the disease was more contagious than had been appreciated. Frost too had observed, in the summer of 1910, an instance of definite contagion, in a rural school in Hancock County in Iowa, but in his article he was cautious about this main issue.

> While it is beyond the scope of this paper to discuss in detail the evidence for and against the contagiousness of epidemic poliomyelitis, it may be said that the best evidence at present available indicates that the disease is *transmissable* from person to person, probably by direct contact. It must be usually rather slightly transmissable, since only a small proportion of persons in intimate contact with cases contract the disease. Under some circumstances, however, it appears to be rather highly contagious, affecting a very considerable proportion of the population of a limited area.[6]

Later Frost temporarily retracted this view about direct personal contagion, but not for long. Within five years it was to become one of his fundamental beliefs.

Also it was in the Hygienic Laboratory, in 1912–13, that Anderson and Frost thought it worthwhile to test the stable fly as a possible vector of poliovirus. It may have been this theory implicating biting insects as vectors in the spread of poliomyelitis which had transiently influenced his views about direct personal contact.

But before the stable fly had come into the picture, during three successive summers Frost had carried out field studies of poliomyelitis epidemics in the tradition of Wickman. These epidemics had occurred in Mason City, Iowa, in 1910; in Cincinnati, Ohio, in 1911; and in Buffalo and Ba-

5. W. H. Frost: Acute anterior poliomyelitis (Infantile Paralysis); A précis. *Publ. Hlth Bull.*, no. 44, 1911.
6. Ibid., p. 15.

tavia, New York, in 1912.[7] He emerged from these investigations with a wealth of experience but a thoroughly cautious attitude. Although the bulk of evidence pointed to contagion as the true method of spread, Frost warned that a rigid conclusion was not permissible at that time.

In the course of the community studies, Frost made innumerable observations on the behavior of the disease in different types of environments: city, village and rural. There had of course been compilations of data on epidemics since the days of Medin and Wickman, but it is fair to say that no other investigator had pursued statistical studies on so many epidemics, or quite so painstakingly, as Frost. Nor had others been in a position to draw conclusions based on the use of not only two, but *three* methods: intimate clinical observations, statistical analyses, and laboratory experiments on the sera he had collected.

Frost made important use of "spot maps" on which the residences of paralytic, abortive, and suspicious cases were plotted according to their dates of onset. With such information it was possible to estimate the monthly rates at which the prevalence of urban versus rural cases progressed and declined. He made use of seasonal and meteorological charts and also conducted extensive investigations of the sanitary conditions of the premises of individual cases, and of the milk and food supply, looking into these matters as only a physician who had been working in a laboratory which had typhoid fever and water pollution as two of its main subjects was able to do. He made observations on the simultaneous occurrence in a given area of cases of paralysis in humans and in domestic animals; and on the presence or absence of flies (biting or otherwise), mosquitoes, and other insects. His conclusions came as a result of years of investigation, after countless clinical observations, using the laborious process of house-to-house surveys, a method which proved so necessary in making the difficult decision as to what was or was not to be considered a suspicious case of poliomyelitis. He thus assembled data which, all in all, strongly confirmed Wickman's view that the disease *was* spread by personal contact.

Along these same lines, Frost also took advantage of his position at the Hygienic Laboratory to see whether he could use laboratory tests to answer some obscure questions which had confronted him during the epidemic in Iowa, the summer of 1910. He said:

> The cases encountered in this epidemic, suspected to be abortive forms of poliomyelitis, but without definite paralytic symptoms, were so numerous and of such apparently great epidemiologic significance that their accurate diagnosis appeared at once to be a most important preliminary to epidemiologic study.[8]

7. W. H. Frost: Epidemiologic studies of acute anterior poliomyelitis. *Hyg. Lab.—Bull.,* no. 90, 1913.

8. Ibid., p. 30.

In attempting to utilize the laboratory to achieve a more accurate diagnosis, he obviously progressed a step beyond Wickman. As it turned out, however, he had chosen a problem which severely taxed the capabilities of the Hygienic Laboratory. Blood specimens were collected from 9 patients in the Mason City epidemic at a time when the patients were well over attacks of what was presumed to be *abortive poliomyelitis*. By rights, the sera of all 9 of these patients should have contained antibodies against poliovirus. The serum neutralization tests were carried out by Anderson and Frost according to the latest and most approved technique,[9] and with the use of various control sera. Luckily, they were not misled into accepting the erroneous but short-lived idea arrived at by Netter and Levaditi in France and by Flexner and Lewis in this country, that sera from the great majority of normal adult persons (similar to normal monkey sera) did not contain poliovirus antibodies; for to the contrary, sera from the great majority of individuals in the United States, who had previously acquired inapparent poliovirus infections *did* indeed contain antibodies. To Anderson and Frost goes the credit for having stumbled upon this finding. Unfortunately they tempered their views with the statement that neutralizing action of the serum "has quantitative limits which clearly differentiate it from the action exercised by the serum of persons who have had poliomyelitis." This statement was incorrect, but the confusion was straightened out in the following year (1912), when investigators at the Hospital of the Rockefeller Institute,[10] who had been alerted to the problem by Anderson and Frost, were able to show that normal adult human sera did indeed contain antibodies against poliovirus in amounts which could be fully as large as in the sera of convalescent paralytic patients. This highly significant observation was one which grew in importance from one generation to the next. The team at the Hygienic Laboratory, after a bit of floundering, had arrived—at last.

Before Frost, no man had gone out into so many communities to deal with epidemic poliomyelitis with such sophisticated weapons; and, it might be added, few investigators were to use these combined approaches in epidemiological research on this disease again, for at least another twenty years. Still, Frost continued to be cautious. In an introduction to the summary of the report on this three-year study of a number of epidemics, he was still undecided as to the means of dissemination; he emphasized that no rigid conclusions were warranted, and in fact the means of dissemination of the infection had not been conclusively established.

It is hard to see how he could have reached this opinion without pondering a number of questions again and again. Were the *people,* more espe-

9. J. F. Anderson and W. H. Frost: Abortive cases of poliomyelitis; An experimental demonstration of specific immune bodies in their blood-serum. *J. Amer. med. Ass.,* 56: 633–69, 1911.

10. F. W. Peabody, G. Draper, and A. R. Dochez: *A Clinical Study of Acute Poliomyelitis.* Monograph no. 4, Rockefeller Inst. Med. Research, New York, 1912.

cially the children, in a given epidemic area infected, or was the whole *place* infected? In other words, could one exclude some sort of concentrated seasonal pollution of the environment with poliovirus which might constitute a special hotbed of infection? Was the presence of an insect vector to be completely ruled out? Few students who have investigated multiple epidemics of poliomyelitis in different environments have not been occasionally haunted, however fleetingly, by such ideas.

However, to go on with Frost's cautious words, he stated his conviction in a summary discussion of his 1913 report.

> The only definite conclusion, then, which is drawn from the epidemiological studies of poliomyelitis is that the infective agent is, during epidemics at least, quite widespread throughout the population affected, the incidence of the clinically recognizable disease being limited by the relatively rare susceptibility to the infection. This conclusion, in the light of our present knowledge, holds equally well whether it is assumed that the route of infection is through contact, through insects, or through dust;[11] whether the ultimate sources of infection are human beings or lower animals.

> As to what constitutes susceptibility or the converse—immunity—practically nothing can be deduced except that age is obviously a factor of importance, susceptibility being generally greatest in the first half decade of life, thereafter progressively diminishing until in adult life there is very general immunity to natural infection.

> The reason for this is at present a matter of speculation. Conceivably the greater immunity of adults may be due to a nonspecific resistance, developing naturally with maturity, without reference to previous exposure to or infection with the specific virus of poliomyelitis.[12]

> On the other hand, there are certain facts which suggest that the very general immunity of adults may be specific, acquired from previous unrecognized infection with the virus of poliomyelitis.[13]

This is a summary of early American (1913) ideas, but not those held in Sweden nor those which Frost held after the study of the 1916 epidemic. Nevertheless in arriving at his 1913 interpretation Frost had been clearly impressed by the views of Wernstedt, which had been reported the year before in Washington. He may also have been influenced by results of his own investigations, and those reported in the Rockefeller Hospital's mono-

11. Two investigators from New York City had claimed to have isolated poliovirus from dust in a sick room (M. Neustaedter and W. C. Thro: Experimental poliomyelitis produced in monkeys from the dust of a sick room; a further contribution. *N.Y. med. J., 94:* 613, 1911). To my knowledge this finding has not been confirmed since.

12. This was a theory that Aycock, whose work will be reviewed in a subsequent chapter, was to seize upon and to pursue avidly.

13. See n. 7, pp. 250–51.

graph, that the sera of virtually all normal adults contain specific neutralizing antibodies against poliovirus. Nevertheless, previous inapparent infection as a source of immunity in adults was an explanation that had been greeted with profound skepticism by other students of poliomyelitis in the United States. Frost was the exception.

To quote again from his 1913 report,

> To even suggest a general immunization of a large population against poliomyelitis, a disease considered quite rare, may seem unjustifiably radical, yet Wernstedt has not hesitated to conclude from the results of epidemiological and experimental studies in Sweden, that such is actually the case.[14]

Suffice it to say that Frost's experiences during the three summers spent in the study of epidemics in the field provided him sufficient food for thought to last a lifetime. It also put him in a position, not shared by others, of being peculiarly prepared and able to jump in and handle the kinds of practical problems which he faced when called upon to deal with the extensive and disastrous epidemic of the summer of 1916. This epidemic involved the entire northeastern area of the United States. In the metropolitan area of New York City alone over 9,000 cases were reported, an urban-incidence rate of 185.2 per 100,000. Frost's contribution to the report that the Public Health Service made on this epidemic is one of the highlights of the early history of the disease in the United States. He had arrived at his views slowly and painfully. But this is a story to be told in a subsequent chapter.

To continue with Frost's career, after 1913 he returned to problems of environmental sanitation and stream pollution, which had been among the Hygienic Laboratory's major concerns until work was interrupted by the 1916 epidemic of poliomyelitis. Another more time-consuming break of an emergency nature which soon came was the participation of the United States in World War I. As his share in public health activities of a military nature, Frost was given an assignment in the American Red Cross. Here his duties were unfortunately interrupted due to a bout of tuberculosis which required an absence of six months for treatment.

By the time he had returned to active duty in late 1918, the pandemic of influenza, which swept around the world, had already reached America. Frost took on the responsibility of an epidemiological and statistical study of that disastrous plague. At least this brought him back once more to the kind of problem in which his heart really lay.

In the meantime, from an entirely different direction, things of another nature were beginning to take shape with regard to Frost's career. The

14. Ibid., p. 211.

radical notion of establishing a school of hygiene and public health at Johns Hopkins University had been in the wind for some time, and the plan was finally consummated in 1919. Dr. William H. Welch, the first director of the school, in his search for a physician capable of developing the scientific potentialities of the epidemiological method, had no difficulty in singling out and appointing Frost as resident lecturer. Later he became professor of epidemiology, and finally head of the Department of Epidemiology and Public Health Administration. Still later, in 1930, Frost became dean of the school.

Thus began a fruitful academic period that endured for twenty years, until the time of Frost's death. In the growth of the young school, which was soon to be imitated by many another elsewhere, he shared a close association with such men as W. H. Welch, W. H. Howell, Raymond Pearl, and Lowell J. Reed of the Department of Biostatistics, who ultimately became president of Johns Hopkins University. Frost's activities during this part of his career quickly set the pace for teaching and research in the field of epidemiology in the United States. Suffice it to say that he succeeded in his teaching position to the extent that a whole generation of students of public health can claim the privilege of having sat at his feet. Most of them boast of this fortunate experience. Many times in those twenty years the author had occasion to make special trips to Baltimore to seek his wise and witty counsel, which he dispensed freely to his friends.

To no man more than Frost is credit due for establishing epidemiology as a biological and statistical science in this country. From the moment he started his teaching career this science began to show signs of belated growth in America which had been denied it before. Today few descriptions of common diseases that find their way into prominent modern textbooks of medicine fail to include a paragraph or a section describing the epidemiology of the illness. And Frost had no small part in implementing this reform. More particularly, the usefulness of the new science (along with microbiology and immunology, which had also burgeoned in the early twentieth century) was soon brought to bear on some of the obscurities of poliomyelitis. Frost's contribution thus becomes an essential part of this history. It was years before another medical scientist of stature and experience who had learned the hard way was to pursue investigation on poliomyelitis with such discernment.

At the time of Frost's untimely death, which occurred after a distressing illness from cancer in 1938, the following editorial appeared in the *Baltimore Sun*.

> One of the fine and rare spirits passed from this earth on Sunday in the death of Wade Hampton Frost. He was a distinguished figure in medical science. . . .

His personality had many facets. He had deep wisdom for the affairs of life, and he had subtle and penetrating wit. He had an austere sense of duty and a fine instinct for leisure. He could be Spartan and he could be a *bon vivant*. No matter which facet he turned to life, it shone as in the sun. No one can recall the mean or malicious as his contribution in any relationship. All who knew him recall at this time the thoughts and the acts that were generous and just, high of mind and mood. He made living a noble adventure.[15]

This was no false eulogy. Frost was singularly able to overcome the aura of remoteness which so often surrounds the serious scientist and college professor who is apt to be preoccupied with his own ideas and with exploring some new and seemingly exotic discipline—such as epidemiology. He was also good company. Accessibility to friends and students alike was his special characteristic. Furthermore he sought to obliterate the differences between Town and Gown. Frost had that rare talent which allowed him to break through the web of a technical vocabulary and express his ideas and himself in amusing words of common usage, to students and laymen alike. This was only one of the personal qualities that never ceased to excite the admiration of his friends.

15. *The Baltimore Sun.* April 30, 1938.

CHAPTER 15

The Epidemic of 1916

In 1916 the northeastern part of the United States suffered one of the most devastating epidemics in the history of poliomyelitis. One might have thought that since New York City had experienced a large outbreak in 1911, it would have been prepared for this new emergency. But the 1916 epidemic so far outstripped in magnitude the earlier ones that the U.S. Public Health Service had to lend a hand to aid the existing municipal services. Added to the city's woes were the drastic quarantine restrictions which local health authorities imposed. An extraordinary degree of anxiety assailed the public, the medical profession, hospitals, and public health officials alike, all of whom were ill prepared to cope with the harrowing problems of a sudden mammoth epidemic.

During the years 1909–15 the maximum annual rate of reported cases in the United States had never exceeded 7.9 per 100,000 population, but in 1916, within the epidemic area, it suddenly leapt to an all-time high of 28.5. In New York City alone there were over 9,000 cases with an urban rate of over six times that in the total epidemic area.

The epidemic of 1916 will go down in history as the high-water mark in attempts at enforcement of isolation and quarantine measures. In many ways health authorities had much on their side, including precedent. Indeed the claim was that there was little else to do in the way of control and here was a visible effort, indicating that at least something was being done about the problem. In several European countries poliomyelitis was one of the diseases in which notification of cases, quarantine, and disinfection were required by law. An epidemic in Nebraska in 1909 had supposedly been checked by imposing an absolute quarantine for three months on all members of affected families with the exception of the breadwinner. An eloquent plea had been delivered in 1910, before the august Association of American Physicians, that poliomyelitis be made a reportable and a quarantinable disease.[1] Infantile paralysis was *contagious*— maybe only slightly contagious, but the proper way to deal with it was by quarantine. The author of this plea, Dr. Joseph Collins of New York City,

1. J. Collins: The epidemiology of poliomyelitis; a plea that it may be considered a reportable quarantinable disease. *Trans. Ass. Amer. Phycns, 25*: 98, 1910; *J. Amer. med. Ass., 54*: 1925, 1910.

apparently had little realization that while the reporting of the paralytic cases was indeed necessary if one wished to keep track of them, the question of quarantine was an entirely different matter. Not only would it be difficult to enforce—but practically impossible, considering the diagnostic difficulties of deciding what was and what was not a case of *bona fide* poliomyelitis. In some quarters, in spite of Dr. Collins' rather convincing remarks, long before 1916 there had been a growing appreciation that the idea of quarantine was not based on sound principles. True, this view was held only by a very small group, of which Wickman had been the pioneer. It included Kling and his Swedish colleagues, and Frost almost as the lone leader in this country. They represented the few who felt that there was little use in such drastic measures since during an epidemic the recognized cases represented less than 10 percent of infected persons.

Dr. Haven Emerson (see fig. 25), at the time commissioner of health of New York City, went about the enforcement of the regulations with that earnest zeal which was to characterize his actions all during his life. He gave to this cause the very best that was in him—according to his own lights. It may be said, nonetheless, that his control measures were subject to constant advice of experts, among whom were numbered such authorities as George Draper, Simon Flexner, W. H. Frost, Hans Zinsser, and many others. Hardly had the epidemic begun when orders were given that all premises housing a case of poliomyelitis should be placarded and the family quarantined; the windows were to be screened, the bed linen disinfected, nurses were to change their clothing immediately after tending any patient, and even household pets were not allowed in any patient's room as they too were considered suspect.

Besides all these restrictions, on July 14 a new order went out, one that caused much adverse public comment. This was the decision to restrict travel, limiting movement out of the epidemic area and requiring the issuance of so-called health certificates, which amounted to travelers' identification cards. Children 16 years of age and under were placed in the restricted category and were not permitted to leave New York City from July 18 until October 3 unless a certificate was produced indicating that the premises they occupied were free from poliomyelitis. This ban on travel was reviewed at a full-scale national conference attended by numerous health officers, which was held in Washington in mid-August 1916.[2] Needless to say, most of those who attended came for purposes of instruction in this matter, not to give advice about travel restrictions, and the meeting seems to have broken up amid a welter of unanswered questions. Nevertheless the travel ban was approved.

2. Transactions of a special conference of state and territorial health officers with the United States Public Health Service, for the prevention of the spread of poliomyelitis. *Publ. Hlth Bull. (Wash.)*, no. 83, 1917.

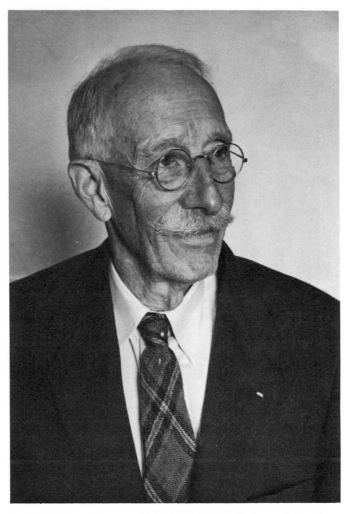

Fig. 25.   Haven Emerson, M.D. (1874–1957). Kindness of Dr. Emerson's daughter, Mrs. Ruth Cooke.

The services of the U.S. Public Health Service had been offered to Mayor Mitchell of New York City early in the epidemic and had been promptly accepted. This enabled a presumably more experienced team to move into the city; its members included epidemiologists, clinicians, sanitary engineers, and even an entomologist. Their arrival posed a certain amount of competition for Dr. Emerson's own working force, but at least the U.S. Public Health Service's jurisdiction covered a wider area, including not only metropolitan New York but also neighboring suburbs, cities, and rural areas. Among the members of the Washington group were such distinguished figures as C. H. Lavinder, Edward Francis, James P. Leake, William F. Draper (not to be confused with George Draper), A. W. Freeman, and, last but not least, W. H. Frost. For some of these men the immediate task was to help with the control measures; for others, to conduct careful sanitary and environmental surveys. Except for Dr. Frost, the group does not seem to have come with any specially prepared questions to answer, other than to start collecting facts and figures on a great variety of clinical, demographic, and environmental aspects of the epidemic. As far as these investigations went, they succeeded in gathering the most extensive amount of significant data that had ever been assembled in any single epidemic of poliomyelitis.

The local New York Health Department, besides being saddled with the task of tending strictly to the medical needs of the community and the overcrowding of contagious disease hospitals, had the overwhelming burden of overseeing various quarantine measures that had been so suddenly and drastically instituted, and of enforcing the travel ban. One can well imagine that any infringements were a constant thorn in Dr. Emerson's side, for he was rigid in seeing that regulations were carried out to the letter.[3]

There were even criminal actions concerning quarantine instituted during the 1916 epidemic. For instance, undue publicity was given to a certain case, and exaggerated reports as to the action and requirements of the department of health were published in the daily newspapers. The parents claimed that the child in question was not suffering from poliomyelitis, and in spite of repeated warnings, instructions, and notifications from the department of health, both written and verbal, they refused, it was said, to isolate the child and take the ordinary precautions to prevent the infection from spreading to other children in the neighborhood. Court action followed, and the child was removed to the Queensboro Hospital.[4]

A word about Dr. Haven Emerson (1874–1957) would not be out of place at this point. He was easily one of the truly great pioneers of public health in this country. Born in New York City, the son of a physician and a grand nephew of Ralph Waldo Emerson, he had graduated from Harvard in 1896 and Columbia's College of Physicians and Surgeons in 1899. Subsequently his professional career in public health covered the first half of the twentieth century. Not only did he treat the last case of cholera that New York City was to see for some time, but he began his career at a time when there was practically no such thing as a profession of public health. Suffice it to say that he changed all this. After a dozen years of medical practice he became, in 1914, sanitary superintendent and a year later, commissioner of health in New York City. He taught at Columbia University from 1922 to 1940, when he became professor emeritus of public health prac-

3. *The Epidemic of Poliomyelitis (Infantile Paralysis) in New York City in 1916.* Based on the official reports of the bureaus of the Department of Health, New York, 1917.
   4. Ibid., p. 60.

tice. The end of his long life of service devoted to public health came in 1957. Imbued with a fervor necessary to awaken lazy members of the medical profession and politicians indifferent to his views, he had preached vigorously that all citizens were entitled to know what public health, as he saw it, had to offer. The causes that he espoused were many and diverse, ranging from the standardization of diagnostic nomenclature to militant campaigns against disease (particularly when the health of children was at stake) to elevation of the health standards of the American Indian; but none of these did he enter into with more tireless zeal than the cause of epidemic poliomyelitis.

In appearance Haven Emerson's tall, almost ascetic figure has epitomized the title which had been bestowed on him, namely, "The last of the great Puritans."

Research Projects during the Epidemic

At the Washington meeting held in mid-August 1916, which had to do primarily with the ban on travel, Dr. Emerson explained that several lines of research were being pursued in New York City. One, laudably enough, was an effort to see whether there was any conceivable connection between the milk supply and poliomyelitis; another, financed by the Rockefeller Foundation, was to document the effect of secondary personal exposure within families or communities—a thankless task indeed; another was a clinical study in which Dr. George Draper must have had a hand, which was designed to determine whether one might detect physical characteristics of those children susceptible to poliomyelitis. "Anybody," said Dr. Emerson, "who goes through a hospital such as the Willard Parker Hospital, with 900 children, will get an impression that these children are different physically from other children." And a final study, admittedly the most practical, was the one concerned with treatment of acute cases by administering serum obtained from patients who were convalescent from poliomyelitis. Was this treatment efficacious? In the words of Dr. Emerson, "The results will take months to work out." He was right in this, for efforts to obtain an answer concerning the usefulness of serum therapy were to last for some twenty-five years.

It is difficult to understand why such tremendous—but misdirected—efforts were made to enforce the travel ban, and yet little or nothing was done in this epidemic toward the collection of information which had to do with poliovirus—its distribution within the body and its distribution in nature. This was in spite of the example set by the Swedish team at least four years previously in an epidemic of almost equal relative proportions. It was all the more surprising considering that on July 27 Dr. Emerson had called a meeting of a research committee, i.e. of acknowledged "investigators in the field of experimental medicine and leaders in the science of prevention of disease," to decide what research work was especially desirable. The suggestion to repeat the Swedish work of 1912 appeared first on the agenda of these proposals, but, incredibly, nothing seems to have been done about it. The six projects listed were:

1. Methods of culture of the virus of poliomyelitis, with especial reference to corroboration of previous work, to simplification of methods, and to the distribution of the virus in the body of patients.
2. The immunologic reactions of patients and supposed carriers of the virus and others.
3. The virulence in animals of the crude virus, in order to determine if possible whether there are any differences in the virus causing outbreaks in different parts of the country as well as to discover perchance more susceptible animals for experimental purposes than are now available.
4. The microscopic study of secretions of the nose and throat and of the intestinal contents of patients suffering from poliomyelitis or persons who have come in close contact with such patients and others.
5. The transmission of the disease by insects and domestic animals and other possible modes of transmission.
6. The study of practical methods of disinfection.[5]

In the framing of the six suggestions for research projects one can see the hands of Drs. Flexner and Noguchi, both of whom were members of the research committee and momentarily hot on the trail of their ill-fated globoid bodies, which they believed would provide a simpler means than the Swedes had used of demonstrating the presence of the virus in various parts of the body. In fact, the wording used in suggestion no. 1 was the "culture of the virus"; and no. 4 contains the implication that the microscope was going to be used for the examination of "secretions of the nose and throat and of the intestinal contents of patients." These statements implied that globoid bodies were as visible in the light microscope as were tiny bacteria.

In spite of the value of these six suggestions, attempts to implement them were never realized, except for no. 5, which was decided in the negative. A study of the distribution of the virus in the body of patients was never carried out, tragically enough (or if so, yielded negative results), in spite of the resources of two or more active local laboratories—New York City Health Department's laboratory, under the direction of W. H. Park, and that of the Rockefeller Institute and its affiliated hospital. To account for this oversight, the zeal for this sort of work and a guiding spirit must have been lacking. Dr. Park had been understandably busy with the collection and preparation of therapeutic sera from convalescent patients, but he did find time to test materials from 40 autopsies of cases of poliomyelitis which had been made available to his laboratory. Specimens from the brain or

5. Ibid., pp. 35–36.

cord from some of these were used for monkey inoculation. However, there is no record that tissues from other parts of the body were tested. The procedure consisted of injecting central nervous system tissue by the then approved method of trephining a hole in the animal's skull and injecting the material directly into the brain. This posed certain difficulties to the unitiated, particularly if the autopsy material had not been collected under sterile conditions. If such was the case, the monkey was likely to succumb with a brain abscess instead of developing experimental poliomyelitis. In any event, the first of these tests made in Dr. Park's laboratory resulted in failure. In the end, when more experience had been gained, 17 monkeys were described as having died of poliomyelitis or having shown signs which were compatible with the experimental disease.[6] It was a credit to the New York laboratory that at least the virus responsible for the epidemic was isolated. Yet in spite of this fact, little was gained except perhaps experience in inoculating monkeys.

After the lapse of fifty or more years it is easy to say what should have been done, namely, to have taken advantage of the large number of cases in an attempt either to confirm or definitely disprove the work of the State Medical Institution of Sweden. But, strange to say, no one was assigned to do any clinical virological work of real importance. The simple truth must have been that there were painfully few well-trained virologists available in the United States at the time.

Frost had been given the role of acting as a mastermind when it came to the solution of epidemiologic problems. As to his ideas about searching for the virus, perhaps he was still mindful of his earlier view, expressed in the report of 1913:

> The technical difficulties in the way of demonstrating the virus, involving the injection of filtrates into monkeys, are such that extensive statistics upon this point can hardly be expected in the near future, unless the technique of the demonstraion can be greatly simplified and the expense reduced.[7]

Frost may have been still misled by the idea that a great many such observations would have to be made to yield the "extensive statistics" that would be necessary; not the comparatively small but still impressive numbers of tests furnished by the Swedish team. The voluminous report of the U.S. Public Health Service on this epidemic[8] deals with virus studies only

6. Ibid., pp. 85–88.

7. W. H. Frost: Epidemiologic studies of acute anterior poliomyelitis. *Hyg. Lab. Bull.*, no. 90, 1913, p. 235.

8. C. H. Lavinder, A. W. Freeman, and W. H. Frost: Epidemiologic studies of poliomyelitis in New York City and the northeastern United States during the year 1916. *Publ. Hlth Bull. (Wash.)*, no. 91, 1918.

in the briefest manner, under a section entitled "Collection of Autopsy Material," and then largely with isolation of virus from the central nervous system alone:

> Ultimately material, in large or small quantities, was secured from about 40 different autopsies in New York City and Newark, N.J. This was all preserved in glycerine and sent to the Hygienic Laboratory for further study.[9]

At least some of this material found its way into the hands of Dr. James P. Leake, who was a member of the Public Health Service's team, although two years were to elapse before his report was made available. Dr. Leake was an experienced field worker in poliomyelitis, having participated with Dr. Frost in observations in Batavia, New York, in 1912, but he was not so experienced in clinical virology. Nevertheless he went to work in the Hygienic Laboratory, testing glycerine-preserved central nervous system tissue from 11 of the 40 New York cases. His experiments succeeded better than those in Dr. Park's laboratory, for virus was recovered from all samples. Possibly the glycerin preservative contributed to this success by exerting a bactericidal effect and thus preventing premature death of the animals from bacterial infection.[10]

To his credit, Dr. Leake also tried inoculating three filtered nasal washings into monkeys by the intraperitoneal route, for the intracerebral route had been found too risky, and the volume of fluid was far too great to be injected into the brain of a monkey. The material he used was decidedly unpromising. One of the washings had been obtained from an adult who had had poliomyelitis six years previously; this could not be expected to have yielded the virus. Another was from a patient of unspecified age who had contracted poliomyelitis eight days previously. The third was from an adult who had been in contact with the second case. Considering all the variegated clinical material which had abounded during this epidemic, these washings represented a sorry lot of specimens indeed, and it was no wonder that none yielded the virus. Nevertheless the trial constituted one of the painfully few early attempts made in America to isolate poliovirus from extraneural sites in living patients during the extensive epidemic of 1916.

Dr. Leake also busied himself transmitting experimental poliomyelitis from monkey to monkey; and in addition he attempted a certain number of neutralization tests, which ended unsuccessfully, or so it would seem. In addition he tried to isolate poliovirus from domestic animals, with entirely negative results.

9. Ibid., p. 208.

10. J. P. Leake: II. Experimental poliomyelitis; Experiments with virus of human origin obtained during epidemics. *Hyg. Lab. Bull.*, *111*: 21–30, 1918.

Two months after the catastrophic epidemic was over, various preliminary scientific observations and opinions were aired at a medical meeting
in New York City.[11] The author, then a second year medical student, can
remember attending this meeting during the Christmas vacation, 1916–17.
Dr. Flexner was in the chair, and the several papers that were read must
have been carefully selected to prevent the discussion from getting out of
hand. Noguchi spoke of work going on at the Rockefeller Institute on
globoid bodies, and, as if to counter them, E. C. Rosenow of the Mayo
Clinic described his findings on the bacterium which he thought was the
responsible agent in poliomyelitis—a special form of streptococcus. Rosenow's presentation was received with prepared skepticism, practically with
scorn. One would think that this would have been enough to silence the
streptococcal theory for all time. But I cannot recall any immediate skepticism being expressed about the globoid bodies, which were eventually to
meet an even earlier oblivion than Rosenow's streptococcus.

As far as the globoid bodies were concerned, it was apparent that Dr.
Flexner, like Rosenow, was after something big, for this research held out
the promise of a simpler method of detecting the agent of poliomyelitis
and of practical immunological tests as well. The manner in which Dr.
Noguchi was introduced at the meeting invested him with an aura of mystery, as a mastermind who was about to clinch a great and useful discovery,
or so it seemed to me.

As early as 1913, Flexner and Noguchi[12] had described their globoid
bodies in terms which intimated that they actually were part of the cycle
of cultivation of the virus of poliomyelitis in vitro. The bodies consisted of
minute formed structures that resembled tiny bacteria, some of which were
able to pass through filters. For their cultivation, a special medium containing human ascitic fluid with a fragment of rabbit kidney was used. In
retrospect, the explanation for this finding may have been that the rich
media containing pieces of tissue, which Flexner and Noguchi used, allowed the poliovirus present in the inoculum to survive, with or without
multiplication, for a limited time. It was unfortunate that these two investigators continued to focus their attention on this apparent bacterial
contaminant for the next five years. Amoss, writing in 1917, described the
globoid bodies as *micro organisms*—not a virus—and how they "had been
shown to have a definite relation to epidemic poliomyelitis," and "to have
fulfilled Koch's law of causation."[13] Ten years later he modified these views

11. This was a meeting of the Federation of American Societies for Experimental Biology
held in New York City on December 27–30, 1916. Dr. Simon Flexner was chairman of the
executive committee and Dr. Peyton Rous, secretary.

12. S. Flexner and H. Noguchi: Experiments on the cultivation of the virus of poliomyelitis.
Fifteenth note. *J. Amer. med. Ass., 60*: 362, 1913.

13. H. L. Amoss: The cultivation and immunological reactions of the globoid bodies in
poliomyelitis. *J. exp. Med., 25*: 545–55, 1917.

with the statement: "In fact the proof that globoid bodies constitute the etiological agent is as yet inadequate."[14] In another few years they were finished.

SUMMATION OF NEW THINGS LEARNED

The 1917 report on this outbreak by the New York City Health Department was the first to appear. By the time the long epidemic was at last over, in the late fall of 1916, the department had probably been taxed almost beyond endurance. It certainly must have been with a sigh of relief that Dr. Emerson wrote his final but unconvincing comments at the end of the report (see n.3). He had tried desperately and, in spite of everything, was able to be optimistic.

> Commentary is unnecessary with such facts as these to prove the efficacy of co-operative sanitation in public health work. Unfortunate as the recent epidemic undoubtedly was, and in some respects unproductive from an epidemiological point of view, this disastrous visitation may yet turn out to have been a blessing in disguise, if it fixes indelibly in our minds one obvious and incontestible truth—that the control not only of poliomyelitis, but of all preventable diseases does not depend upon the mysterious power of any supernatural agency, but the remedy lies largely within ourselves.

It cannot be said that these words have stood the test of time, but they may have been appropriate in 1916–17. Advances in scientific medicine brought about in the laboratory were eventually to provide more effective means for the control of poliomyelitis than "co-operative sanitation." But at the moment Haven Emerson was convinced that control lay in the "obvious and incontestable truth" of his own public health restrictions. Actually, such drastic local restrictions by no means went out with 1916. They continued to be made, at the jurisdiction of local health officers, for a generation, but a national ban on travel was never enforced again. Dr. Emerson had been sorely tried, and the following year he shook the dust of the New York City Health Department from his feet and sought refuge in the position of epidemiologist to the American Expeditionary Force in France —almost as a relief.

By autumn of 1916 leading public health authorities had been sufficiently aroused to put their heads together to see what actually had been learned about the behavior of this dread disease and what to do about it. At the ensuing round table discussion Professor Winslow of Yale University led off with an epidemiological point of view, demonstrating from his

---

14. H. L. Amoss: Is epidemic poliomyelitis preventable and does a specific form of treatment of the disease exist? *Bull. N.Y. Acad. Med.*, 2nd s., 2: 456, 1926.

maps the epidemic's progress. In speaking of the summer incidence of the disease he admitted that he, as almost every other authority in the United States, supported Flexner's theory on the nasopharynx as the portal of entry of the virus; it was indeed "a respiratory disease." But he added:

> All the other phenomena of this disease, as far as I know, are explained by direct contact just like that which occurs in any other respiratory disease, coupled with the existence of a large proportion of immunes. What is not explained is the fact of summer prevalence; for all other nose and throat diseases are winter diseases.[15]

Dr. Winslow went on to say, "Whether it means that the infection is carried by insects, which personally I doubt, or that it is primarily an intestinal infection . . . I do not know." Another thing he especially stressed was that he was "absolutely in accord with all that Doctor Frost has said about human reservoirs and the great importance of the unsuspected carriers." This could only mean that he held a dim view of strict quarantine as an effective control measure in the disease.

One of the redeeming features about the 1916 epidemic, if one can put it in such a way, is that once it was over and done with, it furnished a mass of statistical data the like of which had never been seen. As a result it was possible, among other features, to map out significant characteristics of the behavior of poliomyelitis as it had appeared that year within the northeastern part of the United States—to determine the routes along which it had spread, differences in age-specific rates in urban and rural settings, and differences among individuals of various racial origins—all meticulously recorded with the idea that such information might lead eventually to a better understanding of the kind of infection poliomyelitis was. Granted that the disease was spread by personal contact, a most important thing to discover was whether the environment might exert some controllable influence on the dissemination of the agent; if so, there might be something preventable about the disease after all.

As might be expected, it required a long time to sift through this wealth of data. It was subjected to various analyses not only by the U.S. Public Health Service, but by several municipal and state departments of health as well. The report that contains the most voluminous information, and has a ring of finality about it, is the Public Health Service's monograph (see n. 8). It appeared in 1918, a year after the New York City report, and continues to live in the annals of poliomyelitis epidemics as a model of

---

15. Among those present at this discussion were: Professor C-E. A. Winslow of Yale University; Louis I. Dublin, statistician of the Metropolitan Life Insurance Co., N.Y.C.; Allen W. Freeman and W. H. Frost, both of the U.S. Public Health Service; and W. H. Park and Haven Emerson of New York City's Department of Health. See Infantile Paralysis; a round table discussion. *Amer. J. Publ. Hlth,* 7: 117–43, 1917.

what can be done in the way of extensive statistical analyses of a single outbreak. But it narrowly missed being almost too late. The monograph came out at a time when most people in the affected area had forgotten all about the epidemic, or had their minds on the exigencies of World War I, in which the United States had become involved. Although it did not contain any particularly new revelations, there was an immense number of features of poliomyelitis that were better documented than ever before.

In retrospect, the tragedy was that, in view of the galaxy of talent which had been assembled on advisory committees and working forces alike and the administrational and laboratory facilities that were at their disposal, a golden opportunity to advance knowledge of the clinical virology of poliomyelitis had been allowed to slip by.

What actually was learned from this most extensive epidemic? For one thing the various quarantine restrictions enforced at the time were proved to be ineffective and subsequently have been shown to be not worth enforcing. The idea that domestic animals had anything to do directly with the spread of poliomyelitis to man was disproved and finally laid to rest; and the differences in age-specific incidence among populations living in urban and rural areas was confirmed. Along these same epidemiological lines, the views that Frost had expressed in 1913 with cautious words were now on much more secure ground. These four interpretations were stated in the final summary of the Public Health Service's report:

1. That poliomyelitis is, in nature, exclusively a human infection, transmitted from person to person without the necessary intervention of a lower animal or insect host, the precise mechanism of transmission and avenues of infection being undetermined.
2. That the infection is far more prevalent than is apparent from the incidence of clinically recognized cases, since a large majority of persons infected became "carriers" without clinical manifestations. It is probable that during an epidemic such as that in New York City a very considerable proportion of the population became infected, adults as well as children.
3. That the most important agencies in disseminating the infection are the unrecognized carriers and perhaps mild abortive cases ordinarily escaping recognition. It is fairly certain that frank paralytic cases are a relatively minor factor in the spread of infection.
4. That an epidemic of one to three recognized cases per thousand, or even less, immunizes the general population to such an extent that the epidemic declines spontaneously, due to the exhaustion or thinning out of infectable material. Apparently an epidemic incidence relatively small in comparison to that prevailing in an epidemic may produce a population immunity sufficient to definitely limit the incidence rate in a subsequent epidemic.[16]

An astronomical amount of data had gone into these analyses—without the benefit of the computer. They contained unpopular, but neverthe-

16. See n. 8, p. 214.

less sound, principles to which all the experts in the poliomyelitis field were
to be gradually won over. For these four conclusions, except for a few minor alterations, had the ring of truth about them and were eventually
proved to be correct. Here were the proper guidelines of what to do and
what not to do during epidemics. The public health practice of placarding
the homes and premises of recognized cases and the ultrastrict regulations
about isolating patients became increasingly modified by subsequent health
authorities in due time, in spite of many vigorous even outraged protesta-
tions by a concerned public that felt it should be protected by the usual
safeguards. The truth of the matter was that the infection was simply too
widespread, too hidden for any such measures to be effective. Yet it took a
generation or more for the general public to understand this point of
view that ran counter to everything to which it had become accustomed.

CHAPTER 16

Draper's Clinical Views

Within a year after the epidemic of 1916 Dr. George Draper published his small book entited *Acute Poliomyelitis* in which he brought some novel ideas to this already well described subject. Aside from a book by R. M. Lovett, a Boston orthopedic surgeon, which had appeared the year before and dealt largely with the aftercare of paralyzed patients, Draper's was the first book published in the United States that contained not only sound up-to-date information, but contributed provocative new ideas to the subject of poliomyelitis. It was the first to review the various clinical features and the use of simple laboratory tests in the acute disease in a fashion that practicing physicians might readily appreciate. In the words of Dr. Flexner, it was a timely contribution by a man with considerable previous experience in the clinical and experimental aspects of the disease. As a matter of fact, in 1917 Draper probably had the best qualifications of anyone in the country to engage in such a project, however unusual some of his views might have appeared.

George Draper, of New York, was educated at Harvard College. His immediate family was well known through his sister, that distinguished stage personality and monologuist, Ruth Draper. Dr. Draper's first research assignment was under Dr. Warfield Longcope at the Ayer Laboratory of the Pennsylvania Hospital in Philadelphia, shortly after Dr. Simon Flexner's incumbency there. He then went on to the Rockefeller Hospital and afterward became a clinical professor at the College of Physicians and Surgeons of Columbia University, his alma mater that had granted him his medical degree. He was the only one of the trio of authors of the Rockefeller Hospital's monograph on poliomyelitis who went on with this particular subject as a specialty in his practice and in his writings.

During the poliomyelitis epidemic of 1916, Draper was designated by the New York City Department of Health to take charge of its work on Long Island. Thus he was in the thick of things early in his career, serving frequently on advisory committees in that outbreak, and subsequently.

His unique new ideas centered on constitutional factors in relation to disease in general—and poliomyelitis in particular. He maintained that susceptibility to quite a number of diseases could be recognized by the presence of certain physical traits, and he was convinced that constitutional makeup played a major role in determining the severity of an individual's reaction to a given illness. He was opposed to the thought that differences in response to infections could be attributed entirely to the effects of *acquired* immunity. Of course Draper's views had some truth in them, but the notion that built-in susceptibility could be recognized by physical characteristics was at least problematic. Furthermore, he rode his views too hard, particularly toward the end of his life, and particularly with regard to poliomyelitis.

Draper developed his thesis in many articles and in two books, *Disease and Man* and *Human Constitution,* both of which bear reading. But as far as poliomyelitis was concerned, his theories have gone the way of other hopeful ideas that have been difficult to prove. This should not detract from his other contributions on the whole subject of acute poliomyelitis. During the 1916 epidemic and the years immediately following it, he was for at least a decade the acknowledged *clinical* authority on the acute disease in the United States. His most distinguished patient was Franklin D. Roosevelt.

In the first edition of his *Acute Poliomyelitis,* published in 1917, he said:

> The type of child which seems to be most susceptible to the disease is the large, well-grown, plump individual who has certain definite characteristics of face and jaws, is broad browed, and broad of face. The teeth are particularly interesting. . . . The wide spaced dentition has been a striking feature and frequently involves all the single teeth of both jaws, so that each tooth stands entirely free.[1]

Draper's qualifications for susceptibility altered with age. Among adolescents and young adults, instead of the "large well-nourished children with widely spaced teeth," he noted that "there appeared a more delicately made type."

In a second edition of his book,[2] published almost twenty years later, he went more deeply into this subject, stating that at the Constitution Clinic, which he had established in 1916 at the Presbyterian Hospital in New York, he had made extensive studies between 1916 and 1931, using an elaborate and dependable technique which enabled him "to perceive distinguishing particularities which had previously escaped notice." In addition to the characteristics just given, he maintained that scattered pigmentation of the skin was another feature which "marks poliomyelitis susceptible children." Most physicians who came before and after Draper were, however, unable to perceive these subtle physical features which spelled susceptibility to poliomyelitis. The method of measuring body susceptibility to illness had not developed into the discipline that it became later.

1. G. Draper: *Acute Poliomyelitis.* Philadelphia, P. Blakiston's, 1917, p. 8.
2. G. Draper: *Infantile Paralysis.* New York, Appleton-Century, 1935, pp. 52–73.

In 1912, five years before the first edition of Draper's book appeared, Wernstedt had expressed rather different views of how resistance was acquired by the general population. Lavinder, Freeman, and Frost had confirmed these views in 1918, but it was not until some two or three decades later, when new virologic techniques were available, that they were universally accepted. In the meantime, in the 1920s and 1930s, a number of curious hypotheses on the subject of immunity to poliomyelitis enjoyed temporary popularity, particularly those of Aycock. Draper's ideas of constitutional susceptibility were taken so seriously that it was widely believed that if and when effective prophylactic measures became available they should be reserved for the ultrasusceptible child, who could be identified on the basis of certain features in his appearance.

Afterward, Jungeblut and Engle introduced another theory complementing that of Draper. Early in the 1930s, Jungeblut was a professor under Dochez in the Department of Bacteriology at the College of Physicians and Surgeons in New York. He and his colleague Engle maintained that "the mass protection enjoyed by the adult human population rests primarily on the normal function of endocrine balances characteristic of mature age.[3] This interpretation immediately received widespread publicity in the daily press and elsewhere. No less an authority than Haven Emerson, also a member of the faculty of the College of Physicians and Surgeons, was so enthusiastic that at a meeting of the American Epidemiological Society in New Haven in 1931 he requested an unscheduled place on an already crowded program in order to deliver a paper describing the revolutionary concepts of his colleagues—Jungeblut and Engle. These authors maintained that any hypothesis postulating that the resistance of adults was due to universal subclinical immunization as a result of infection was inconsistent with their epidemiologic observations. They claimed that they had demonstrated virus-neutralizing substances in the blood of immature monkeys which had been treated with extracts from the anterior pituitary gland or similar substances recovered from the urine of pregnant women.

In correspondence which I had with Dr. Draper on this point in 1933 he summed up his own ideas about immunity against poliomyelitis as well as commenting on the hypotheses of others:

> Aycock's figures on the number of adults with immune blood serum who have not had paralysis in some way also points to a high non-paralyzed incidence. But this work of his may be questioned in view of the recent work of Jungeblut and Engle which supposes the strong possibility of a non-specific immunity which is related to the phenomena of growth and development generally. My own recent studies on the

3. C. W. Jungeblut and E. T. Engle: Resistance to poliomyelitis; the relative importance of physiologic and immunologic factors. *J. Amer. med. Ass., 99*: 2091, 1932.

constitutional types of infantile paralysis cases, lead me to feel that the type of child which is capable of developing the disease is just as specific a living organism as is the virus. Consequently the constitutional factor emerges as a very important one in the problem.[4]

I can recall participating as a speaker, with Dr. James Trask, at a meeting of the New York Academy of Medicine either in 1932 or early 1933. A packed audience listened to different ideas on the subject of how immunity to poliomyelitis was acquired in the general population. At this session the two members of the Yale Poliomyelitis Study Unit (Trask and Paul) who tried to support Wernstedt's views came off decidedly second best. They were greatly outnumbered by those in favor of the "new and exciting" physiological explanation.

Although Draper's theories have not stood the test of time, they marked an important chapter in the history of American medicine. His ideas went along with a growing body of evidence that of all the factors involved in familial clusters of certain diseases, the genetic influence is one which is most pervasive.

In dealing with a completely different aspect, Draper made a singularly telling clinical observation. This had to do with the early stages of the acute illness, and appears in the first edition of his book. Similar findings had been noted in the monograph from the Hospital of the Rockefeller Institute published in 1912, but five years later Draper had had much more experience which enabled him to pay more attention to the occurrence of minor symptoms that preceded the onset of the paralytic phase. These might clear up entirely so that in a day or so the child appeared to have recovered. "Nevertheless," runs the text at this point, "one or two days later, and perhaps without warning, the child becomes paralyzed."

Of the two distinct phases in the clinical course, Draper emphasized that, "though previously recognized by us, the full significance of the phenomenon was but vaguely appreciated." He then went on to describe these early systemic symptoms and illustrated his interpretation with the diagram shown in figure 26, reproduced from the first edition of his book.[5] He wrote:

> Because of the two definite masses or humps of symptoms, the analogy to the arrangement of the dromedary's back was taken to express the type figuratively. The temperature curve may show one or two elevations but the figure refers to all the signs and symptoms of each group or hump whether there is an associated rise of temperature or not.[6]

4. Personal letter to the author from Dr. George Draper (dated January 19, 1933).
5. See n. 1, p. 43.
6. Ibid., p. 40.

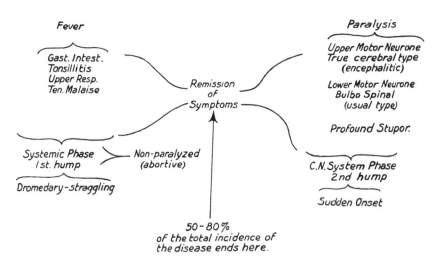

Fig. 26. Draper's diagram illustrative of his concept of the "dromedary" form of the acute disease. Reproduced from Draper (see n. 1) by permission of the Mc-Graw Hill Book Co.

Draper was on the right track about the symptomatology, but somewhat off in his terminology, for the dromedary (*Camelus dromedarius*) has a single hump. In spite of this terminological slip, however, his concept of the two phases of acute poliomyelitis is still occasionally referred to as "the dromedary form" of the disease. The important feature was not the nomenclature but the concept, which he expressed as follows:

> Obviously then we are dealing with a disease which has two distinct phases, one of general systemic nature and another of specialized expression in the form of central nervous system disorder. Furthermore, there may be a variety of symptom complexes representing the systemic phase.[7]

This interpretation was more or less in line with views expressed by Rissler, Medin, and Wickman, beginning some twenty years earlier, although they had not illustrated their ideas with any kind of a diagram. As a matter of fact Draper was more accurate than he appreciated when he implied that the early phase was of a "general systemic nature." And he had the added laboratory evidence to back him up for he had already discovered that when the spinal fluid was tested during the first phase (or hump) the cell count and protein levels could be normal, a sign that the central nervous system was not yet involved.

In modern parlance it seems clear that Draper was speaking of the minor illness of poliomyelitis when he described the first phase, which according

7. Ibid., p. 39.

to his calculations represented the entire course of the illness in 50–80 percent of infections.

In summary, Draper's real contribution to the history of poliomyelitis was his success in impressing clinicians around the world with the importance of the dromedary form of the clinical course and his interpretation of it. In any event, the term stuck.

In keeping with many a physician of the first third of the twentieth century Draper entertained a hearty distrust of statistical measurements. In the same letter quoted above, which he wrote to me in 1933, he expressed his views on this point—somewhat eloquently:

> I do not believe that you can prove anything about the incidence of the disease and the distribution of paralyzed and non-paralyzed cases by statistics. There are too many variables and subtle factors which we do not as yet fully understand. My own impression about susceptible types is that one finds a pretty close parallel between the severity of the disease and the degree of constitutional markings. I appreciate very much your desire to get an accurate numerical evaluation because it would be a great help to know; but I suspect that you will never be able to do it because both sides of the disease-producing mechanism, namely the virus on the one hand and the susceptibility of the individual on the other, are constantly changing with the seasons and with the years. It is a little like trying to apply a mathematical formula to the alternations of shadows cast upon the surface of a sea which is calm, or slightly ruffled, or boisterous, by clouds which float past the sun in masses of irregular shape and size.

By and large, physicians of a later generation do not take such a dim view of biostatistics. A modern champion of the opposite side, Dr. Warren Weaver, ex-director of the Division of Natural Sciences of the Rockefeller Foundation, severely took to task those members of the medical, biological, and agricultural professions who disparaged the use of statistical methods.[8] But Draper cannot be blamed for his views on the subject, for such an attitude was almost universally held in his day.

8. W. Weaver: The disparagement of statistical evidence. *Science, 123*: 1859, 1960.

CHAPTER 17

Other "Virus" Diseases of the Central Nervous System

Earlier in this book it was stated that poliomyelitis is almost the only disease with the unfortunate capacity to precipitate sudden paralysis in a previously healthy infant or child. This characteristic alone might enable one to identify it—even historically. Yet, as in any disease, there are always atypical cases, and in poliomyelitis there may be a variety of clinical patterns, depending on the location of the lesions in the central nervous system. Since hundreds of thousands of cells in the brain and spinal cord may be attacked by the virus, the symptoms and signs reflect those sites, or combinations of sites, which happen to be involved in a given patient. Thus, encephalitic signs such as drowsiness and coma may occasionally predominate; paralysis may be limited to ocular or facial or other muscles; or, if only a few scattered motor nerve cells are affected, there may be no muscle weakness, the clinical picture being limited to the aseptic meningitis syndrome. As physicians began to recognize other acute varieties of illness involving the central nervous system, there were bound to be occasional difficulties in the differential diagnosis of poliomyelitis. Particularly was this true since quite a number of diseases share a similar pattern of onset, viz. fever, drowsiness, and stiff neck, sometimes followed by paralyses. The problem came into focus after World War I, when several apparently "new" diseases of the central nervous system appeared, and at the same time poliomyelitis epidemics began to occur with disturbing frequency.

To begin with, in the late summer and fall of 1918, during the closing months of World War I, a pandemic of influenza erupted.[1] For a time it was dubbed the "Spanish influenza," because it has always been found both convenient and expedient to blame certain diseases on one's neighbors, and the attitude of Europeans proved no exception. But gradually the influenza epidemic of 1918 became so widespread and lasted so long that its hypothetical geographical source was forgotten. Volumes have been written about this catastrophic pandemic in which untold numbers of persons, young and old alike, died. It was a pestilence which, in the words of Dr. William H. Welch, came close to resembling the "black death" of the Middle Ages—a type of calamity that was not supposed to happen in the twen-

---

1. A *pandemic* is worldwide in distribution in contrast to the more circumscribed geographical distribution of an *epidemic*.

tieth century. My account will have to forego any description of this pandemic except as the story contains threads of a tenuous relationship with encephalitis lethargica, or "sleeping sickness." This disease had also begun at about the same time and was to drag on for the next few years. Because of this overlap in time, to this day it is believed that there may have been some sort of a connection between pandemic influenza and lethargic encephalitis.

Be that as it may, in the early 1920s another and more alarming thought began to take root and grow in the minds of physicians, amounting to an obsession among some—even some in high places. This was the idea that the human race was becoming more vulnerable than it had ever been before to infections of the central nervous system. It was a frightening concept. Where was it to end? What with poliomyelitis epidemics becoming ever more numerous and more severe; and, on the opposite side of the world, with large epidemics of Japanese encephalitis occurring with increasing frequency; with the sudden appearance of the mysterious Australian X disease; and now—last, but far from least, lethargic encephalitis —what was the world coming to? It was enough to set people thinking. Were all of these infections that had similar clinical features related in some way? Was the whole world to suffer the hazards of ever-increasing vulnerability of the brain and spinal cord to infection? However farfetched some of these thoughts may sound today, they were not so ridiculous in the 1920s. Even Simon Flexner had something to say on the subject in an address before the College of Physicians of Philadelphia in 1923.

> The reappearance of cases of epidemic encephalitis in Europe and America in the last few months has served to emphasize the sinister character, as well as our imperfect knowledge, of the disease. Moreover, it has served to remind us of the notable fact that within a period of about twenty years, several epidemic diseases having their chief seat of injury in the central nervous organs have prevailed widely in America and in other parts of the world.[2]

Among the diseases to which Flexner was referring was Japanese encephalitis, which, although it had been described in the latter part of the nineteenth century, had not attracted serious international attention.

JAPANESE ENCEPHALITIS

Beginning in 1871, seasonal summer epidemics of encephalitis had appeared several times in Japan. Fifty or sixty years later, in 1924 and 1935, two of the largest outbreaks occurred. During the 1924 epidemic more

---

2. S. Flexner: Epidemic (lethargica) encephalitis and allied conditions. *J. Amer. med. Ass.*, *81*: 1688–93 and 1785–89, 1923.

than 6000 cases were listed, and the death rate, particularly in older age groups, was extremely high. Epidemics usually were restricted to the southern half of the country and were especially prone to occur in the region surrounding the Inland Sea, notably around the city of Okayama.

As to symptoms and signs, these were terrifying enough, but not quite the same as those of poliomyelitis. Only occasionally were the two diseases confused. In the initial phases the patients frequently suffered from alternate periods of delirium and somnolence, and occasionally a maniacal state. Facial and other types of paralysis often appeared, especially in the fatal cases, but fortunately they were apt to be transient in those patients who recovered from the acute disease, unlike the paralyses of poliomyelitis. Fortunately, also, the majority of the seriously ill patients recovered without suffering residual mental damage. However, by and large it was a serious and frightening disease, and the hope was that it would not spread to other lands, as poliomyelitis was erroneously supposed to have spread from Scandinavia. In the 1920s there was hardly an inkling of what the cause of the disease was or how it was transmitted.

THE AUSTRALIAN X DISEASE

In 1917, another epidemic disease of the central nervous system—a new plague—had come out of the blue. This was the Australian X disease. Nothing like it had been seen, or at least reported, before. It appeared in the Murray Valley region of Australia in the spring of 1917, and during the ensuing hot dry season 134 cases occurred. The age group of those clinically affected was much younger than with Japanese encephalitis; 50 percent of the patients were under five years old. The disease was accompanied by somewhat the same symptoms as those of Japanese encephalitis: high fever, muscular rigidity, mental confusion, and coma. The mortality was very high. But this type of encephalitis was unique in that a viral etiology was discovered quite promptly. Cleland and Campbell were successful in isolating the responsible virus from the central nervous system of three fatal cases.[3] This was a triumph for it marked the first time that any specific virus had been isolated from a case of human epidemic encephalitis. Unfortunately the agent was lost after a few years, but enough studies had been done to determine with certainty that the virus was not that of poliomyelitis. It is said that this mysterious X disease appeared in Australia again in 1922 and again in 1926, but actually very little was found out about it until many years later.

3. J. B. Cleland and A. W. Campbell: The Australian epidemic of acute encephalo-myelitis; a consideration of the lesion. *J. nerv. ment. Dis., 51*: 137, 1920. It would seem that isolation of the etiologic agent of this epidemic marked the first, though short-lived discovery of any virus identifiable as a *human arbovirus*. The virus of yellow fever was not to be discovered for another eight years.

Encephalitis Lethargica

By far the most devastating and widespread of the three "new diseases of the brain" which attained prominence in the early twentieth century was encephalitis lethargica, or von Economo's disease, named for the Viennese physician who first described it in 1917. The possibility of a direct relationship between pandemic influenza and lethargic encephalitis, largely because the two diseases were more or less contemporaneous in time and place during 1917–20 and for some years thereafter, has already been mentioned. Some felt that an attack of influenza might render a person more susceptible to encephalitis. Unlike Japanese B and Australian X disease, von Economo's encephalitis had a distinct tendency to chronicity, often with the distressing features of gradually increasing mental and physical deterioration which became manifest after an interval of some months or several years. Tremors and double vision, present early in the course, might clear up only to recur months or even years later and be accompanied by distinct personality changes coupled with speech defects and mental deterioration that were so characteristic of this disease. In the author's own experience lethargic encephalitis proved to be such a common disease in 1920–21 that during a year's medical internship at the Pennsylvania Hospital in Philadelphia, the hospital wards seemed never to be free from chronic cases, with new acute ones being admitted almost every month. Happily this period of prevalence is now long since past. Lethargic encephalitis came and went during the period between 1917 and 1927.

It is understandable that in the 1920s physicians and epidemiologists alike were alarmed by what seemed like the sudden emergence of devastating new diseases and began to look around for the causes. The idea had barely occurred to them, however, that perhaps they were dealing with old diseases which only occasionally came to the surface, at intervals of many years.

In any event no etiological agent was discovered for lethargic encephalitis. Numerous viruses were proposed, prominent among them being the common herpes virus, but an association with it was never established. The disease gradually sank into oblivion within a decade without anyone knowing whence it came, what caused it, or where it went,[4] although the redoubtable E. C. Rosenow of the Mayo Clinic felt that it was due to a neurotropic streptococcus. Its demise was accompanied with many sighs of relief. It has not returned to plague the world in any recognizable form during the forty some years which have elapsed since 1927. But that is by no means an indication that it will not raise its ugly head anew; indeed, it is likely to do so.

---

4. For an account of this disease the reader is referred to: Josephine B. Neal: *Encephalitis; A Clinical Study*. New York, Grune & Stratton, 1942.

SEROUS MENINGITIS

Still another polio-like illness was for a time, especially in the 1920s and 30s, pushed into the foreground. There was considerable stir among internists and pediatricians when a Swedish pediatrician, Arvid Wallgren, described in 1925, under the name of "acute aseptic meningitis," a clinical syndrome which he felt could serve to unify a group of illnesses that all had the same symptoms.[5] In popular parlance the syndrome soon became known as "serous meningitis."

Inasmuch as aseptic or serous meningitis resembled mild poliomyelitis so closely, it was inevitable that some physicians began to question whether cases of Wallgren's syndrome had not been confused with nonparalytic poliomyelitis all along. Perhaps Wickman and later observers had been incorrect in their assumption that during an epidemic of poliomyelitis the abortive and nonparalytic cases had all been due to the as yet undiscovered poliovirus.

For a time "aseptic meningitis" seemed to be a convenient label and was immediately taken up by Europeans and Americans. And yet the syndrome was obviously a nonspecific one that included a hodgepodge of viral and other infections. As its usual mild course had many of the clinical features of nonparalytic poliomyelitis, doctors began to use it as a convenient substitute diagnosis, and incidentally as a subterfuge in mild cases of poliomyelitis, telling parents that their child only had serous meningitis instead of "polio." This popular usage was decidedly a backward step.

This then was the state of affairs during the early 1920s with regard to three or four diseases of the central nervous system, all of which posed diagnostic difficulties in relation to poliomyelitis, and for only one of which an etiologic agent was known. The subsequent story of these diseases may be briefly stated. Beginning with the oldest one, Japanese encephalitis, in the early 1920s when lethargic encephalitis came upon the scene as an additional plague, physicians in Japan felt it incumbent to differentiate it from their own native type; and so the former was designated as Type A, the latter as Type B, a term (Japanese B encephalitis) which has lasted to this day. But soon enough, the B type began to reassume its erstwhile major position, with extensive epidemics occurring in 1924 and 1935. Long before the mid-1930s a number of Japanese scientists had begun to suspect their national affliction was a virus disease, and in 1935 they were able to prove it. Not only did they establish the viral etiology, but they found that they could transmit the infection to sheep, goats, and smaller animals. As to the manner of spread, for a number of years before the onset of World

5. A. Wallgren: Une nouvelle maladie infectiose du system nervous centrale. *Acta pedriatrica (Upsala)*, *4*: 158, 1925. The term *aseptic* or *serous* meningitis was used to imply a nonbacterial etiology and to distinguish it from the purulent meningitis caused by meningococci and other pathogenic bacteria.

War II, Japanese epidemiologists were in a quandary about this. Most of them claimed that the disease was disseminated in the manner of polio-myelitis—by personal contact. One team of scientists (consisting of Drs. Mitamura and Kitaoka) maintained that it was spread by special varieties of *Culex* mosquitoes, while others felt that the manner of spread was entirely unknown.

To appreciate even part of the story we must retrace our steps and recount a bit of medical history, largely enacted in the United States. In 1930, a disease long known among shepherds in Scotland as *louping ill* (the leaping sickness) was shown to be due to a virus which affected the central nervous system of sheep. Shortly thereafter, in the early 1930s, in the United States, epidemic encephalitis of horses was shown to be due to two different and distinct viruses. It was in 1931 that Karl F. Meyer of the University of California isolated the virus of western equine encephalo-myelitis (WEE) from the brain of a horse sacrificed during the acute disease. Later Dr. Carl Ten Broeck of the Rockefeller Institute at Princeton, New Jersey found that eastern encephalitis virus could be readily distinguished from WEE virus. The diseases for which these two agents were responsible were regarded at the time as primarily, if not entirely, limited to horses. A manifestation of interest by the U.S. Army in this matter was the report in 1934 by Lt. Col. (later Brig. Gen.) Raymond A. Kelser, V C (Veterinary Corps), that one of these viruses could be transmitted from horse to horse by certain species of mosquitoes. Thus the role of culex mosquitoes was established in the transmission of the western type of equine encephalitis, and there was an obvious similarity to the insect-borne disease of sheep in Scotland. So far it was thought that only large animals were subject to attack. And for a time, it was thought that this class of serious diseases belonged wholly in the field of veterinary medicine.

But at this point (1933) in the United States, a totally unprecedented event took place. This was an extensive epidemic of human encephalitis that broke out in and around the city of St. Louis, Missouri. Before it was over more than 1,000 cases had occurred. From the brains of fatal cases an agent was promptly isolated and given the name *St. Louis encephalitis* virus. But the manner in which the infection was disseminated remained a mystery, despite the efforts of a whole battery of experts from the Public Health Service and the Harvard Infantile Paralysis Commission. Nevertheless, with the discovery of a new encephalitis virus that attacked humans, gradually the implication dawned that, besides Japanese and St. Louis varieties of encephalitis, there might be a number of other viruses affecting man and animals simultaneously, each causing somewhat similar lesions.

Events had by now begun to move rapidly; in Russia and in Siberia a very widespread and serious form of both human and animal viral encephalitis carried by ticks was recognized in 1937 and given a name reflecting its seasonal occurrence, Russian spring-summer encephalitis. A more revealing discovery came in New England in the summer of 1938, when it was found that the disease identified as eastern equine encephalomyelitis (EEE) was not limited to horses, but that this infection also was capable of attacking man in epidemic form! The obvious manner of spread was via the mosquito. At least this was the manner in which the disease spread among horses. By this time evidence pointed to the existence of a whole family of encephalitis viruses which might be spread through the agency of insects, and these viruses affected both animals and man. As a matter of fact, by 1938 another new member with similar characteristics had already cropped up in Venezuela, and Venezuelan equine encephalitis virus was added to the growing list.

It remained for Dr. W. McD. Hammon and K. F. Meyer of the Hooper Foundation of the University of California as well as several other investigators in the years 1939–42 to establish beyond a doubt the mosquito transmission of both western equine and St. Louis encephalitis in man, horses, and even in birds. They also recognized the dependence of these infections upon certain ecological relationships within the geographical areas where they are prevalent, involving entomological, avian, and mammalian cycles of infection.

In the meantime World War II had broken out, and all scientific and other forms of communication had been cut off from Japan. Also, the claims of the two virologists Mitamura and Kitaoka, who had certainly been among the first to suggest that human encephalitis could be mosquito borne, went unheeded; presumably they had lost face for the time being with Japanese university authorities. Mitamura, at least, had retired to his home an ill man.

In the spring of the final year of World War II, and at the time of the United States occupation of the Pacific islands northwest of Guam, the medical department of the army recognized that American troops were entering territory where Japanese encephalitis lurked. It was reasonable to assume that these men would be susceptible to a disease to which they had never before been exposed. This had already become a matter of some concern to the Preventive Medicine Department of the Medical Corps during the years of army occupation of Japan. So, the sudden appearance of an epidemic of Japanese encephalitis on Okinawa during combat there did not come as a great surprise. The final count was 127 cases, the great majority being in the native population;[6] there were 11 unequivocal cases

6. A. B. Sabin: Outbreak of encephalitis on Okinawa in 1945; preliminary report on status as of August 21, 1945. *J. Mil. Med. in Pacific, 1*: 79–84, 1945; also, Epidemic encephalitis in military personnel; isolation of Japanese B virus on Okinawa in 1945; serologic diagnosis, clinical manifestations, epidemiologic aspects and use of mouse brain vaccine. *J. Amer. med. Ass., 133*: 281–93, 1947.

in military personnel, and it is highly probable that more than this number occurred. The Okinawan outbreak did not allay fears as to what was going to happen later.

Apprehension on this score had already been communicated to the Neurotropic Virus Disease Commission of the Army Epidemiological Board, which went to some pains to prepare in February 1945 a monograph[7] containing all available information the members could lay their hands on about this exotic disease, including bits of information gleaned from two Russian virologists who visited the United States early in 1944, and were encouraged to tell of their experiences with Japanese encephalitis in eastern Siberia. They indicated that this disease was indeed a serious menace that should be guarded against with all possible means, especially by vaccination.[8]

So when the war with Japan suddenly came to a halt in August 1945, United States military medical authorities lost no time in dispatching a small two-man commission, consisting of Dr. Hammon and myself, to make a preliminary investigation of this very question. What were the actual chances of American troops becoming a prey to this disease, and what might and could be done about it?

Among the commission's first duties was to call upon Drs. Mitamura and Kitaoka in Tokyo, whose culex mosquito theory of transmission had gradually been discounted by Japanese medical and university authorities. Mitamura and Kitaoka were understandingly fearful about the commission's visit. Japanese war criminals were currently under trial; the two scientists naturally feared the worst. To their immense relief, however, it gradually dawned on them in the course of the interview that the members of the commission had come not to punish them for their scientific crimes, but to congratulate them for having been the first to have seen the light and to have maintained that a particular epidemic form of human viral encephalitis was mosquito borne. To say the least, the meeting was a moving experience (see fig. 27).

As an anticlimactic sequel to the story of Japanese encephalitis in occupied Japan, during the decade following 1945 it turned out that the disease, with all of its ugly implications, did not prove to be the serious menace to American soldiers that was expected. Nevertheless the U.S. military medical officers lost no time in taking advantage of the opportunity to study this important infection in its native environment, and to prepare and use for a time, a formalinized (inactivated) vaccine on civilian and

7. Commission on Neurotropic Virus Diseases: Japanese B Encephalitis. Part I. The Disease. Part II. Control Measures with particular reference to Vaccination. Submitted to the surgeon general of the U.S. Army Feb. 1945, unpublished.

8. To Russian microbiologists of that day the virus of Japanese B encephalitis went under the name of *Far Eastern encephalitis virus*.

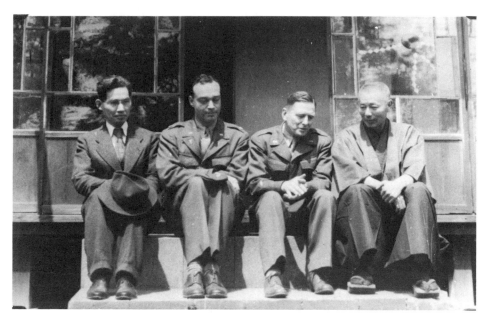

FIG. 27. First post–World War II Conference on Japanese B encephalitis between U.S. and Japanese medical scientists, Tokyo, Feb. 1946. Left to right: M. Kitaoka, Maj. S. E. Moolton, MC, the author, T. Mitamura. Photograph taken by Dr. W. McD. Hammon, in the author's collection.

military personnel alike.[9] This was almost the first time that such a vaccine was used by U.S. military authorities against a potentially epidemic viral disease of the central nervous system and accordingly had all the aspects of a field trial. One of the first stumbling blocks to the success of the program was the low antigenicity of the material and the consequently feeble antibody responses of the vaccinated troops. Because of this, and because the disease did not eventually prove to be such a serious threat to U.S. forces occupying Japan between 1946 and the early 1950s as had been anticipated, the vaccine was abandoned. Instead, reliance was placed on environmental measures such as screening and other types of mosquito control as means of protection.

In the ensuing years, in addition to the encephalitis viruses discussed above, close to 200 agents belonging to the heterogeneous arthropod-borne (or, as it was eventually called, arbovirus) group have been identified in

9. Several types of inactivated vaccines were tried over a period of several years. None proved particularly promising. In this connection four members, W. McD. Hammon, H. A. Howe, J. R. Paul, and A. B. Sabin, who had served on various commissions of the AFEB from 1941 to 1956 had served likewise on the National Foundation's Immunization Committee and taken part in discussions of poliovirus vaccines when a choice between an inactivated and an attenuated vaccine was brought up before the NFIP's Committee on Immunization in Oct. 1953. However, by that time the formalinized (inactivated) Salk-type vaccine had already received its early testing, whereas the attenuated poliovirus vaccine was in an embryonic stage.

various parts of the world, including Asia, Africa, and Australia. Some of these viruses cause disease in man; others are not known to do so, but all have one common characteristic, transmission by insect vectors.

As a final postscript to the story of the mysterious Australian X disease, for which a virus had been discovered as early as 1917 only to have been lost again, it too became a respected member of the arbovirus family. Following that first epidemic the disease apparently smoldered along for many years in Australia and was finally recognized again as a definite entity in 1950. This time it was identified under a geographical name, Murray Valley encephalitis, and the virus was rediscovered in 1951.

Over the years, as more was learned about the arbovirus family, the realization came that certain environmental conditions were much more conducive to the spread of such infections than any hypothetical increase in susceptibility of the human central nervous system. Also, the increased availability of protective measures against insects, including screening, the control of breeding places, and the use of more powerful insecticides, contributed to keeping arbovirus infections in check.

In terms of poliomyelitis, it turned out that the various arbovirus infections and other diseases of the central nervous system were separate and unrelated; the main similarity was that occasionally the symptoms were similar and that arbovirus infections also tend to appear in the summer, at least in warm weather. Yet by and large poliomyelitis emerged more than ever in the light of a distinct and separate entity with its own special characteristics and diagnostic tests.

CHAPTER 18

Aycock's Autarcesis Theory

Dr. W. Lloyd Aycock had established an enduring interest in poliomyelitis when as a young man he participated in therapeutic trials during the epidemic of 1916. Seven years later he was able to continue this interest as a member of the Harvard Infantile Paralysis Commission. Indeed, during the decade from 1920 to 1930 he was almost the only American medical scientist besides Dr. Flexner who took it upon himself to blaze the trail in poliomyelitis, if that is at all an apt simile, because the trail led up some blind alleys during that comparatively unproductive period. He was nevertheless described by one of his biographers at the time of his death in 1951 as a man "who in the course of the past thirty-five years contributed more to our understanding of poliomyelitis than any living scientist."[1] Perhaps the reason Aycock was able to embark on this quest so vigorously was that he had acquired an early zeal for discovery in matters pertaining to poliomyelitis and also had the financial backing adequate to maintain a well-equipped laboratory. This enabled him and his small team to carry on experiments which required the purchase and care of monkeys, so necessary then and subsequently for any kind of experimental work in poliomyelitis.

Not that things were particularly easy for Aycock, but in the 1920s, as distinct from later years, when many more laboratories were able to engage in poliomyelitis research, he was able to work largely as a self-trained explorer in an uncrowded field with very little competition. He could make his way freely without the inevitable claims that his experimental work needed repeating or that he had been wrong in his observations and theories. He is also described by one who knew him well as being at his best among a group of students; "in informal seminar teaching or even every day conversation about a common interest. . . . They met a keen mind, adept at argument and repartee." In any event Aycock was to have wide and salutary influences on the direction of thought about poliomyelitis in this country in terms of its epidemiological and therapeutic aspects; yet eventually not in the way that he had hoped.

A native of Georgia, Lloyd Aycock obtained his medical degree at the University of Louisville in 1941. For a short time thereafter he became a

1. Obituary note; William Lloyd Aycock 1889–1951. *New Engl. J. Med., 246*: 158–59, 1952.

bacteriologist at the New York Post-Graduate Medical School in that city. It was here, during the large poliomyelitis epidemic of 1916 in New York, that Aycock first had his interest in this infection aroused. He was called into emergency service at the Westchester Isolation Hospital of New York, and here he also came in contact with leaders in the field of poliomyelitis research.

Within a year, however, with the outbreak of World War I, he entered the U.S. Army for a brief tour of duty as laboratory director at Base Hospital No. 8, at Savenay, near the port of St. Nazaire, France.[2]

After the war, Aycock became director of the privately endowed Poliomyelitis Research Laboratory of the Vermont State Board of Health. In 1923 he was put in charge of the Harvard Infantile Paralysis Commission but was also able to continue his collaborative association in field and laboratory investigations with the Vermont State Board of Health, a board which, owing to guidance by Dr. Caverly, had been interested in poliomyelitis for almost thirty years. Coincidentally Aycock was appointed associate professor (later professor) of preventive medicine and hygiene under Milton J. Rosenau at the Harvard Medical School.

One of Aycock's outstanding characteristics was a readiness to indulge in spirited argument in order to defend his theories. Woe to the opponent who was not quite certain of his ground or not very clever, because he was sure to be worsted. Unfortunately, throughout his professional career, and particularly toward the end of it, he suffered from a hip ailment which forced him to walk with a sturdy cane, but this disability in no way dampened his spirit. The illustration in figure 28 shows him in a characteristic posture, his right hand on the cane and looking as though he has just gotten the best of an argument.

During the 1920s and 1930s Aycock became an acknowledged authority on the epidemiology of poliomyelitis, and as such his views were in line with those expressed in the voluminous 175-page chapter on Epidemiology in the "Polio Bible" of 1932,[3] published under the editorship of W. H. Park.

But Aycock had other qualities besides those of an articulate debater. In the mid-1920s he had become interested in a somewhat unique aspect of the epidemiology of poliomyelitis, that of milk-borne epidemics. In this cause he had joined forces in 1926 with the New York State Health Department in its efforts to investigate an epidemic which had occurred in Courtland, New York. Among the conclusions he and his colleagues reached was that "the chain of circumstances is as complete as is found in the ma-

2. For a time, particularly in 1917, St. Nazaire was the chief port of disembarkation in France for the American Expeditionary Force.

3. "Epidemiology," chap. 7, in *Poliomyelitis*. International Committee for the Study of Infantile Paralysis, Baltimore, Williams & Wilkins, 1932, pp. 306–47, 452–57.

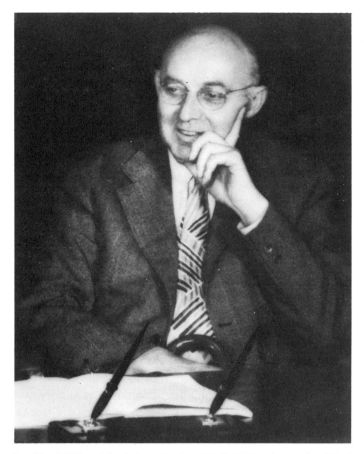

Fig 28. William Lloyd Aycock, M.D. (1889–1951). Picture furnished by the Dept. of Preventive Medicine, Harvard Medical School, kindness of Dr. David Rutstein.

jority of milk-borne outbreaks of other diseases." But the authors add cautiously: "While this outbreak points to transmission through milk, we are not of the opinion that this is the usual mode of spread of poliomyelitis."[4]

Within a very few months another opportunity presented itself to Aycock, this time in the form of an epidemic at Broadstairs, England, and he immediately set out to investigate this new and exciting lead.[5] Indeed it looked then that this manner of spread was going to turn out to be more important than had been previously suspected. The British epidemic totaled 71 cases and furnished evidence that strongly pointed to the milk furnished by one dealer as a common source of infection. The circumstances further suggested that contamination of only one grade of the deal-

4. A. C. Knapp, E. S. Godfrey, Jr., and W. L. Aycock: An outbreak of poliomyelitis, apparently milk-borne. *J. Amer. med. Ass., 87*: 635–39, 1926.

5. W. L. Aycock: Milk-borne epidemic of poliomyelitis. *Amer. J. Hyg., 7*: 791–803, 1927.

er's milk, which came from a single farm, was responsible. But in spite of this impressive support for the theory of milk-borne epidemics, Aycock abandoned this lead just as suddenly as he had taken it up. He even abandoned the point of view that environmental, as opposed to endogenous, influences[6] played a major or minor part in the way children acquired poliomyelitis. This change in direction marked an end for Aycock of community or house-to-house investigations, which he had begun so enthusiastically two or three years before. Nevertheless, it is to his credit that he pursued this type of detective work in epidemiology as far as he did. His word certainly was not the last one to be heard on the subject of poliomyelitis epidemics spread by milk.

In subsequent years, before the era of vaccination and particularly between 1925 and 1955, along with a variety of other ways in which this disease is transmitted, suspicion has fallen time and again upon contaminated milk as a source of poliovirus infection. Yet few have claimed that this has been definitely proved; fewer still believed it to be a *common* way that the virus is spread, and no one considered the situation comparable to the milk- or waterborne epidemics of typhoid fever or viral hepatitis. Nevertheless, in at least two of several explosive outbreaks reported in detail by A. B. Sabin in his record of poliomyelitis in the U.S. Army in World War II, milk was suspected as a possible or probable source of infection.[7] One of these outbreaks occurred in a U.S. naval receiving station at Portland, Oregon, during the fall of 1944.[8] In another, equally explosive one in 1946, at a U.S. naval flight preparatory school in San Luis Obispo, California, the evidence also pointed to transmission by milk; in a group of 730 officers and enlisted men, 17 cases of poliomyelitis occurred, 9 of them paralytic.[9]

It is my own belief that poliovirus has been in the past and still is capable of being transmitted through the agency of milk in some instances and

6. Endogenous: meaning influences arising within the body of the host.

7. A. B. Sabin: "Poliomyelitis," in *Preventive Medicine in World War II, Vol. 5, Communicable Diseases.* Medical Dept. U.S. Army, Gov. Printing Office, 1960, pp. 367–400.

8. The epidemic consisted of 11 paralytic cases which occurred in a total military population of 1,400. See D. M. Goldstein, W. M. Hammon, and H. R. Viets: An outbreak of polioencephalitis among navy cadets, possibly food borne. *J. Amer. med. Ass., 131*: 569–73, 1946; and F. P. Mathews: Poliomyelitis epidemic, possibly milk-borne, in a naval station, Portland, Oregon. *Amer. J. Hyg., 49*: 1–7, 1949.

9. Sixteen of the cases occurred between the 1st and 8th of September, 1946. Here again the explosive character of the epidemic indicated a common food-borne source of infection. Epidemiologic data pointed to milk contaminated by flies, but no conclusive evidence was available.

Also in the author's files are several unpublished reports of small epidemics which due to their explosive character and to the attendant circumstances could very well have been caused by milk contaminated with poliovirus.

some places; but outbreaks are less frequent in developed countries because the opportunity for milk to become contaminated has been greatly decreased since pasteurization has become more widespread and efficient. Moreover, the urgency, from a practical standpoint, of testing this theory has diminished almost to the vanishing point in countries with high levels of sanitary standards coupled with an increasing use of vaccination.[10]

But to return to Dr. Aycock, he had more strings to his bow than the study of milk-borne epidemics. From an altogether different point of view, he had begun to develop some novel theoretical ideas about the epidemiology of poliomyelitis, which curiously enough he never relinquished. He had become concerned, as Draper had before him, with questions as to how children gained their natural immunity against poliomyelitis, and he set about devising theories to explain this phenomenon. These theories represented a repudiation, or a compromise, with the long-established belief that inapparent specific infections, occurring in the summertime either sporadically or during epidemics, are responsible for the natural immunization of the great majority of children. But Aycock and his colleague Eaton claimed that the process of acquiring immunity involved not only multiple infections, which they believed were going on all the time during childhood, winter and summer, but there also was a normal growth phenomenon contributing to immunity as well.[11] By such means he claimed that a solid resistance was eventually built up through a mysterious process that merited the name of immunological maturity. Although Aycock considered infection with poliovirus to be prevalent all the year round, the great majority of overt cases only came to the surface during epidemic times, usually in the summer. His explanation of this was that the child who developed paralysis was one that had somehow failed to acquire immunologic maturity and was therefore unable to cope with the infection adequately.

At least the process of acquiring nonspecific resistance was vivid enough in Aycock's mind for him to give it to the descriptive term of *autarcesis,* from the Greek words ἀυτος, self, and 'αρκέω, keep off. It is said, and I believe it thoroughly, that Aycock himself was the only one who really knew how to pronounce this term correctly. Be that as it may, in his own words autarcesis was meant to imply that power to resist infection which lies within oneself, or at least operates without outside assistance, as dis-

10. As a postscript to this story, there have been many attempts in the laboratory to test the degrees of heat required to render milk safe when poliovirus has been artificially introduced into it. By and large, depending upon the concentration of poliovirus, pasteurization temperatures that will completely destroy the virus when diluted in water and milk will allow traces to survive, if the virus is diluted in cream.

11. W. L. Aycock and P. Eaton: The seasonal prevalance of infantile paralysis; seasonal variation in case fatality rate. *Amer. J. Hyg., 4*: 681–90, 1924.

tinguished from specific immunity, which is built up as a result of invasion of the body by the disease-producing agent.[12]

Essentially Aycock's autarcesis doctrine was at odds with the idea that
had been originally proposed by Wernstedt in 1912, to which Frost was
partial. Wernstedt believed that whenever and wherever poliovirus existed, even for a short time, and whenever and wherever susceptible children were exposed to it, they became infected and gained lasting immunity
from this experience. When the virus was not present, immunity was not
acquired. Aycock believed, on the other hand, that the mechanism was
not so simple as the Swedish scientist claimed, and that there was something more to the process which could only be explained by *immunological
maturity*. His theories underwent various alterations from time to time
and were elaborated upon by other investigators who maintained that the
imbalance of certain endocrine glands contributed to the susceptibility
or resistance of the child. Vitamin deficiency, it was said, might also contribute in a similar manner. This maturation theory occupied a respectable place among poliomyelitis workers for fully a decade or more.

It is certainly agreed that resistance may exist in some instances in the
absence of demonstrable specific poliovirus antibodies, and also that immunological immaturity has been demonstrated many times in the first few
days or even weeks of life when some mammals, including humans, have
not yet developed their full capacity to handle infections. But Aycock's
view that this transient inadequacy may continue after the age of one or
two years in man, up to and even through the years of puberty, has so far
not been proved. Certainly, high levels of poliovirus antibodies are consistently acquired in the second and third years of life and even much
earlier in some populations. But whether some ideas regarding hereditary
and "immunological maturity" as applied to poliomyelitis will be revived
again is a different matter. Indeed it is likely that this will happen, but
hardly in the terms that Aycock conceived of the process.

Aycock, who was fundamentally interested in the nature of poliomyelitis,
had hoped to give an entirely new slant to concepts of its immunity and
epidemiology. He was also concerned, as was natural, with doing something effective about prophylaxis. But the doctrine of autarcesis must have
presented difficulties for him. It was as if one were trying to prevent a disease which possessed a built-in (inherited) physiological mechanism of
susceptibility. Yet despite his belief that acquired immunity only represented part of the problem, he and his colleague Kagan did make a series
of attempts to immunize monkeys with various inactivated poliovirus an-

12. W. L. Aycock: A study of the significance of geographic and seasonal variations in the
incidence of poliomyelitis. *J. prev. Med., 3*: 245–78, 1929.

tigens.[13] Their efforts unfortunately met with no success, so this line of research was quickly abandoned for what was considered at the time a much more promising approach—that of treatment of the acute disease with convalescent serum. This will be reviewed in the next chapter.

Despite the fact that Aycock had devised his own pet theories about the disease, which he was more than anxious to defend, actually he was partially convinced of the correctness of Wernstedt's point of view. Indeed, I for one could never understand how he could have possibly deviated from it; he seemed to agree so completely with Wernstedt's interpretations in almost every detail. Certainly Aycock's experimental work on serological epidemiology tended to bear out the essential role of specific acquired immunity. His aberrant stand was a point about which we had numerous personal arguments—in which I invariably came off second best. Not that Wernstedt's facts were not solid enough, but simply because I suffered from inferior powers of argument in defending them against Aycock's convictions and eloquence.

And yet, paradoxically and remarkably enough, Aycock himself conducted a convincing series of experiments designed to prove that immunity to poliovirus was actually acquired through natural exposure and infection, usually at a subclinical level, i.e. through a process of subclinical immunization.[14] In a statement made in 1928, that immunization against infectious diseases was acquired subclinically, Aycock gave almost as clear an explanation of the manner in which poliomyelitis is both disseminated and controlled by a natural process of immunization as that made by Wernstedt. This makes it all the more puzzling that he should have taken up the cudgels in defense of his autarcesis theory. My explanation is that his problem had to do with the multiplicity of antigenic types of poliovirus, about which there was no knowledge when his theory was in the making.

The reason Aycock should have supported Wernstedt's theory is that he soon became (in 1930) a pioneer in experimental work on serological epidemiology. With his partner Kramer, he was among the first to use this method as an epidemiologic tool in poliomyelitis.[15] This approach involves the examination of sera from many individuals in different age groups for specific antibodies against poliovirus (or other agents) in order to deter-

13. W. L. Aycock and J. R. Kagan: Experimental immunization in poliomyelitis. *J. Immunol., 14*: 85, 1927.

14. W. L. Aycock: The significance of the age distribution of poliomyelitis; evidence of transmission through contact. *Amer. J. Hyg., 8*: 35–54, 1928.

15. W. L. Aycock and S. D. Kramer: Immunity to poliomyelitis in normal individuals in urban and rural communities as indicated by the neutralization test. *J. prev. Med., 4*: 189–200, 1930.

mine whether the infection had ever been present in the particular population and, if so, how prevalent it had been. This is possible only when such antibodies persist in the individual's serum for life, as is the case with poliovirus-neutralizing antibodies. Under such circumstances they constitute "footprints" of past experience, indicating that certain infections have passed that way. Although antibodies and immunity are clearly not synonymous, particularly as demonstrated by the crude tests used in Aycock's day, still it does follow that the presence of type-specific neutralizing antibody in a given individual's serum correlates well with immunity to poliovirus infection due to that particular type.

Aycock and Kramer employed the cumbersome, tricky, and expensive method of performing neutralization tests in monkeys. This was the only technique available to them to demonstrate man's immunity to poliomyelitis. The tests were crude for several reasons; among them, that the actual presence of antibody rested on interpretations based on a sliding scale, in which it was the contemporary fashion to consider the category of "partial immunity." Furthermore, in the 1920s, investigators had no conception of the different antigenic types of polioviruses. This inevitably resulted in confusion amounting almost to disaster. But since theirs was one of the first serum surveys, these pioneers can certainly be excused for a few errors in technique and in principle.

Using this method, Aycock and Kramer set out to search for reasons that would explain differences in the ages at which rural versus urban individuals acquired poliovirus antibodies within the same general geographical area, i.e. Massachusetts and Vermont. It was not a simple experiment, and that they succeeded in it as well as they did was a stroke of luck. The results, transcribed from their paper, are shown in Table 4.

The data suffer from lack of adequate numbers in each age group; the samples were so small that by today's standards the results would not seem particularly significant. But by and large the trend is for a higher percentage of antibody-positive persons to appear in the urban population as compared to its rural counterpart, particularly in the younger age groups. These differences are what might have been expected. Aycock and Kramer rightfully interpreted them as proof that the juvenile immunity patterns in the two types of population depended upon differences in their relative exposures to poliovirus. Such exposure they considered to be heavier at a relatively early age in urban environments than in rural areas. It might have seemed a body blow to the autarcesis theory. In the light of present-day findings obtained by the use of more sophisticated methods, one would have expected that, with increasing age, immunity levels in the two adult groups (urban and rural) might have approximated one another.

Aycock and Kramer went further in their interpretations and compared

TABLE 4. Neutralization tests for "immunity" to poliomyelitis in sera
from urban and rural individuals: by age groups

Age Groups	Urban No.	Rural No.	Urban Percent Immune	Rural Percent Immune
Adult	8	5	87.5	40.0
15–19	7	4	85.7	50.0
10–14	9	8	66.7	25.0
5–9	10	8	80.0	0.0
0–4	12	4	41.7	0.0
Total	46	29	69.6	20.7

Data transcribed from W. L. Aycock and D. Kramer (see n. 15).

these two curves (urban and rural) with results of Schick tests for immunity to diphtheria (see fig. 29).[16] From this comparison they concluded that, in view of the parallelism of both series of tests, the manner in which man naturally acquired immunity to the two diseases must be the same. After giving one exception, they said (see n. 15):

> We have the same grounds in poliomyelitis as in diphtheria for maintaining that immunity is the result of exposure to the causal agent, and we may consider that immunity to poliomyelitis as shown by the neutralization test is due to previous exposure to the poliomyelitis virus and not to autarcesis.

This use of serological epidemiological methods to demonstrate the manner in which a population achieves its immunity to a given infection was in later years to be further perfected and to become almost a routine procedure. In time, it contributed mightily to the control of poliomyelitis. The authors' tenacity in clinging to autarcesis in spite of their seemingly convincing evidence to the contrary is astounding.

Aycock and Kramer's investigations marked the beginning of measurements of age-specific susceptibility to the disease in areas where the immune status of the population was unknown. It is doubtful whether they realized at the time what a crucial experiment they had performed or how fundamental their results were to prove. But Aycock himself realized it later, and in 1949, after a lapse of almost twenty years, in a small book for

16. A skin test known as the Schick test is used as a means of determining whether an individual possesses immunity to diphtheria. The test, named for Bela Schick, an Austro-American pediatrician who attained great respect and popularity in this country, has the advantage of simplicity, whereas the poliovirus neutralization test was quite complicated in Aycock's time.

which he himself set the type, which he printed and bound by hand,[17] he indicated his belief that this comparison between immunity to diphtheria and to poliomyelitis was sufficiently important—as indeed it was—to deserve a key place among his lifelong contributions to epidemiology. As such the chart illustrative of this concept occupies the frontispiece of his little book (see fig. 29).

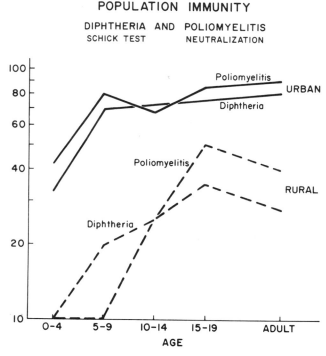

FIG. 29. This chart originally appeared in 1930 in an article by Aycock and Kramer (see n. 15). Almost twenty years later Aycock reproduced it in a small privately printed book (see n. 17) as one of his special achievements in epidemiology. It has been redrawn for purposes of reproduction.

Aycock and Kramer carried out further serum surveys in 1930 before going on to various other kinds of investigation. In one they measured the antibody status of 21 adults from Atlanta, Georgia, as contrasted to the findings in sera of adults from Massachusetts and Vermont. Results in the northern population, they conceded, confirmed the Wernstedt theory of widespread naturally acquired specific immunization; but, the authors added that this type of immunity was not to be confused with nonspecific (autarcesis) immunity. Somewhat to their surprise Aycock and Kramer found that the sera of practically all (90.5 percent) of the 21 adults from

17. W. L. Aycock: *A Sketch of Epidemiology.* Privately printed, 1949.

Atlanta also contained poliovirus-neutralizing antibodies. This level was even higher than the 83.3 percent exhibited by the northern population, and this in spite of the fact that overt poliomyelitis cases were far more uncommon in the deep South. Indeed there had not been an epidemic in Georgia in recent years, and all of the individuals tested denied ever having had an illness resembling poliomyelitis. "These tests," Aycock and Kramer said, "indicate that immunity to poliomyelitis is equally extensive in warmer and cooler climates, and therefore suggest that the extent of the distribution of virus is equal to that in cooler climates."[18] Why did these impressive results not turn Aycock from preoccupation with his favorite autarcesis theory? It is an example of having one's theories at odds with one's experimental results and yet trying doggedly to reconcile the two.

With all this burgeoning enthusiasm for the neutralization test in the 1930s it would be logical to expect that more and more serologic surveys would have been attempted, and that serological epidemiology should promptly have gone on to the bright future that was in store for it. Yet such was not the case, and this approach shortly fell into a decline. The reasons were complex (see chap. 34). A major one was that the multiplicity of poliovirus types was unknown at the time; the test as performed in monkeys was expensive, relatively imprecise, and limited by statistical inadequacies. Not until the 1940s, when many of these difficulties had been overcome and murine-adapted poliovirus of the Lansing type made available for use in the test, was interest in serologic epidemiology revived and put on a sound basis.

In the meantime, Aycock already was busy with other investigations. With his colleague Luther he set out to evaluate the effectiveness of convalescent serum therapy in poliomyelitis. This we shall hear much about in a subsequent chapter. In addition, however, in 1929 the team of Aycock and Luther was to make another highly important and discerning discovery. They were among the first to observe that severe cases of poliomyelitis were apt to follow recent tonsillectomy.[19] They reported 36 patients whose tonsils had been removed within a year before onset of the disease. Of these, 16 developed the acute disease within 7 to 18 days after the operation. The frequency with which this occurred suggested that poliomyelitis was in some way associated with recent tonsillectomy.

This same clinical observation had been made thirteen years earlier by a nose-and-throat surgeon, who, as a specialist in this field and therefore too close to it, might have seemed an unlikely candidate to suspect any such correlation. But in 1916, during the year of the great epidemic in

18. W. L. Aycock and S. D. Kramer: Immunity to poliomyelitis in a southern population as shown by the neutralization test. *J. prev. Med., 4*: 201–06, 1930.

19. W. L. Aycock and E. H. Luther: The occurence of poliomyelitis following tonsillectomy. *New Engl. J. Med., 200*: 164, 1929.

New York City, Dr. Max Talmey, a surgeon at the Harlem Eye, Ear, and Throat Infirmary, had stated his belief that tonsillectomy acted as a predisposing factor in infantile paralysis. Writing in 1916, he said:

> The campaign to exterminate the tonsils, started ten or twelve years ago, has been carried on relentlessly ever since, and has succeeded in making the well meaning general practitioner and even the lay public dread a piece of tonsillar tissue left back between the palatine arches after operation, as much as the cobra's venom.
>
> There are two ways in which predisposition to poliomyelitis may develop from tonsillectomy, one of considerable and another of utmost importance. The first is the trauma, psychical and physical, caused by the operation. . . .
>
> The second way for the predisposition to develop from tonsillectomy, which I have stated to be of the utmost importance, is the elimination from the system of a valuable protective substance the nature of which is yet unknown.[20]

Dr. Talmey was anxious to see whether his view on tonsillectomy and poliomyelitis was correct and suggested that a questionnaire be sent to every physician attending a case of infantile paralysis—to investigate this point and see whether the theory could be proved statistically. He concluded with the statement:

> It is possible that statistical as well as experimental data may prove my views on tonsillectomy to be entirely fallacious and even the operation to be beneficial. . . .
>
> I will brave the storm of criticism that may break out over this article with the quotation from Horace:
>
> *si fractus illabatur orbis*
> *impavidum ferient ruinae.*[21]

Talmey's astute observations were apparently lost sight of, and the relation between tonsillectomy and poliomyelitis was not rediscovered again until Aycock and Luther's paper was published in 1929. Aycock again reviewed the subject in 1942,[22] stating that the preponderance of posttonsillectomy cases were of the most serious variety, the bulbar form.

20. M. Talmey: Reflections on predisposing factors in infantile paralysis. *N.Y. med. J., 104:* 202, 1916.

I am indebted to Dr. Aaron Lerner, professor of dermatology, Yale University School of Medicine, for having brought this reference to my attention.

21. *Odes* of Horace. Book III, No. 3, lines 7 and 8. "Were the vault of heaven to break and fall upon him, Its ruins would smite him undismayed." C. E. Bennett, trans. Horace, *Odes,* 337–8.

22. W. L. Aycock: Tonsillectomy and poliomyelitis; epidemiologic considerations. *Medicine, 21:* 65, 1942.

In recent years, in spite of vigorous denials made in the 1940s by some laryngologists, the evidence that recent tonsillectomy does prepare the ground for severe infection with poliovirus has been borne out many times. Confirmatory epidemiological observations were subsequently made by Thomas Francis and his team at the University of Michigan and by Gaylord Anderson at the University of Minnesota. Experimentally, Sabin was the first to show, in 1938, that rhesus monkeys, when inoculated with poliovirus in the tonsillopharyngeal region, developed poliomyelitis with greater frequency than when inoculated by other routes. Ten years later, von Magnus and Melnick demonstrated that the susceptibility of cynomolgus monkeys became greatly enhanced in animals which had had their tonsils recently removed. But to Aycock belongs the credit for having forcibly drawn the attention of the medical profession to this relationship; he also made the suggestion that the menace could be controlled, partially at least, by avoiding the performance of tonsillectomies during the poliomyelitis season.

Dr. Talmey, too, deserves a place in this story for he was the first to recognize tonsillectomy as a precipitating factor in poliomyelitis. The fate of his proposed campaign to prove his point statistically is unknown; very likely it got nowhere, but the echoes of his courageous voice could still be heard crying out at the height of the senseless stampede to "exterminate the tonsils" in all children, healthy or unhealthy. Today that stampede has mercifully declined to a more reasonable and rational pace.

As a final and significant postscript to Aycock's continued vigorous defense of his position on the importance of physiological imbalances as one basis of susceptibility in poliomyelitis, he was among the first to note an increase in the incidence of poliomyelitis in pregnant women. This he maintained, correctly it would seem, may depend on hormonal influences, and on this note his autarcesis theory at last came to rest.

CHAPTER 19

Convalescent Serum Therapy

Comparable to the manner in which almost the entire interest in polio-myelitis was to be directed toward the subject of vaccination in the early 1950s, interest in the 1920s settled upon the therapeutic use of convalescent serum. Although this type of treatment had represented the culmination of a year or more of effort when it was launched, it was felt that neither the right technique nor the right answer had been achieved—yet that it would somehow all come out correctly in due time. At first the idea of overall planning in the design of trials of serum therapy seems to have been thrown to the winds. Instead, there were frantic efforts to establish through ill-conceived field trials that convalescent serum was a satisfactory treat-ment for the acute disease. It was a matter of such desperation that the sub-ject was to dwarf all other considerations about poliomyelitis for a long time.

Primarily, convalescent serum therapy had been recommended in 1915, by Netter in France.[1] It was hailed at first as a discovery of the first magni-tude, for which the genius of France was responsible. Netter was of the opinion that the series of 30 cases which he had treated after onset of paral-ysis had subsequently recovered with a speed and completeness that did not occur in patients who had not received serum. Doubters, including Draper, claimed it was controversial whether Netter's case reports really bore out this contention, since his interpretations had been based largely on clinical impressions.

Nevertheless, when the 1916 New York epidemic came along a year later, Netter's treatment was taken up promptly by physicians in this coun-try. The use of serum became a new and popular approach, especially in-asmuch as Flexner and his associates at the Rockefeller Institute had re-cently been successful in treating meningococcal meningitis by a similar method. Besides, there was added support from the experiments of Flexner and Lewis, Levaditi and Netter, and others which indicated that the serum of monkeys recently recovered from paralytic poliomyelitis (as well as human convalescent serum) possessed virucidal properties against polio-virus. Flexner and Lewis had also demonstrated that injections of serum

1. A. Netter: La Sérothérapie de la poliomyélite; nos résultats chez 30 malades; indications, techniques; incidents possibles. *Gaz. méd. Paris, 86*: 88, 1915.

from recovered animals would sometimes prevent paralysis in monkeys which were then inoculated with virulent poliovirus.[2]

The first of several therapeutic trials in humans to be reported in the United States came in 1916. This was a series of 21 cases treated by Schwarz,[3] who concluded that not too much could be expected from this form of therapy. It would have been wiser if the whole business could have been dropped at this point, but that was obviously impossible, for far more extensive trials were under way that same year, including one by the New York City Health Department under the direction of W. H. Park.[4] Acting according to Netter's evidence, serum was collected from patients recently convalescent from poliomyelitis at New York City's Willard Parker Hospital and in some instances from patients at other hospitals. The trials were started with the laudable premise that

> it is only by comparing a large group of early cases treated with immune serum, with normal serum, and no serum at all that we shall be able to arrive at any certain data as to the efficiency of the serum treatment.[5]

In attempting to follow these principles, however, the investigators fell down badly. The New York City trial was doomed to failure almost from the start because of the lack of uniformity and a failure to adhere to approved plans, not only at the various hospitals but particularly by some private physicians. Also, by the time the trial had progressed very far it had shrunk to a comparison of two groups, not three, and these were of unequal size (119 versus 43). In any event a comparison between the two would have been meaningless. It was a situation to be repeated over and over again.

In those early days the techniques of administration of serum were cumbersome and time-consuming. The recommended method was to inoculate it intrathecally in a manner similar to that employed in the treatment of meningococcal meningitis.[6] The dose, while not specified as to amount, was supposed to be repeated every 20–24 hours until two or three had been given. Also, a major problem was the decision as to which patients were to be treated. Here the crucial point was the detection of a "positive"

2. S. Flexner and P. A. Lewis: Experimental poliomyelitis in monkeys; active immunization and passive protection. *J. Amer. med. Ass., 54*: 1780, 1910; and further contributions to the subjects of immunization and serum therapy. *J. Amer. med. Ass., 55*: 662, 1910.

3. H. Schwarz: The treatment of poliomyelitis, prophylactic and curative. *Arch. Pediat., 33*: 859, 1916.

4. W. W. Oliver: *The Man Who Lived for Tomorrow; A Biography of William Halleck Park, M.D.* New York, E. P. Dutton, 1941, pp. 356–57.

5. *The Epidemic of Poliomyelitis (Infantile Paralysis) in New York City in 1916.* New York City Department of Health, 1917, p. 265.

6. *Intrathecally:* meaning an injection into the spinal canal.

spinal fluid. This was considered requisite for the initiation of serum treatment. It made it difficult to assemble a group of untreated controls, for any physician who performed a lumbar puncture and found the characteristic spinal fluid changes was more than likely to use the serum and equally likely to incur the wrath of the patient's parents if he withheld it.

Draper had not yet clearly enunciated his concept of the biphasic nature of the acute disease at this time but nevertheless he was correct in his opinion that only in the first phase of illness is the spinal fluid still normal; and, as a result his practice was to withhold serum at this stage, pending a decision as to whether the child did indeed have poliomyelitis or was in the acute phase of some other illness. This turned on an important point. Patients in the New York City series, as others treated at this time, were for the most part in the second phase (the major illness phase) of their disease, for positive spinal fluid findings indicated that the virus had already penetrated the central nervous system and probably produced lesions there. Interpretations of the effect of any therapy should take into account that although a far higher percentage of patients with negative spinal fluid findings (presumably an indication of the minor illness) recover uneventfully, a smaller but appreciable proportion of those with central nervous system involvement (the major illness) also recover spontaneously without residual paralysis; in many of the latter, muscle weakness is extremely transient, or absent altogether.

In the face of these complexities in the clinical course of the disease and in view of the way the clinical trial of the New York City Health Department was carried out, with all its woeful inadequacies, it is surprising that the investigators were able to arrive at any conclusions at all. What came out was the observation, clearly not a discovery, that cases treated early in the acute disease had a better chance of recovery than the more serious and advanced cases treated later. This did not mean that the treatment had anything to do with the outcome, but it seemed enough to warrant the following statement:

> While no absolute judgment of the value of a serum can be based as yet upon the results obtained, they are, nevertheless, encouraging and justify a continuation of the serum treatment in acute poliomyelitis until in the course of time, more definite data be available.[7]

The failure of these efforts stemmed from a lack of appreciation of the necessity for carefully matched treated and control groups in the evaluation of serum or any other form of therapy. It was a pity that the plan of this crude experiment set the fashion for similar subsequent trials. The 1916 New York City trial had reflected a point of view then almost uni-

7. See n. 5, p. 279.

versal among physicians—that it was not mandatory that strict rules be applied for the testing of any particular form of new treatment. Such rules were *required* in subsequent years if a trial was to be published. But in 1916 the physician made his own rules. He naturally had the welfare of his patients at heart, and particularly in the early years of the twentieth century he found it difficult, almost immoral, to withhold serum therapy in order to assemble a suitable control group. He also could not help but give himself every benefit of the doubt, aided by a certain amount of wishfulness when it came to seeing improvement as a result of this new and "promising" treatment in which both he and his patient's family had faith. But inevitably this kind of judgment meant the postponement of an accurate decision on the real value of such treatment. It caused a delay which dragged on for years and years.

The data from the New York City Health Department was further analyzed in 1917 by Zingher, whose interpretations differed slightly from those given in Dr. Haven Emerson's official report. Zingher expressed a somewhat more favorable point of view, although it was a toss-up as to how one was to deal with the results. It seemed to him, however, "that the action of serum in poliomyelitis is beneficial . . . and is indicated in the treatment of the acute stages especially in the preparalytic period of the disease."[8]

In Boston, Francis Peabody also treated a series of 51 cases during the 1916 epidemic, employing the same diagnostic criteria used in New York —that the spinal fluid should be "positive" before the serum was given. He gave only one intrathecal injection. However, his interpretations were much more guarded than those of Zingher. Peabody's trial was of necessity an emergency measure and had scanty planning, as had the others. But at least he recognized its inadequacies. He was accordingly cautious about the significance of his results. Had his wisdom prevailed, the obscurities might have ended sooner.

> For the proper interpretation of the results of treatment it is essential that we should have a much more complete knowledge of the natural history of the disease. At the present time we have only an imperfect idea as to what proportion of persons affected with the disease became paralyzed even if no treatment is instituted. Nevertheless there is apparently general agreement among those who have used immune serum as to its harmlessness, and as to the fact that in certain, possibly in numerous instances its administration is beneficial.[9]

8. A. Zingher: The diagnosis and serum treatment of anterior poliomyelitis. *J. Amer. med. Ass., 68*: 817–23, 1917.

9. F. W. Peabody: A report of the Harvard Infantile Paralysis Commission on the diagnosis and treatment of acute cases of the disease during the year 1916. *Boston med. surg. J., 176*: 637–42, 1917.

Only one of the other therapeutic trials performed in this epidemic year deserves mention. This was carried out by Amoss and Chesney,[10] and it did not have the disadvantages of having quite such hasty planning as the others. Nevertheless it also suffered from a similar lack of an adequate control group.

Harold Amoss had already become Dr. Flexner's right-hand man. He and Alan Chesney, who eventually became the dean of the Johns Hopkins Medical School, were members of the staff of the Rockefeller Institute

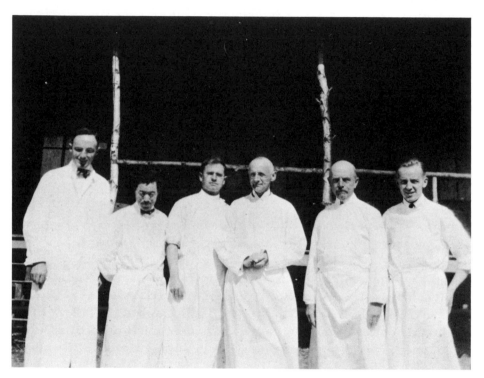

Fig. 30. Picture taken at the Westchester County Hospital, summer 1916. Left to right: Drs. W. L. Aycock, H. Noguchi, H. L. Amoss, S. Flexner, Hubbard, A. M. Chesney. Permission to reproduce this photograph was kindly given by Dr. Thomas H. Weller of the Harvard School of Public Health.

and its hospital respectively, in 1916–17. Most of the actual work on the serum therapy project, however, was conducted at the Westchester County Isolation Hospital, where Aycock also had been a participant. A picture of the group that supervised this project appears in figure 30. All of the 26 patients in the series who underwent treatment with immune serum were bona fide cases of poliomyelitis, verified according to the criterion of show-

10. H. L. Amoss and A. M. Chesney: A report on the serum treatment of twenty-six cases of epidemic poliomyelitis. *J. exp. Med., 25*: 581–608, 1917.

ing characteristic spinal fluid abnormalities. The investigators made one important innovation by deviating from the practice of introducing the serum only into the spinal canal; in 3 of their patients it was also administered intravenously, and in 25 it was given intrathecally and subcutaneously. This was done for the ostensible purpose of increasing the quantity of serum which could be safely given to a child. Apparently a second or a third dose, as used in the New York City health department study, was not considered necessary.

Amoss and Chesney were ultracautious in expressing a favorable opinion of the efficacy of serum therapy. They too emphasized the familiar point that best results were obtained when the patient was treated within 48 hours of the onset of symptoms, the earlier the better. But they also suggested that good results might be expected when more than 30 cc of serum was given and concluded that serum obtained from recently recovered cases of poliomyelitis was probably the most effective.

When Draper had had sufficient time to consider these results he inserted a chapter on serum therapy in the first edition of his book (1917), in which he drew heavily on Amoss and Chesney's data. Here, he was not so hesitant as he had formerly been about advocating the use of serum treatment. Indeed he maintained that in the organization of a campaign to combat epidemic poliomyelitis there should be a "sufficient number of doctors with clinical and laboratory experience working from a central office or laboratory, to go on call ready to do lumbar punctures and give serum."[11] Each man was to carry a microscope and the necessary laboratory equipment for examining the cerebrospinal fluid. This elaborate scheme must have been hard to implement and is one which has seldom been used.

Draper had considerably more knowledge than others of the natural history of the disease, and he understood the difficult diagnostic decisions that had to be faced; he was aware that many cases of poliomyelitis came to a favorable end with no paralysis. In his own series he had assembled a group of 32 untreated control patients for comparison with 45 who had received serum treatment. Yet he rightly maintained that there were too many variables involved to make a valid comparison possible. Actually, in his two groups the untreated ended up with a 28 percent paralytic rate whereas the treated fared considerably worse—51 percent developed paralysis! Nevertheless he stated with conviction that best results were obtained when the cases were treated in the preparalytic stage or in the intermission between the two phases (see fig. 26).

All these early trials of serum therapy were carried out some thirty years before Sir George Pickering, subsequently Regius Professor of Medicine at Oxford, outlined the strict scientific premise on which he felt that clini-

11. G. Draper: *Acute Poliomyelitis.* Philadelphia, P. Blakiston's, 1917, pp. 87–88.

cal therapeutic trials should be based. In his 1949 presidential address before the Section of Experimental Medicine and Therapeutics of the Royal
Society of Medicine, he said:

> Therapeutics is the branch of medicine that, by its very nature, should
> be experimental. For if we take a patient affected with a malady, and
> we alter his conditions of life, either by dieting him, or by putting him
> to bed, or by administering to him a drug, or by performing an opera-
> tion, we are performing an experiment. And if we are scientifically
> minded we should record the results. Before concluding that the
> change for better or for worse in the patient is due to the specific treat-
> ment employed, we must ascertain whether the result can be repeated
> a significant number of times in similar patients, whether the result
> was merely due to the natural history of the disease or in other words
> to the lapse of time, or whether it was due to some other factor which
> was necessarily associated with the therapeutic measure in question. . . .
> This would seem the procedure to be expected of men with six years
> of scientific training behind them. But it has not been followed. Had
> it been done we should have gained a fairly precise knowledge of the
> place of individual methods of therapy in disease, and our efficiency
> as doctors would have been enormously enhanced.[12]

Needless to say no one was aware of this judgment in 1916 or in the early
1920s. Indeed the failure to observe any rules of this kind prolonged the
search for an answer to the question of whether or not convalescent serum
therapy for poliomyelitis was effective until the early 1930s. By this time,
although more attention was beginning to be paid to the design of adequately controlled trials, results were unnecessarily obscure. They were
hampered by the fact that just that type of scientific discipline described
by Pickering was lacking. It was equally unfortunate that during the period 1928–33 the major energies of most poliomyelitis laboratories in the
United States were expended on this confusing issue instead of on one
of the more critical questions.

In the summer of 1927 Aycock and Luther published results on the
most carefully controlled study yet undertaken.[13] They had treated 106
patients who already had spinal fluid changes, but had not yet developed
any muscle weakness. Some 482 similar patients from whom serum had
been withheld served as controls. Serum was given intrathecally and intravenously. The outcome in treated and control groups was measured by an
elaborate scoring system to determine the degree of paralysis in a quantitative manner not attempted in earlier studies. They found that 19 per-

---

12. Quoted by A. Bradford Hill, in *Principles of Medical Statistics,* 7th ed. New York,
Oxford University Press, 1961, p. 243.
13. W. L. Aycock and E. H. Luther: Preparalytic poliomyelitis; observations in one hundred
and six cases in which convalescent serum was used. *J. Amer. med. Ass., 91*: 387–93, 1928.

cent of the patients who had received serum developed significant paralysis as compared with 63 percent in the untreated controls. It was a good study for its time, but it prolonged the agony and even set the stage for another five years of trials.

After a decade or more of observation from the sidelines, Flexner, no doubt encouraged by Aycock and Luther's results, cautiously entered the arena and threw his personal weight in favor of the administration of serum not only prophylactically but also therapeutically. In the paper by Flexner and Stewart delivered before the Association of American Physicians in 1928 they leaned heavily on their experimental work with monkeys but in speaking of clinical cases in man, concluded: "It would seem advisable, theoretically at least, that one intraspinal injection of the convalescent should be given at the earliest practicable moment."[14]

By his stand, Flexner in effect said that at last the Rockefeller Institute, almost the highest scientific authority in the nation, was giving the nod to practicing doctors to use serum therapy. Such scientific backing was a boon to the physician who had not yet made up his mind on the subject. At least, Flexner's views were a great help to Aycock, who warmly welcomed his support.[15]

Support also came from investigators in such widely separated parts of the world as Canada and Australia, where Dr. Jean Macnamara (later Dame Macnamara), of whom we shall be hearing more later, carried on an ardent campaign.

In the midst of these not too convincing opinions about the value of human convalescent serum, treatment with serum from horses (or other large animals) that had been hyperimmunized was also taken up. This followed the example of hyperimmune horse serum therapy then being used successfully for meningococcal meningitis and lobar pneumonia. Early in the history of experimental poliomyelitis (1910) Flexner had attempted unsuccessfully to produce high-titered neutralizing serum in horses. Others had also failed, but Pettit, at the Pasteur Institute in Paris, reported that his efforts, initiated in 1917–18 during the trying period of World War I, had been crowned with some success.[16] Twelve years later investigators in W. H. Park's New York City Health Department Laboratory, taking a leaf from Pettit's book, were able to make a presumably potent antipoliomyelitic horse serum[17] that was tried out extensively on patients during the 1931 epidemic in New York City, but to no avail.

To sum it all up, in 1930 hopes for serum therapy still ran high. Con-

14. S. Flexner and F. W. Stewart: Specific prevention and treatment of epidemic poliomyelitis. *Trans. Ass. Amer. Phycns, 43*: 252–57, 1928.

15. Ibid., page 257.

16. A Pettit: Sur la préparation d'un sérum neutralisant le virus de la poliomyélite. *C. R. Soc. Biol. (Paris), 81*: 1087, 1918.

17. E. R. Weyer, W. H. Park, and E. J. Banzhaf: A potent antipoliomyelitic horse serum concentrate and its experimental use in infected monkeys. *J. exp. Med., 53*: 553, 1931.

valescent serum and, to a lesser extent, horse serum continued to be used for another five years, chiefly because it seemed to be the only therapy available. But by late 1931 a reaction set in. Some leading figures had begun to express grave doubts about the value of serum therapy in poliomyelitis. The first major upset came from a group that had hitherto supported this form of treatment, the Harvard Infantile Paralysis Commission. In trials conducted during the 1931 outbreak in the northeastern United States, Aycock's team[18] reported that results of a well-controlled trial provided no statistical evidence that convalescent serum was of any value; nor could the reverse conclusion be drawn. It must have required some courage for Aycock, a former enthusiastic supporter of serum therapy, to reverse himself and to repudiate earlier claims by many authorities, himself included. Similar conclusions were reached the same year by other eminent investigators, viz. Park and his associates, who conducted trials in New York and Connecticut. They reported that both horse serum and convalescent human serum had yielded discouraging results; the following year reports from Germany followed suit. In 1933 an outstanding authority on infectious diseases from Harvard Medical School's clinical faculty, Dr. C. Wesselhoeft, joined the chorus, in stating:

> There is no positive proof from this compilation of statistics or from controlled clinical experiments that such sera (convalescent, or normal adult) are efficacious. . . .[19]

The demise of serum therapy after so many years of crude trials in which claims of its value had been made by so many physicians, a number of whom were acknowledged authorities and occupied high places in the medical hierarchy, must have been a bitter pill for the medical profession to swallow—if such a metaphor is at all appropriate. It was like so many forms of treatment that had been all the rage in one generation but dropped out of fashion in the next. After 1935, the less said by the medical profession about their past enthusiasms for serum, the better. And yet serum treatment in poliomyelitis was not to die a sudden death; it was used on quite a large scale in the Los Angeles epidemic of 1934. After that it fell into oblivion in the United States. Almost its last supporter was its originator, Netter of France, who wrote his final paper in favor of serum therapy in 1937.

So after two decades of hopeful efforts this form of treatment was finally recognized as ineffective. One thing that could be said of it was that apparently it did little harm to the patient. Subsequently, in the 1940s, when the

18. S. D. Kramer, W. L. Aycock, C. I. Solomon, and C. L. Thenebe: Convalescent serum therapy in preparalytic poliomyelitis. *New Engl. J. Med., 206:* 432, 1932.

19. C. Wesselhoeft: The present status of serum treatment in acute poliomyelitis. *J. Pediat., 3:* 330, 1933.

antibody-containing gamma globulin fraction of serum had been concentrated and separated out, the quantitative inadequacy of even administering 20 or 30 ml of unconcentrated convalescent serum became more apparent. Furthermore, an important observation was made at this time by Hammon and Roberts,[20] that by the time the patient is admitted to the hospital with signs of central nervous system involvement, he is apt to have already produced his own antibodies to the infecting virus. The amount of antibody added by the administration of convalescent serum, viewed in this light, was very insignificant. But such information was available neither in 1916 nor in the fifteen years thereafter, during which investigators and clinicians struggled to find in serum some help in dealing with the desperate problem of treating paralytic poliomyelitis. To justify this action the claim rightfully was maintained that antibodies might not be the only substances in serum that were beneficial, but other unknown essentials as well might contribute to the patient's recovery.

As a matter of fact the principle on which the use of convalescent serum was based both as a therapeutic and a prophylactic measure was fundamentally correct. Failure came partially as a result of the homeopathic doses that were used, most of them too late in the infection to do any good. In defense of Dr. Flexner's prediction of its use for prophylaxis, this was tried in 1932, and it came decidedly into its own shortly after World War II when gamma globulin (concentrated immune globulin) was introduced. This provided a vindication of earlier views when, in the early 1950s, Dr. W. McD. Hammon and his colleagues showed that the large-scale administration of this vastly superior product in appropriate doses was of some benefit in reducing cases in an epidemic. These events will be described more fully in chapter 36. But from 1916 until the early 1930s the application of a method of treatment which was sound in principle went wrong because its enthusiastic implementers were to all intents and purposes amateurs when it came to proving their point. In retrospect of such efforts, Sir George Pickering proved to be the real professional.

20. W. McD. Hammon and E. C. Roberts: Serum neutralizing antibodies to the infecting strain of virus in poliomyelitis patients. *Proc. Soc. exp. Biol. Med. (N.Y.), 69*: 256–58, 1948.

CHAPTER 20

Investigations in Clinical Virology, 1931

During ten years preceding 1931 hardly a single case of poliomyelitis had been seen on the adult medical service of the New Haven Hospital, but at midnight on June 15, 1931, a girl of seventeen was admitted with complaints of fever, drowsiness, pain in the back, and generalized weakness. The interns were puzzled about the diagnosis. It was considered too early in the season for polio, and besides, cases in adolescents even at that time were uncommon. On ward rounds the next morning, I, as the attending physician, was also uncertain as to the diagnosis until the patient volunteered this bit of information: "I don't seem to be able to move my legs at all." It was the first case of poliomyelitis ever to be entrusted to my care. But other cases came thick and fast, and in a few days we realized that we had an epidemic on our hands.

The 1931 epidemic in the northeastern part of the United States was almost but not quite so severe as the one of 1916. In Connecticut the case rates ran a pretty close parallel in those two epidemic years. In the city of New Haven there were 149 cases in 1931 as against 95 in 1916, even though the population had increased only from 150,000 to 162,000. The epidemic certainly kept the hospital busy throughout the summer. It also prompted the formation of a new poliomyelitis research organization in the United States, one which persists to this day. This was known as the Yale Poliomyelitis Commission (later, the Yale Poliomyelitis Study Unit), and its first director was Dr. James D. Trask.[1]

A word is in order about this remarkable man—James D. Trask (see fig. 31). He was born in Astoria, New York in 1890, the son of a physician. He attended Lawrenceville School and the Yale Sheffield Scientific School, where he barely squeaked through, and Cornell University Medical College, where he did better and received his M.D. degree in 1917. After serving on abbreviated wartime internship at Bellevue Hospital in New York City, he joined the Medical Corps of the U.S. Army in the closing months of World War I. Most of his time in military service was spent in per-

---

1. In 1931 the original members of the Yale Poliomyelitis Commission consisted of the following: from the pediatric staff, James D. Trask, director, Robert Salinger, and Paul Harper; from the internal medicine staff, John R. Paul and one fourth year medical student, Mr. Jack Leonard.

forming physical examinations to determine the cardiac status of thousands of army recruits at Camp Wadsworth in Spartanburg, South Carolina.

But whether due to his army tour of duty or not, by the time his military service was over in 1919, he had had enough of performing physical ex-

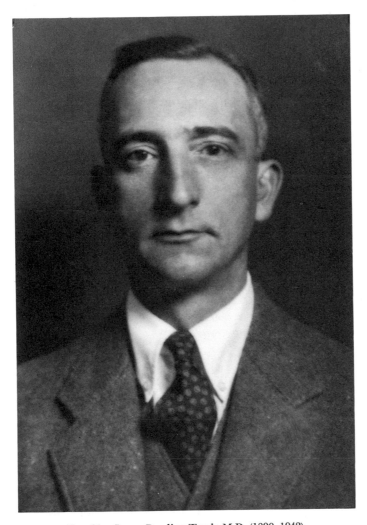

FIG. 31.   James Dowling Trask, M.D. (1890–1942).

aminations for the time being, and the thought of entering private practice was also unappealing. So, although he had had little training and less experience in research work, he decided to try it just the same and seek an academic career. Accordingly he went to the top in an effort to secure a place for himself and applied to Dr. Rufus Cole for a position on the staff of the Hospital of the Rockefeller Institute. He was promptly turned down because all available positions were filled. Six months later, however, Dr.

Cole wrote him that a vacancy had just come up and if he were still available he could take it that day, or next week at the latest, for in those postwar months there were innumerable young doctors just out of military service, who were seeking extra training. To this lucky break Dr. Trask responded with alacrity. At the Rockefeller Hospital he had the good fortune to come under the influence of as vigorous a small group of clinical investigators as had ever been gathered under one roof at one time—men such as Oswald T. Avery, A. R. Dochez, Thomas M. Rivers, Homer F. Swift, Alfred Cohn, Donald Van Slyke, John P. Peters, W. T. Stadie, and, last but far from least, Francis G. Blake.

Almost immediately upon his arrival the team of Blake and Trask embarked on an ambitious project to determine whether measles was due to a specific virus or, as some claimed, to a streptococcus. Dr. Blake had worked during World War I and for a year thereafter on influenza at the Walter Reed Hospital in Washington. He had been thwarted in his attempts to discover the etiology of influenza (the virus was not isolated until fifteen years later), but he had gained valuable experience in the use of monkeys for research purposes. So, the first decision of the two investigators was to try to infect rhesus monkeys with throat washings from children who were presumably in the infectious stage of measles.

The team of Blake and Trask succeeded admirably in this work. They quickly established the fact that measles is indeed due to a virus that can be recovered from children who are just coming down with the disease. Their results, while not extensive, were absolutely definite and have stood the test of time.

Reasons for the failure of previous attempts to isolate measles virus, which Blake and Trask were able to achieve so easily, arose from a feature that was little understood at the time and was not clarified until some twenty-five years later. This had to do with the susceptibility of monkeys to the virus. It is now clear that in the wild state rhesus monkeys are highly susceptible to measles, and once they have been caught and herded together in collecting points within villages, they frequently are exposed to measles virus and become infected. So, by the time a group of animals has been shipped overseas in the usual crowded conditions, the infection will have spread among them so that when they arrive at their destination in a research laboratory they are already immune. It was just by luck that Blake and Trask happened to acquire a shipment of monkeys recently arrived from India that were still susceptible. Otherwise they would have failed in their attempts to recover the virus, as did so many others who came after them. The experience gave the young Dr. Trask a sense of confidence in his newfound research activity.

In 1921, Francis Blake accepted the chair of internal medicine at the Yale Medical School in New Haven, Connecticut, which had been recently reorganized on a full-time clinical basis.[2] Dr. Trask, who had developed an ardent hero worship coupled with respect and affection for Dr. Blake, always claimed that although no position had been offered him on the Yale faculty, he was going to stick with Dr. Blake. And so, in due course the team of Blake and Trask moved to New Haven.

Five years later, in 1927, Trask made the decision to specialize in infectious disease and, in line with this move, decided to switch to the Department of Pediatrics at Yale. The shift was prompted by a desire to gain greater experience in the study of acute infections, which are more common in pediatric patients than in adults, and to indulge in his favorite subject of clinical microbiology.

Trask also deviated from orthodoxy by developing interests beyond his immediate teaching and clinical responsibilities, beyond those of the individual case at hand. He was concerned, as a clinician ought to be concerned, not only with the patient but also with the patient's family and with the circumstances under which the individual had become ill. Because of this interest, he was well qualified to serve as a member of the Board of Health of the City of New Haven, a post to which he was appointed in 1939 and held until his death.

As a full-time associate professor of pediatrics, Trask's duties in the early 1930s included teaching, the practice of hospital medicine, and the running of a large research unit. Any one of these three activities would have been a full-time job for most men, but he was still able to find time for extracurricular activities, such as duck hunting, trout fishing, and sailing, all in their appropriate seasons. His enthusiasm for these three sports knew no bounds. Among his endearing qualities was his generosity to fellow workers. It is difficult not to dwell almost rhapsodically on the all-too-short career of Dr. Trask.

His was an untimely death, due to a severe bacterial infection, which occurred in the spring of 1942 when he was only fifty-two years old. World War II was in progress, and Trask was engaged in carrying out a military mission as a member of the Commission on Hemolytic Streptococci of the U.S. Army Epidemiological Board. It was a scant month after he had received the John Phillips Memorial Medal of the American College of Physicians honoring him for his work on poliomyelitis.

In the spring of 1944, with the war still on, a memorial ceremony took place on the occasion of the launching of a 10,000-ton liberty ship named

2. This reorganization was among the early educational reforms wrought in the medical schools of this country that went along with the general policies of the Abraham Flexner Report. Following the example of Johns Hopkins, the Yale Medical School established its clinical departments on a full-time basis much as the preclinical departments of anatomy, physiology, etc. had been for many years. Yale was only one of several medical schools that were similarly reorganized in the early 1920s with the help of the Rockefeller Foundation.

in his honor—the *James D. Trask.* Basil O'Connor, president of the National Foundation for Infantile Paralysis, who had been responsible for
this project and for choosing the name of the ship, can be quoted on this
occasion somewhat as follows: "If this fine ship succeeds in getting half as
far in its voyages and in assisting the war effort, as well as Dr. Trask has
succeeded in his voyages charted for the purpose of carrying on the fight
against polio, it will have gone far indeed."

But to return once more to 1931, when the severe epidemic of that year
began in Connecticut early in the summer, it was by no means immediately apparent what the members of the pediatric and internal medicine
departments at the Yale University School of Medicine were going to do
about it. As the only research unit in the state with experience in the clinical investigation of virus diseases it was unthinkable that it should undertake no research at all on the subject of poliomyelitis, particularly when
such men as Francis Blake and James Trask were on the faculty. But at
the moment the school was ill prepared to handle virus research. The purchase of equipment and monkeys, particularly on an emergency basis,
was going to be expensive. The epidemic might soon be over, before investigations could be gotten under way. There were other difficulties, too,
such as the canceling of vacations by certain key people. Indeed, the emergency nature of poliomyelitis epidemics, coming in the summertime (as
they nearly always do), just when staff members are about to go on holiday,
has invariably posed vexatious problems.

But when it appeared that the epidemic would probably last for some
time, the Yale Poliomyelitis Commission was created under the able direction of James Trask. A month-long sailing cruise had to be cancelled, which
had included both of us. Emergency funds amounting to about $1500 were
hastily scraped up from various sources, and the work of the commission
got under way.

After a few false starts it was decided to take on the study of clinical
virology. Apparently no one had made a serious attempt to repeat the 1912
investigations of Kling, Pettersson, and Wernstedt since the small but uneasy trial of Taylor and Amoss back in 1917. So, following along in the
manner that had succeeded in the measles work and taking advantage of
the experience and skill in the use of rhesus monkeys that Dr. Trask possessed, it was decided that the first project of the Yale Poliomyelitis Commission was to be an attempt to clear up the old problem of isolating the
virus from acutely ill patients, particularly from abortive cases.

It might seem that the existence of abortive poliomyelitis would have
been settled long ago; the detection of virus in such cases was an old—but
still unconvincing—finding. In any event it had all but been forgotten by
the rank and file for when a veritable deluge of "minor illnesses" struck
Connecticut at the height of the 1931 epidemic, many local physicians
could not believe that such illnesses were indeed examples of abortive

poliomyelitis. In a way this incredulity and negativism was understandable, for the conventional doctor of the 1930s knew what the public's reaction would be. The majority of American parents considered themselves to be much more knowledgeable about infantile paralysis than they were about most diseases, and if told that cases with only slight fever and no paralysis were examples of the disease, they would have considered the idea ridiculous and might immediately have turned to a new doctor.

Also in 1931, modified rules for isolation of paralytic cases and their families were still being enforced. Since it was obviously impossible to quarantine all patients with minor illnesses or abortive forms of the disease, physicians were understandably perplexed as to what to do. The proper procedure, which was subsequently adopted, was to point out to parents and the public the futility of isolating the few frank cases of paralytic disease, when a far greater number of infected persons, either asymptomatic or with minor symptoms only, were allowed to move about freely in the community. Yet such advice was far from satisfactory to the general public, which continued to believe that quarantine offered some degree of security.

So, as a starter, the Yale Commission decided to attack the question of what actually was a "case" of poliomyelitis. Could poliovirus be recovered from patients with the abortive form—or its new name, the minor illness? Were such cases infectious? The plan at first was to limit the study to individual families in which one child had suffered from a frank paralytic or nonparalytic attack, while other members of the family had simultaneously experienced only minor illnesses; and to attempt to recover the virus from oropharyngeal washings collected from the latter type of case—as the Swedes had done twenty years before.

Such a family, encountered at the height of the 1931 epidemic, is shown diagrammatically in figure 32. One frank case of poliomyelitis in the child Corinda occurred in this Rn family in which there were four children. This was followed closely by two cases of characteristic minor illness in the other children. In the youngest child, Michael, the symptoms were sufficiently suggestive to warrant a lumbar puncture, which proved negative yet poliovirus was isolated from his oropharyngeal washings. The family doctor was adamant in claiming that the child Michael did *not* have poliomyelitis. In fact, he said: "If that's what you call polio, I for one, am heartily in disagreement with you."

Of course it could be speciously argued that the child had been merely a chance carrier of the virus, and his symptoms had nothing to do with poliovirus. However, enough similar situations were to crop up during that severe epidemic to indicate that such minor febrile illnesses were more than apt to be mild manifestations due to infection with poliovirus.

Another opportunity for virologic investigation of children suffering from the minor illness of poliomyelitis came when Dr. M. P. Rindge ex-

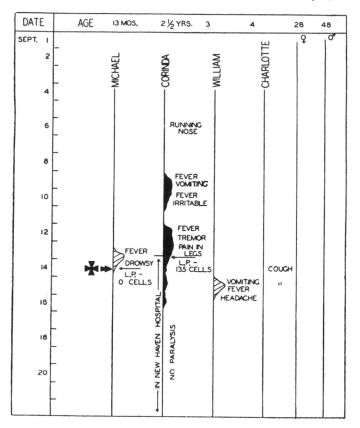

Fig. 32. Schematic diagram of family Rn. Vertical lines portray the different members; their ages appear at the top. The solid black areas indicate the course of a major illness in the second child (Corinda). Shaded areas indicate minor illnesses which occurred in the other two children. L. P. surmounted by an arrow denotes that lumbar punctures were performed.

tended an invitation to the Yale group to study a group of his patients. Dr. Rindge was at the time the most prominent practitioner of the town of Madison, Connecticut, which regularly had a large summer population occupying cottages on the shore of Long Island Sound. From mid-July to mid-August in that summer of 1931, several cases of mild illness, characterized by sore throat, fever, vomiting, and headache, appeared among the children of this summer colony; they were almost the exact counterpart of patients that Wickman had described in his account of the disease in Swedish villages in the epidemic in 1905 (see fig. 16). There had been considerable apprehension on the part of Dr. Rindge (and the community itself) as to whether these illnesses might be poliomyelitis, but none of the children seemed to show symptoms which would warrant a definite diagnosis, so they were designated for the moment as cases of "summer grippe." It was at this point on August 10 that the Yale Poliomyelitis Commission was called in.

Dr. Rindge was not satisfied with this vague diagnosis of summer grippe, and his suspicions were well founded, for on August 20 a child who had left the summer colony the week before developed paralytic poliomyelitis, and shortly thereafter three other paralytic cases appeared in the colony in rapid succession. In all, there were 29 instances of acute illness between July 15 and September 22, and 4 of them turned out to be frank poliomyelitis. It was possible to obtain oropharyngeal washings from 5 of the children among the 25 who did not develop paralysis, and from one of these poliovirus was isolated.

A final review of the findings of the Yale Unit during that eventful summer of 1931 revealed that out of twelve oropharyngeal washings obtained from children who were in the early and mid stages of suspected abortive poliomyelitis, two yielded poliovirus when injected into monkeys.[3] The positive specimens came from a child in the Rn family and from a 5-year-old resident of the summer colony. It was not a particularly spectacular or impressive result, but it was a demonstration that our approach was practical.[4] Furthermore, if these experiments accomplished nothing else, they allayed some of the fears which had been engendered by earlier work of Taylor and Amoss, that irrigation of the oropharyngeal passages of an ill child was dangerous (Chapter 23), and that virus isolations were not as expensive as had been anticipated. For instance some baleful critics had predicted that it would take $10,000 or more to demonstrate virus in either a carrier or a single case, abortive or otherwise. And yet our two positive virus isolations had been successful at a price of about $750.00 apiece.

By and large, these experiments marked a revival of virologic studies on patients, an approach that had been begun by Kling's team some twenty years previously but had gradually lapsed into obscurity. In addition, it was a reminder to local and perhaps other members of the medical profession in the United States, of what the clinical picture of abortive poliomyelitis might really be like. In doing so, the principle was reestablished that a poliomyelitis epidemic is not restricted to the diagnosed and officially

3. J. R. Paul and J. D. Trask: The detection of poliomyelitis virus in so-called abortive types of the disease. *J. exp. Med., 56*: 319–43, 1932; also J. R. Paul, R. Salinger, and J. D. Trask: "Abortive" poliomyelitis. *J. Amer. med. Ass., 98*: 2262–68, 1932.

4. The techniques used in these attempts were those employed by Taylor and Amoss, not those of Kling, Pettersson, and Wernstedt. Had the latter been followed we might well have had better success. The Yale technique was to mix oropharyngeal washings with 10 percent ether, which had been found to be detrimental to bacteria but not to poliovirus, and to centrifuge this mixture. A small amount (1.0–1.5 ml) of the supernatant fluid of the etherized material was then injected into the brain of a rhesus monkey. In contrast, in 1912 the Swedish workers had inoculated 10–15 ml of filtered washings into the peritoneal cavity and a smaller amount intraneurally into the sciatic nerves.

reported cases, but that actual infections far exceed this number. It might have been difficult for the local medical profession to accept this view without a convincing demonstration that poliovirus could indeed be isolated from patients with minor illnesses.

As a postscript to this work, it was at a meeting of the Society of American Bacteriologists in Baltimore during the Christmas holidays that Trask gave a preliminary report of the findings, which evoked plenty of discussion. Following his presentation, some of the participants adjourned for lunch at the Hotel Belvedere to continue talking. In the group were Drs. Warfield Longcope, professor of medicine at the Johns Hopkins School of Medicine, Hans Zinsser, professor of bacteriology at Harvard, Simon Flexner, Trask, myself, and several others. In the course of the luncheon Dr. Flexner turned to me and asked whether our Yale group needed any money. I was ill prepared for this question, so much so that I immediately choked on a glass of water. By the time I had recovered, the conversation had taken a different turn. But Dr. Flexner did reopen the subject later and in fact contributed one thousand dollars to the Yale unit, which enabled its work to be continued the subsequent year.

The investigations of the Yale Poliomyelitis Commission in 1931 started a trend that was to continue for many years. After 1931, several laboratories in the United States became interested in pursuing similar studies, and soon it was a legitimate practice during poliomyelitis epidemics for the health officer of the affected area to call on a team of "experts" to study the local cases and perhaps to make recommendations as to what to do. It is difficult today to realize how helpless physicians and particularly health authorities were in the face of a severe epidemic of poliomyelitis in those prevaccination days. Having issued weak guidelines to the public, warning that children should stay away from crowds, and quarantining households (a useless practice), there was little else they could do but watch as the number of cases mounted. The arrival of consultants from some distant place gave the impression that at least *something* was being done. As a rule, not much else than the bolstering of public morale was expected from the visiting investigators; nonetheless, often these requests for assistance were made in the honest belief that a real opportunity had arisen for advancing research in poliomyelitis. University and U.S. Public Health Service research teams were generally willing to cooperate,[5] for they recognized that here was a valuable chance to test theories and techniques under

5. The experience of the Yale Poliomyelitis Study Unit was an example of the frequency of calls for assistance from health officers between 1932 and 1941. The unit was invited, often urged, to visit, study, and advise at epidemics in Philadelphia, Pennsylvania, 1932; Los Angeles, California, 1934; Toronto, Canada, 1937; Charleston, South Carolina, 1939; Buffalo, New York, 1939; Detroit, Michigan, 1940; Miami, Florida, 1941; Cordova, Alabama, 1941; Winnipeg, Manitoba, Canada, 1941; and Huntington, West Virginia, 1941. All of these were large outbreaks which required from a fortnight to several months of work on the part of different numbers of the unit.

epidemic circumstances. One of the hazards of such undertakings, however, was having to contend with the misguided publicity that attended certain aspects of these operations. This was before the day of carefully edited press releases, and the investigators themselves were constantly hounded by reporters who visited their laboratories daily for news of discoveries or information to use in writing feature stories about the epidemic. It was not exactly an atmosphere in which careful laboratory work could be carried out.

For instance, an early request to the Yale group for such a study of an epidemic came in 1932 from Dr. J. Norman Henry, the health officer of Philadelphia. This city and the area surrounding it had escaped the epidemic of 1931 but was hard hit the following summer and fall. Among the tasks which the Yale Poliomyelitis Study Unit set out to accomplish in 1932 was the isolation of poliovirus from intestinal as well as oropharyngeal washings collected from acutely ill patients.[6] In this quest we were to suffer a sharp disappointment. The reason was that the wrong method of testing intestinal washings was used. The material was inoculated intracerebrally into monkeys, and although it had been treated with ether to remove bacteria, it was not rendered sufficiently sterile for this kind of an injection. Inevitably the monkeys developed brain abscesses before there was time for them to come down with paralytic poliomyelitis. The use of the intracerebral route of inoculation was understandable, for it was the only one deemed feasible in the United States at the time, but this slavish adherence to current research fashions of the day was certainly unwarranted—and indeed indefensible.

It was an expensive and discouraging lesson that the Yale group learned in Philadelphia that autumn of 1932. Oropharyngeal specimens from 8 patients and intestinal washings from 6 were tested without adding a single poliovirus isolation from either of these sources. The newsmen who had visited our laboratory almost daily were particularly disgusted. They felt that we had let them down and reminded us that funds to support this useless research on the Philadelphia epidemic had been quickly and enthusiastically raised by a group of public-spirited local citizens; also, the community had been generous in granting laboratory and other facilities at the Bryn Mawr Hospital—all to no avail.

In the meantime, during the years since 1912, Kling, with the help of others, had recently reported on a 17-year summary of their successes and failures in isolating poliovirus from clinical cases and from individuals with inapparent poliovirus infections.[7] Almost the same technique had been employed in these trials as had been used in 1912. But their success with

6. J. R. Paul and J. D. Trask: Observations on the epidemiology of poliomyelitis. *Trans. Coll. Phycns. Philad., 54*: 158–63, 1932.

7. C. Kling: Recherches sur l'épidémiologie de la poliomyélite. *Acta Soc. med. Suecanae, 55*: 1, 1929.

nasopharyngeal washings was, to say the least, even less spectacular than that achieved by Taylor and Amoss in 1917 and by Trask and Paul in 1931, for of 84 attempts made with such washings, only 3 had yielded the virus (3.5 percent)—considerably less than the 9.1 percent achieved by the Yale unit in 1931 and 1932. However, Kling also reported a more significant finding. Out of 54 tests on filtered intestinal washings carried out during the same period, 5 positive results had been obtained, yielding a 9.2 percent isolation rate.

To return to the previous year, three other papers were published by the Yale Commission during that summer of 1931, on a variety of subjects.[8] While objectives varied, it can truly be said that as a result of the 1931 epidemic this unit had been precipitously launched upon a long-term general study of poliomyelitis, particularly its clinical aspects, virology, pathogenesis, and manner of spread—studies which were to continue for forty years. At the start, little concentrated thought was given either to questions of prevention or of cure; attention to the former was to come much later. For the time being, members of the commission were to settle on more basic problems of clinical epidemiology.

But now I must hasten to avoid the impression that little was accomplished during the 1931 epidemic outside of New Haven. Obviously this was not the case. Some of the most important contributions of that epidemic year were controlled trials to determine whether convalescent, normal, or hyperimmune horse serum therapy was effective in the *treatment* of poliomyelitis. The large numbers of cases enabled two important groups of investigators to reexamine this question in a statistically adequate fashion. The answers obtained represented an almost complete about-face on this, the main issue of the day. For in spite of favorable opinions that had been expressed about the use of serum in the past, this treatment had proved ineffective and that was that. One result was that research could now move in a variety of other directions, because so much progress in poliomyelitis investigations had been sorely held up for many years over controversies on the use of serum.

Another landmark was the extensive study of the pathology of extraneural lesions in the human disease that Lawrence W. Smith at the Cornell University Medical College in New York was able to make as a result of the unprecedented number of autopsies performed that year on poliomyelitis cases. He published his findings three years later as a chapter in a text-

<hr>

8. J. C. Leonard: *An epidemiological study on poliomyelitis in summer camps in Connecticut in 1931.* Unpublished thesis submitted as a requirement for the degree of Doctor of Medicine in the Yale University School of Medicine, 1932; J. D. Trask and P. A. Harper: A diagnostic problem in poliomyelitis; a consideration of typical and suggestive cases showing normal spinal fluid. *Yale J. Biol. Med.*, 5: 155–63, 1932; J. R. Paul, J. D. Trask, and R. Salinger: Comparative statistical analyses of the 1916 and 1931 epidemics of poliomyelitis in and about the city of New Haven. *Yale J. Biol. Med.*, 5: 39–54, 1932.

book on poliomyelitis by Landon and Smith.[9] On the basis of examination of these fatal cases, Smith was able to strengthen the evidence that poliomyelitis is indeed a systemic infection, for he showed that beginning early in the disease there is a general lymph node enlargement, particularly of the mesenteric (intestinal) nodes. Rissler had been the first to document this, and Burrows had recognized it in 1916 but had only recently gotten around to the publication of his findings.

Smith also directed attention to the question of lesions in the olfactory bulbs in human fatal cases. He collected material from about 40 cases and stated that his examinations had shown "a surprisingly small amount of pathological change." This observation was soon picked up by Dr. Sabin and will be discussed in a subsequent chapter as a revolutionary finding.

There were activities of a totally different kind in a different part of the world, for 1931 was the year in which Burnet and Macnamara in Australia announced the signal discovery that immunological (antigenic) differences between different strains of poliovirus actually did exist. This finding was of such importance that it also deserves a separate chapter.

9. J. F. Landon and L. W. Smith: *Poliomyelitis; A Handbook for Physicians and Medical Students based on a Study of the 1931 Epidemic in New York City*. New York, Macmillan, 1934, p. 50.

CHAPTER 21

The Los Angeles Epidemic of 1934

Among the first few epidemics that the Yale Poliomyelitis Unit investigated was a remarkable one which hit the city of Los Angeles, California in the spring of 1934. In retrospect this outbreak has been accused of not being due to poliovirus at all; the stage was possibly shared by another disease, although it is certain that at least some of the cases were examples of poliomyelitis. In any event, a striking feature of the outbreak was that although most of the cases were mild, an atmosphere of stark dread prevailed, particularly among hospital personnel who had the task of caring for patients. This was in spite of information which had been available for a generation, indicating that poliomyelitis is not transmitted primarily from one paralytic or frank case to another but is spread far more frequently through the agency of abortive cases or inapparent infections, many thousands of which exist (unrecognized, of course) during a sizable urban epidemic. The medical or public health profession, it would seem, should have attempted to educate the Los Angeles public along these lines. Anyway, whether it did or not, the local population refused to accept the facts, preferring a simpler explanation that focused on the obviously ill patient as the main source of danger. It was as if plague had invaded the city, and the place where cases were assembled and cared for was to be shunned as a veritable pest house. The brunt of this fear fell particularly upon the Contagious Unit of the Los Angeles County General Hospital, where physicians, nurses, attendants, etc. were all caught in the same noisome net. The dramatic aspects of the 1934 epidemic were certainly exaggerated, probably because Los Angeles is by no means a typical American city.

In any event, shortly after the epidemic broke, in June 1934, Dr. George Parrish, health officer of Los Angeles, got in touch with Dr. Flexner in New York with the request that he immediately dispatch one of his staff members, or anyone else whom he saw fit, to make a study and propose recommendations. The upshot was that Dr. Leslie T. Webster, who had been on the staff of the Rockefeller Institute for some fifteen years but had only recently been appointed to full membership there, was given the assignment of heading a commission of three—the other two being Drs. Trask and Paul, who were recruited on an emergency basis from the Yale School of Medicine.

Dr. Webster was an old friend of both of the Yale members of this commission. Born in Mt. Vernon, New York, he had attended Amherst College and had been a fellow classmate of the author at the Johns Hopkins Medical School. After spending a year in the Department of Pathology at Johns Hopkins, Webster joined the staff of the Rockefeller Institute in 1920 and remained there until his untimely death in 1943 at the age of forty-nine.

Leslie Webster was well qualified to head a commission slated to investigate the Los Angeles epidemic, even though the choice may have seemed strange, for he had had no previous experience with poliomyelitis, either on the clinical or the experimental side. He had become an assistant to Dr. Flexner almost immediately upon his arrival at the institute and had carried on a program which Flexner and Amoss had started on *experimental epidemiology,* using mouse typhoid among murine populations as models. During the course of this work Webster had succeeded in breeding special strains of mice which were either highly susceptible or highly resistant to both bacterial and viral agents. Only recently had he become interested in human neurotropic virus infections, for in the previous year he had been sent by Dr. Flexner to deal with the extensive 1933 epidemic of encephalitis that had broken out in St. Louis. On this trip, Webster, using one of his susceptible strains of mice, had promptly isolated the causative virus—a discovery which was simultaneously made by a local team headed by Muckenfuss. The new agent was named St. Louis encephalitis virus. So what could have been more natural than to suggest that a trial of these highly susceptible mice be made in an attempt to isolate a viral agent from patients in the Los Angeles epidemic?

Our commission left for Los Angeles well equipped with apparatus, as well as monkeys and Webster's susceptible mice. All of this livestock demanded a certain amount of care on the four-day train ride from New York to the West Coast. Even so, there was ample time to discuss plans and techniques. The decision was to stick closely to attempts to isolate poliovirus from the oropharyngeal washings collected from clinical cases or subclinical infections, and to inoculate these (as well as some CNS material from fatal cases) not only into monkeys but also into Webster's highly susceptible mice. The Yale Unit's disappointing 1932 trial with intestinal washings was all too fresh in our minds to bear repeating, especially since the supply of monkeys that we could take along was limited. Also, some radical deviations in technique were decided upon. One portion of each oral washing was to be filtered through a bacteria-tight (Seitz) filter, and another portion of each specimen was to be rendered bacteria-free by treatment with 0.5

percent phenol—techniques with which we had had no previous experience. In retrospect, several of these decisions were unfortunate. It was all
too clear that we had not used the proper gambit. The filtration process,
while it removed all bacteria, also reduced the virus content and correspondingly lessened chances of a positive result. The decision not to try
intestinal washings was also a great mistake, considering that the larger
volumes which could be injected intraperitoneally might have contained
enough virus to infect monkeys successfully. But careful planning along
orthodox lines was the order of the day. The background presence of Dr.
Flexner was in the minds of all of us. He was intent on isolating some sort
of virus. We did not want to let him down.

Our arrival in Los Angeles had been preceded by a certain amount of
advance publicity. The announcement that a team of visiting scientists
was coming, from Rockefeller Center it was said, and included two Yale
men who were ostensibly going to solve the city's epidemic problems,
found newsmen agog. "Why," they said to us upon our arrival, in a letdown
tone of voice, "we thought you were going to be wonderful looking people!" One reporter confided in me that his image was that in the true tradition of a *team* from Yale College, no matter what its function, it at least
should have made its first appearance appropriately garbed with sweaters
or blazers, adorned with the proper insignia. We were to prove a great disappointment to them not only in our appearance but also in our reluctance
to talk.

To mention one incident of what I mean about the Los Angeles epidemic being atypical: soon after the arrival of our group, a meeting was
called of local physicians, public health officials, and newspapermen, ostensibly to give information about the current epidemic. We thought that
clinical and epidemiological features would receive their fair share in this
discussion, but, to the contrary, the specter of the epidemic had become so
dominant that it overshadowed other aspects in the discussion. Dr. A. G.
Bower led off before a packed hall; he described how, early in the epidemic,
he had been taken ill with symptoms that might have been poliomyelitis—
but happily, he had recovered. During the course of his illness his thoughts
had turned not unnaturally on his future. He recounted his apprehension
over whether in the event of his becoming paralyzed he would be legally
justified in claiming compensation for disability received "in line of
duty." The discussion then became animated and focused on questions as
to whether doctors and nurses generally deserved compensation if they
became ill as a result of efforts spent in caring for poliomyelitis patients.
The majority decision was in favor. There was little time left for a dispassionate discussion about the nature of the epidemic, except to emphasize
that a strange variety of poliomyelitis indeed had visited the city.

In order to give contemporary color to the story, parts of letters that Dr.

Webster wrote to his wife during our one-month stay in Los Angeles are included here.[1] They convey more vividly that I am able to do some of the atmosphere and some of the intimate problems which beset us in our work.

June 15, 1934
Biltmore Hotel
Los Angeles

Somewhat in a fog, I pen my first letter from that greatest, biggest, largest, most—and other superlatives, according to those inhabiting it—city of dreams.

Our trip out was quite ideal—the best train food I have ever eaten. As we commenced to get Los Angeles papers, we realized we had newspaper troubles ahead. A telegram was received requesting that we disembark at Pasadena. There we were met by the City Health Commissioner, Dr. Parrish and his aides. We were told that they had sidetracked us at Pasadena because of the crowd at the terminal. Then they said the Mayor was waiting to receive us and award us the Freedom of the City. I said "Positively we will not give out statements, we came to work: leave us alone."

The mayor had been called to quell a riot but we met his brother—then in came about 15 reporters and 10 cameras. We smiled and said NOTHING! as Parrish tried to explain the basis for our unpopular and noncommittal attitude. Pictures were taken in various poses—then they shouted "Now for the monkeys." "Nothing doing!" said we. "My God," said they—"what's the matter, Doc. Ain't you goin' to give us a break?"—but we were adamant about this.

Then to the Health Department to inspect the space, which was good. We were assigned a brand new Plymouth car and driver, and taken to the largest hotel in the City and put up at ½ rates.

After dinner we went to a Medical Meeting and renewed some old Johns Hopkins acquaintances.[2] Next noon, the mayor gave us a lunch and the entire Board of Health were present to assure us that everything would be done to make us feel at home. Invitations for each hour in the day were showered upon us. After dinner, the Police Commissioner of Los Angeles gave us his private car and we were driven at breakneck speed with red lights, policeman's radio, and siren going full blast. We skipped all traffic stops and just roared 18 miles to Hollywood's Greatest Premier Movie Theater, where the great owner, Sam Grauman, gave us complimentary seats. He held up the main show 3 minutes to meet us. My feelings cannot be committed to paper! ! !

No more engagements will be made—Not even lunch with the Police Chief and Grauman—at the pistol point ! !

1. I am indebted to Mrs. Harold T. White, of Katonah, New York, the widow of the late Dr. Leslie T. Webster, for her gracious permission to transcribe certain portions of letters which Dr. Webster wrote to her during this expedition to Los Angeles. The parts that I have selected have been transcribed verbatim with only a minor amount of editing, and with the addition of a few footnotes.

2. This was a meeting of local alumni of the Medical School of Johns Hopkins University at which Dr. Alan Chesney was the speaker. Chesney had worked on the serum treatment of poliomyelitis in the 1916 epidemic in New York. Now he was the dean of the Johns Hopkins Medical School.

In the meantime—and since, we set up our lab and cared for our animals. We are waiting for the crosscurrents of local jealousies to straighten out and to receive formal permission to do as we wish.

As for the epidemic—50 cases a day—20 nurses and 4 of the doctors in charge, down, one after another. Must stop here.

June 20, 1934

What a week! But now we have our first quiet evening and are ready to commence our investigations to-morrow.

Considerable has been accomplished. In the first place, we have convinced the Health Commissioner that we wish to avoid publicity. So he turns away news reporters, and magazine reporters, and photographers daily. That does not prevent some absurd statement about us from appearing in all issues of all papers, but in this city, that just *must* be. In the second place, we have gone over and beyond the very real jealousies between city, county, state officials, Hospital and attending physicians, and have their enthusiastic cooperation to the extent of allowing us to direct the procedures which bear upon our work.

In the third place we have set up and equipped our laboratory, set machinery going for making media, washing, sterilizing, special procedures,—all with the enthusiastic help of the municipal health department. We have a full time stenographer, a lab man with experience, a car and chauffeur. And lastly we have had our animal quarters constructed entirely to our specifications on the roof of the Health Building—25 cages for 75 monkeys. By Friday we shall have 40. Today we found a good animal man—so that very important problem is settled. That makes us ready to start in tomorrow to *find the virus.*

I wish I felt sure of success but although I am very much excited and eager about it all, too many others have failed, to make the job look easy. We have already injected brain tissue from fatal cases into monkeys and mice but that is known to be successful in about 20% of trials. The real trick is to find the virus in living people. Only 7 successful attempts on cases and 4 on carriers recorded![3]

So tomorrow we go to the admitting rooms of the hospital and collect nasal washings from patients just coming to the hospital. And what a place that hospital is:![4] 50 polio admissions per day,—30 nurses and 6 doctors down with the disease and all those now taking care of patients nervous and frightened and tired. The technique is poor, there is crowding, and no time for good nursing. But the old spirit of adventure is strong within us and the tougher the job the more we want to get at it.

June 23, 1934

Now we are well on our way. All the preliminary hurdles have been crossed and it is decidedly up to us. It is a difficult job. People are hysterical, the internes, nurses, and helpers are scared to death and have one or two cases among themselves each day. 50 admissions every day—everyone strained and worried. We, our-

3. Here Dr. Webster slightly underestimated the number of positive isolations of poliovirus that had been obtained from clinical cases.
4. The Los Angeles County General Hospital.

selves, are only just now commencing to sleep nights—nervous tension. We are at the lab at 8 A.M., get lunch for ½ hour any time between 1 and 3 P.M. and stop at 6–8 P.M. We have worked all day Saturday and Sunday and have not yet taken one minute of daytime recreation. But do not get the idea that it is drudgery. On the contrary we are thrilled and regard this opportunity as unique.

Perhaps I'm not such a poor diplomat after all—or perhaps some people understand down-right honesty. At any rate, these people are turning themselves inside out.

June 25, 1934

Last night, Sunday, we stopped work at 10:05 P.M. after working from 8:00 A.M., running up and down 11 flights, elevator not running on Sundays.

We are doing experiments rapidly and soon will be getting results—negative, I fear.

Rosenow arrives tomorrow! Leake is here.[5] All goes well with us.

June 29, 1934

Nine-thirty, work done for the day, tired but not exhausted. So here goes for the first decent letter to you.

As for the epidemic, adults continue chiefly to be affected, contagion is more evident than ever before, people are panicky. But although we are in hot sweaty cubicles, on wards, examining patients most of the time, unless we are in the laboratories preparing the hoped for virus containing material, we have no thought or intention of becoming ill ourselves.

Now that things are under way, Jim (Dr. Trask) spends the greater part of his time in the hospital, getting acquainted, helping internes, talking with the older men. In this way, he is invaluable. It rather falls upon me to crystallize what we want to do, plan the experiments in a logical, progressive and exact manner. This is indeed a most difficult—I may say impossible—task. The reason is this: poliovirus can be obtained from fatal cases, in about 25% of trials. From living cases, late or early or suspected or from contacts, it has only been obtained a total of 9 times in thousands of trials by hundreds of workers. Why? Is it because it isn't there, as Rosenow says—(who is here, by the way, and doing and saying precisely what he did in St. Louis)[6] or because the methods are inadequate to demonstrate small amounts?

The only thing to do here in the field is to go on the latter assumption, then do two things: i) Search for the virus (by monkey inoculation) under the most favorable conditions—theoretically, that is, from fatal cases; then under next most favorable, that is, from early cases; and lastly from abortive cases and contacts. At the same time; ii) Test or compare the most likely methods of isolation.

Then, of course, I'm making a valiant effort to transmit the disease to smaller animals, mice, rabbits, 250 gram, and guinea pigs, 100 gram.

5. E. C. Rosenow of the Mayo Clinic, who was an ardent and colorful proponent of a neurotropic streptococcus as the cause of poliomyelitis.

J. P. Leake, medical director of the U.S. Public Health Service, of whom we have heard previously, arrived accompanied by his assistant, Dr. A. G. Gilliam.

6. Both Drs. Webster and Rosenow had been together in St. Louis, Mo., during the previous summer working on the epidemic of encephalitis that had struck that city in 1933.

To-date, we have obtained poliovirus from one fatal case,[7,8] so the disease or epidemic is probably polio, in spite of many opinions to the contrary.

Also, if by a 1:1,000,000 chance I can get a take in smaller animals from human material, the door will be open for a quick solution of the mode of spread of the disease.

Frankly though, I feel that all I will get is a grasp of the problem, a clear understanding of what had been done, and what needs to be tried. I'm not going to quit, though, until I've wracked my brains and tried everything to the utmost. People here are so hopeful, so eager to help, and every one has been so good, that one feels as though one could not entirely fail. So with our several irons in the fire, we hope and hope and hope.

July 4, 1934

No faint ray brightens the murky sky. Aside from getting poliovirus from two fatal cases, nothing has developed. All experiments must be made by July 15 as the animals must be watched at least two weeks. Jim must be on duty at New Haven August 1, John (Dr. Paul) August 15 at the latest. I must confess to being discouraged although really one must not expect to succeed at once where everyone else has failed. One thing I've learned—*a method is needed*—a method of *proved adequacy*. Whether or not that can ever be worked out with monkeys, I do not know.

I think, however, that we can work out a method with the encephalitis virus and the epidemiology of the two diseases appears similar.

No one knows how much of this disease is polio—nearly all adults—nurses and doctors still coming down—much pain and weakness—very few deaths—not nearly the amount of paralysis that one expects. So I'm covering the possibility of this being a new or somewhat different virus.

We all feel terribly stodgy. A one hour swim on Saturday and one hour swim today are absolutely all the exercise we've had. No time off Saturdays, Sundays, or holidays. Soon, however, when we've finished setting up our experiments, there will be nothing but the watching of the animals—then we shall get some time off.

July 8, 1934

Nearly four weeks since I left home! Four weeks of turmoil, battle, and a great deal of shouting. But nature still clutches her secret tightly and we haven't made a dent.

Not a dent and I'm quite certain now that we are not going to this trip. None

7. From this fatal case, the Wfd. strain of poliovirus was isolated. It was to take its place among important strains isolated in the 1930s, and it also exhibited in our laboratory in 1934 tantalizing signs of causing a paralytic disease in mice—an almost unheard of feature up to that time. Years later David Bodian succeeded in successfully adapting this strain to mice and designating it as a Lansing (Type II) strain.

8. It might be recounted that in the performance of the autopsy on the Wfd. case at the Los Angeles County General Hospital, our team was assisted by a young medical student from the University of Southern California, one Norman H. Topping by name. This same medical student was subsequently to become the president of the University of Southern California. He served for a long time on the Board of Scientific Advisers of the National Foundation for Infantile Paralysis.

of our animals given nasal washings has turned a hair—none of the smaller animals has seen fit to respond, so here we are, high and dry.

But this experience has put some ideas in my head about encephalitis—the whole picture of which is so similar, you know, that it isn't even funny,—and those ideas I believe will result in *establishing a technique,* learning about the *mode of spread of encephalitis,* and learning about the *behaviour of related viruses.*

So although frustrated for the moment, I'm far from discouraged. Also I've learned more about people. An epidemic like this is almost like the battlefront—in the one case, "shell shock" develops, in the other "queer polio."

Well, let's see—Our daily routine might interest you, so regular it is:—up at 7:00, bath, breakfast 7:30, into waiting auto at 8:00, Lab at 8:00, 8:15–8:45 let out monkeys and examine all animals, 9:00 to hospital, laboratory work, or visiting polio families and institutions. Probably I see and am in contact with 100–200 polio patients a day—but remember hardly any of them are sick. So it isn't as terrible as it sounds. If John and Jim are right, they are the cases which are spreading the virus, if I am right 90% are not *polio.* But I'm no doctor!

We went to the beach yesterday and go again today. The weather has been marvelous,—dry, invigorating, breezy air, sunshine, temperature 85–65.

July 9, 1934

As things stand now, we shall probably be up and away the last week in July. That is of course if *nothing* continues to happen as it is happening now at a discouraging pace. That should bring me home on or just before August first. Our experiments on searching for a new susceptible animal are discouraging, on searching for a virus in the nasal passages, discouraging,—all quite discouraging.

However, as the problem clarifies, I am not a bit surprised, so do not think that I am discouraged.

July 10, 1934

Just a few minutes here on the "Contagious Disease" admitting floor (of the Los Angeles General Hospital) to sit down and send along a note. We are commencing the last phase of the work, testing for virus in the nasal washings of children with mild symptoms of less than six hours' duration, in a family in which one case of diagnosed polio has already occurred. We use the Health Board Doctors and see all admissions here at the Hospital in order to run down these cases. Aside from that, I am trying to make some reason in the epidemic among nurses and doctors—which by the way still persists. Personally, I question whether it is polio—but that is a matter of opinion, purely.

In about ten days our intensive work will be finished,—we then wait around and watch the animals—which are amazingly well.

This problem is amazingly complex. First, there is fear and interest on the part of the public. Infantile (it isn't infantile, ordinarily), paralysis (it doesn't paralyze ordinarily). There is the notoriety to be gained from working with this disease. Anything is news. There is hysteria of the populace due to a *fear* of getting the disease, hysteria on the part of the profession in not daring to say a disease isn't polio and refusing the absolutely useless protective serum—that has become evident

once again—and the treatment serum.[9] Then gradually getting down to the problem—what method is good? Where is the virus other than in the nervous tissue of
fatal cases?

We know that there is polio here (some question even that).

Guinea pigs and rabbits are still doing strange things but I am not at all impressed.

July 11, 1934

We find ourselves pensive, rather discouraged, reading about notoriety seekers
with a certain cynicism and waiting for Rosenow's announcement that he has discovered the cause and mode of spread of the disease. We are already being criticized; Parrish bet on the wrong horses, etc., etc.

But *time, time,* does strange things, and he who keeps his own council and works
alone has at least the satisfaction of not making a fool of himself.

This evening we have a monkey that looks very odd, one that received material
from a healthy person in contact with cases. It's only one chance in one hundred
but we are excited and hoping.

Suffice it to say that the "monkey that looks very odd," mentioned in Dr.
Webster's letter of July 11, 1934, was one of two monkeys in which a positive result was finally obtained from a child with a minor illness. Only one
of the trials with oral washings from 26 frank clinical cases and minor illnesses yielded a positive result, although, as already mentioned, several
isolations were made from fatal cases.

A published description of the patient's clinical picture and technical
details on the one recovery of virus from oral washings obtained from a
living patient (the McC. child) appeared in 1935.[10] The virus isolate as
well as all those from the fatal cases turned out eventually to be Type II
strains.

In addition, a valuable technical discovery was made after the completion of this expedition. This was the observation that oral washings, consisting of ropy fluid containing a few flakes of mucus and debris, could be
preserved for months. The sediment from such specimens could be spun
down in the centrifuge and after being preserved in glycerin over a period
of at least 101 days, could still yield the virus. This meant that the clinical
investigator did not need to transport a whole menagerie of monkeys and
mice to the scene of an epidemic; instead, the sediments from oral washings
could be brought back to the base laboratory for testing. Not only was
there no apparent loss of potency of the virus under these circumstances,
but there was the added advantage that the contaminating bacteria were
inhibited by the glycerin. The glycerin method of preserving oral washings

9. This reference is to the use of parents' blood, employed on a large scale in Los Angeles
both as a prophylactic and as a therapeutic measure (see chap. 19).

10. J. R. Paul, J. D. Trask, and L. T. Webster: Isolation of poliomyelitis virus from the
nasopharynx. *J. exp. Med., 62:* 245–57, 1935.

was short lived, being largely abandoned when dry ice and deepfreeze refrigerators came on the scene. Nevertheless, it was successfully applied for a few years in investigations of a number of viruses, including influenza, for which it proved singularly useful.

To sum up various opinions about the Los Angeles epidemic, there seems to be little question that Los Angeles County was visited by an epidemic of poliomyelitis in the summer of 1934, although even this fact has been denied in some quarters. But a major question has been whether there was not some other, unrecognized illness combined with the poliomyelitis cases, as Dr. Webster had suspected almost at the start of our virologic studies, and perhaps he was correct.

It is doubtful whether this question will ever be satisfactorily answered. All sorts of speculations have been offered. Might the disease have been due to some other member of the enterovirus family, either a Coxsackie or echovirus—agents that were not discovered until some years later? This would seem unlikely. Might it have been due to the unknown agent which causes an exotic neurologic disease first noted in 1948 in Iceland by Sigurdsson?[11] Or might it not have been due to hysteria, as has been repeatedly suggested?

In any event, during the months of May through November 2,499 cases suspected of being poliomyelitis were treated at the Los Angeles County General Hospital. Slightly more than half of these (1,301) were actually diagnosed and reported as poliomyelitis. That some few were indeed bona fide cases was established by the isolation of poliovirus from the spinal cord of the fatal ones, not only by our team but also by a team headed by John F. Kessel and his collaborators, who were then at the University of Southern California. Surprisingly, all of these isolates subsequently turned out to be Type II strains; Type II epidemics have been rare indeed and, when they have occurred, have involved the youngest age group almost exclusively, except in a highly susceptible population in the Arctic to be described in chapter 34.

According to the report of Dr. M. F. Bigler, who had been on duty at the Los Angeles General Hospital the summer of 1934 before she herself fell ill, the epidemic *was* poliomyelitis "affecting children but also adults of nearly all ages."[12]

By far the most authoritative account was prepared by Dr. A. G. Gilliam of the U.S. Public Health Service. He had spent all of that summer in Los Angeles and had conducted an extensive statistical survey, almost entirely devoted to the cases among personnel of the Los Angeles County General

11. B. Sigurdsson: Disease epidemic in Iceland simulating poliomyelitis. *Amer. J. Hyg., 52*: 222–38, 1950.

12. M. F. Bigler and J. M. Neilson: Poliomyelitis in Los Angeles in 1934; neurologic characteristics of the disease in adults. *Bull. Los Angeles neurol. Soc., 2*: 47, 1937.

Hospital, especially the resident doctors and nurses.[13] After examining the difficult questions as to whether or not the disease was poliomyelitis and whether there had been another, coincidental disease, he left the matter open. In his report he mentioned that among the hospital population as a whole there was an attack rate of 4.4 percent, but the nurses and physicians suffered even higher rates, 10.7 and 5.4 respectively.

Dr. James P. Leake of the U.S. Public Health Service characterized the Gilliam report in a foreword as follows:

> [an] epidemiological account of the remarkable occurrence of a neurological disorder among the personnel of the Los Angeles County Hospital . . . [which] is greatly appreciated by all who have been puzzled by this epidemic. The evidence is clear that the cases were conditioned by employment at the hospital where the great bulk of patients with undoubted poliomyelitis occurring in Los Angeles County were treated.[14]

Gilliam recorded relatively little fever among these 198 cases in nurses and physicians, and no deaths. Other clinical and epidemiological characteristics which differentiated their illnesses from typical cases of poliomyelitis included the age of the patients (most of whom were young adults); the extraordinarily few patients with abnormal spinal fluid findings (only 2 out of 59); and the dearth of cases with frank paralysis. The majority of atypical symptoms could be described as being "rheumatoidal or influenzal" in character, as well as those with striking emotional overtones.

One feature that may well have affected the atmosphere in which these hospital personnel cases found themselves was that the epidemic occurred at the height of that unfortunate era in the orthopedic treatment of the disease when it was the fashion to handle even a slight degree of weakness of a limb by rigid immobilization in a plaster cast (see chap. 32). Furthermore, it was a time when the common practice was to erect an elaborate system of frames and pulleys over the beds, which gave the poliomyelitis ward the appearance of a ward occupied by patients who had suffered extensive trauma inflicted in a disaster area, whereas in actuality very few patients turned out to have any paralysis at all.[15] In describing the illness

---

13. A. G. Gilliam: Epidemiological study of an epidemic diagnosed as poliomyelitis occurring among the personnel of the Los Angeles County General Hospital during the summer 1934. *Publ. Hlth Bull. (Wash.)*, no. 240, 1938, pp. 1–90.

14. J. P. Leake: See foreword in n. 13.

15. See n. 13, p. 26. The interns on these wards used to tell me that after encasing one or more limbs of a given patient in plaster casts, the patient's symptoms were very apt to worsen from the standpoint of pain, and they ascribed this, probably rightfully, to the effect of rigid immobilization. It is hard to imagine that a more unhappy form of treatment could have been instituted. But whatever the causes of the illness may have been, the interns cannot

and its treatment among hospital employees, Gilliam mentioned that one or more limbs were splinted in three-quarters of the patients, and half of them were immobilized on a Bradford frame, making the evaluation of weakness difficult; actually, paralysis in these patients had not been mentioned.

Added to this dramatic picture was the fact that some of the interns on duty were not getting proper guidance. The reason for this was that several attending physicians had decided to forego daily rounds on the poliomyelitis wards at the height of the epidemic, preferring to consult with the interns by telephone. This resulted partially from a feeling that was running high in the community, that the hospital was a "pest house"; a doctor who was visiting daily on the contagious disease wards at the Los Angeles County General Hospital was not welcome in many private homes. Public opinion it seemed was strong enough to have dictated this rule. So for a time interns and nurses on the contagious disease wards who needed the clinical judgment of the attending staff were not getting it.

In regard to another infection which had been spreading among the Los Angeles County Hospital personnel, Dr. Gilliam said:

> Whatever may have been the actual origin and mechanism of spread of this infection, the distribution of the disease was such, both in intensity of risk of attack and in time sequence, as might be expected . . . had it been an epidemic of a disease such as scarlet fever, spread by direct personal contact with cases and carriers.

He also included:

> Irrespective of the actual mechanism of spread and the identity of the disease, this outbreak has no parallel in the history of poliomyelitis or in other central nervous system infections.
>
> It should, however, be pointed out that certain observers were of the privately expressed opinion that hysteria played a large role in this outbreak. While it cannot be denied that hysteria was an important factor in some cases it appears extremely unlikely that many of the cases were purely hysterical in nature.[16]

In retrospect, many years later, the cases among personnel of the Los Angeles County General Hospital were likened to a strange disease which occurred in the remote Akureyri district of Iceland in epidemic form during the winter of 1948, a disease which has apparently been noted in sev-

---

be blamed for their handling of these cases. When faced with an incipient weakness of a limb in poliomyelitis, rigid splinting was the medical fashion and the teachings of the day.

16. Usually such hysterical cases encountered during poliomyelitis epidemics can be identified as having very little fever, a dearth of spinal fluid changes, little permanent weakness, and no deaths.

eral other places since. Indeed there have been numerous accounts of outbreaks and individual cases of an illness similar to that which prevailed
during the Los Angeles epidemic of 1934. To one of these illnesses that occurred in an epidemic in 1954 the name *benign myalgic encephalomyelitis*
was given. Later some thirteen outbreaks were described—the majority under the name of *epidemic neuromyasthenia*.[17] In any event, to the author
at least, the similarity between the Icelandic disease and that which occurred in Los Angeles seemed insufficient to characterize the two epidemics
as being unequivocally alike.[18]

Interpretation of the nature of the Los Angeles outbreak is almost as
difficult now as it was in 1934, and this is the reason that it has been described in more than usual detail. It was a striking example of what can
happen in almost any epidemic of poliomyelitis. Recently two British
psychiatrists have described it as an example of mass hysteria and have
quoted similar examples. They summarized their reasonable views:

> We believe that a lot of these epidemics were psycho-social phenomena
> caused by one of two mechanisms, either by mass hysteria on the part
> of the patients or altered medical perception of the community.[19]

Nonetheless the Los Angeles episode is a reminder that even those who
believe themselves to be experts occasionally ride for a fall, although they
may be extremely loathe to admit it, especially to their patients. It is sometimes the bitterest pill they have to swallow. The members of our team of
investigators had somehow failed to recognize the treachery of the situation
and had not emphasized sufficiently the possibility of a hysterical element
or the intrusion of another polio-like illness on the scene. As a weak excuse, it may be said that we had our hearts so set on isolating poliovirus
that we could think of little else. The events also illustrate the part that
the character and attitude of the community can play in distorting the accepted textbook picture of a common disease—almost beyond recognition.

17. These outbreaks have been listed in the columns of correspondence in the *New Engl.
J. Med., 280*: 1131, 1969; and *281*: 105–06, 1969.

18. My opinion is based on experiences gained in the course of several weeks spent in Iceland during the summer of 1950, when it was possible to learn about the Akureyri epidemic
firsthand from the late Dr. Bjorn Sigurdsson, whose report on the outbreak had appeared
that same year (see n. 11).

19. C. P. McEverdy and A. W. Beard: Concept of benign myalgic encephalomyelitis. *Brit.
med. J., 1*: 11–15, 1970.

CHAPTER 22

Immunological Differences among Polioviruses

Up to the early 1930s there had been only intimations that the family of polioviruses did not represent a single homogeneous strain of virus, the differences among the members being only those of virulence or neurotropism. Indeed, prior to 1931, it had been suggested by several investigators, as a result of immunity tests, that regardless of whether the virus came from Austria, France, Germany, or several sections of the United States, complete similarity existed among different strains.

From 1931 on, however, history took a new turn. In that year a major discovery was announced by two Australians[1] that was to change the whole course of the poliomyelitis story—the discovery that fundamental antigenic differences existed between at least two strains of poliovirus.[2] Even the nomenclature used from now on to describe poliovirus in this book will be different; for what was thought to have been a single virus will now be considered as a family of individual serotypes. From this time forward this history would be unintelligible if the situation with regard to the three component members of the poliovirus family were not explained.

Two features tended to belittle the importance of this fundamental discovery: the full significance of the observation was not appreciated for some years because it was regarded as just something that had come out of that far-off continent of Australia; and the splintering of the family of polioviruses was hardly a subject to interest the rank and file of the medical profession and particularly the general public, which by this time had begun to follow eagerly the advances made in the field of poliomyelitis. To medical scientists, however, especially to immunologists, its impact can hardly be overestimated. Because Aycock had assumed in the 1920s that all poliovirus strains were alike, he was led into the vagaries of his autoarcesis theory; other theories about immunologic maturity also foundered on this very point. Appreciation of the differences between strains of polio-

1. I am indebted to the late Lord Florey of Oxford University and to the late Prof. Sydney D. Rubbo of Melbourne University, Australia for certain of the items in this chapter dealing with Australia. Also, to Dr. W. McD. Hammon of the University of Pittsburgh for review of this chapter.

2. F. M. Burnet and J. Macnamara: Immunological differences between strains of poliomyelitic virus. *Brit. J. exp. Path., 12*: 57–61, 1931.

virus was fundamental to any attempt to vaccinate against the disease or to develop serologic tests for detecting immunity. Eventually the demonstration that the family of polioviruses is composed of three types, each endowed not only with its special antigenic but characteristic biologic attributes, changed most concepts about the virology and immunology of the disease. The failure of two eager investigators to grasp the significance of the discovery of multiple types in their ill-fated vaccination attempts in 1935 turned out to be one of their major mistakes.

Before 1931, even though the original discovery of poliovirus by Landsteiner and Popper had been made some twenty-three years earlier, surprisingly few strains of the virus had been "established" as satisfactory ones for use in the laboratory. A strain was established after its isolation by keeping it going in continuous intracerebral passage in monkeys. After an unknown number of such transfers, some strains had a tendency to die out whereas others increased in virulence and neurotropism. Such a process of adaptation was an expensive procedure. Only when a given strain reacted consistently and had reached a certain level of virulence was it considered adequate for use. Thus it became an early belief, indeed a doctrine, that if differences did exist among poliovirus strains, these had been artificially *induced* due to continuous passage in the monkey and were not attributable to any inherent property of the strain. But Burnet and Macnamara's observation in Australia established that these differences were in fact of an antigenic and genetic nature, and as such were much more significant than artificial changes induced in the laboratory.

During this period and long afterward, if one wished to do research on poliovirus, the approved procedure was to write to an established investigator in one of the few laboratories that maintained these "standard" strains, asking for one or more of them. Then you could start working with the assurance that this was the proper way to begin. In 1930 so-called standard strains of poliovirus in the United States were:

1. The "MA" strain, which had been originally isolated by Dr. Flexner and his colleagues from a fatal human case as early as 1909 and had been kept in continuous passage at the Rockefeller Institute ever since.
2. The "MV" strain, whose origin and qualifications as a type-specific strain left much to be desired, as it was of *mixed* origin. The date of its first isolation and actual number of passages were unknown. Its most outstanding property was that it was highly virulent (highly neurotropic for monkeys on intracerebral injection). Almost all animals succumbed with complete paralysis of all four limbs. It was the most popular of the three strains.
3. The Aycock strain, which had been isolated from a fatal case in Vermont in 1920 and had been passed many times.

Early investigators argued as to whether the differences between newly isolated and passage strains of poliovirus were *entirely* due to alterations induced by continuous intracerebral transfer in monkeys. It was a tough question, practically unanswerable. In 1929, Stewart and Rhoads at the Rockefeller Institute had given some intimation of differences between strains when they compared the MA, Aycock, and MV strains, but this work did not lead to any clear-cut conclusions. Two years later, Weyer in Park's laboratory had contrasted a "passage" strain (MV) with a "human" strain, isolated in 1931 in New York City, and had concluded that differences between the two were quantitative—not qualitative. So the bulk of American opinion did not favor a family of strains.

By 1931, however, Burnet and Macnamara proceeded to examine this question with a thoroughness which was to characterize Burnet's work throughout his long and productive career. In brief, they compared the MV strain (received from Dr. Flexner) with their Victoria strain, derived from a fatal case that had occurred in 1928 in Melbourne, Australia, and found distinct differences, demonstrable by cross-immunity experiments and by serological (neutralization) tests. In three instances, monkeys that had recovered from typical experimental attacks induced by the Victoria strain, and accordingly should have been immune to the disease, had succumbed to paralytic poliomyelitis after injection of MV virus. It was another landmark in the history of poliovirus and of poliomyelitis.

The report by Burnet and Macnamara was greeted with a certain amount of skepticism by microbiological authorities in the United States. Burnet was a comparatively unknown figure who had done little in the poliovirus field and Australia was remote; anything, it was argued, might come out of that far-off continent, including an exotic variety of poliovirus. Nevertheless, the report did receive some attention, although far less than it deserved.

Dr. Frank M. Burnet, subsequently Sir Macfarlane Burnet (see fig. 33), was to have a particularly distinguished career.[3] Born in Australia, in 1899, he was educated at the University of Melbourne, served as intern and resident at the Melbourne Hospital between 1922 and 1924, as a Beit fellow at the Lister Institute in London during 1926–27, and again at the National Institute for Medical Research, in London, in 1932–33.

It used to be claimed, especially before the air age, that medical scientists in Australia and New Zealand, being remote from the mainstream of thought, were at a serious disadvantage in not knowing what was going on elsewhere. But Burnet was enough of a genius not to regard this as a handicap. He had schooled himself from the start to figure out on his own what he considered to be the most important problems in the field in which he was interested; and above all—what was *not* important. This put him in the

---

3. Sir Macfarlane Burnet: *Changing Patterns; An Atypical Autobiography.* Melbourne, William Heinemann, 1968.

unique class of independent thinkers who are often liable to come up with
ideas of extraordinary originality.

This has remained Burnet's major characteristic during all of his scientific career, which, except for the brief period of early training in London,

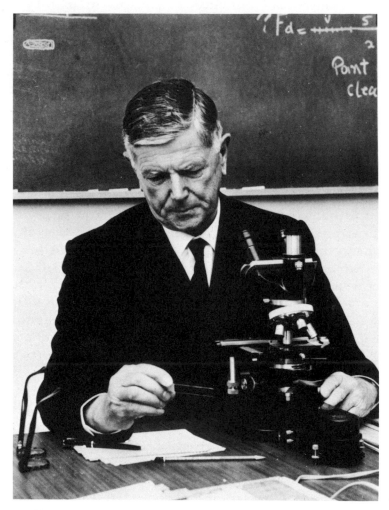

FIG. 33.   Sir Macfarlane Burnet, M.D., F.R.S. From a photograph in the
author's possession.

has been spent at the Walter and Eliza Hall Institute of Medical Research
of the University of Melbourne, where for many years he was the director.
His work has covered several broad fields, but at the start and for almost
twenty-five years he was concerned with infectious disease, particularly virus infections. In this period he showed a degree of discernment far more
penetrating than that of the usual virologist or immunologist. It was a

characteristic that never failed to impress me during his many visits to this country. His remarkable insight enabled him to view the natural history of a given disease—its immunology, pathogenesis, and epidemiology—as a whole. This creed was epitomized early, in his *Biological Aspects of Infectious Disease,* which first appeared in 1940 and has run through three editions, under different titles.

From 1957, Burnet became deeply interested in theoretical immunology and the phylogenetic approach—interests which were to win him the Nobel Prize in Physiology and Medicine in 1960. He retired as director of the Walter and Eliza Hall Institute in 1965, full of well-deserved honors.

With regard to Dame Jean Macnamara, Burnet's partner who shared in the discovery that antigenic differences between strains of poliovirus actually existed, her career, though distinguished enough, followed a completely different course. For a time she was associated with the Walter and Eliza Hall Institute primarily as a fieldworker in poliomyelitis. But she was first and last a crusader for worthy causes who carried on, among other enterprises, an enthusiastic fight for the promotion of "better" care of patients with paralytic poliomyelitis in her own native land of Australia— and according to her own ideas. Typical of her tenacity in this fight was that she became a staunch advocate of serum therapy of poliomyelitis long after it had been given up elsewhere. Her orthopedic advice on how best to care for patients in the early stages of paralysis was given freely in the 1930s; this included recommendations for early and continued splinting of the limbs of a paralyzed patient. She was also active in the promotion of organizations supported by community funds whose objective was to aid patients who needed aftercare. In these endeavors she antedated the establishment of the National Foundation for Infantile Paralysis in the United States by at least five years.

So zealous was Dame Macnamara in her efforts to promote early splinting of the limbs in a patient suffering from paralytic poliomyelitis that it is alleged that her campaigns eventually, and almost inevitably, led to a reaction in which opposite points of view about this treatment were taken. Thus in the 1940s rigid immobilization of weak limbs was decried by some in a movement that for a time led to a lively controversy. The leader of this movement was another Australian lady, the redoubtable Sister Kenny.

The impact in America created by Burnet and Macnamara's discovery of antigenic differences between two poliovirus strains (or, what was more significant, the interpretation of this finding) remained, in spite of the convincing nature of the evidence, lukewarm. It was argued that the Victoria strain of poliovirus might not be poliovirus at all; it was recalled that the Australian X disease, still a mystery in 1931, had come and apparently gone from that continent. Those were the days when statements by Burnet were not greeted with the respect that they were to be accorded in his later life. Flexner had great difficulty in believing in a family of polioviruses as long as he lived.

Yet in spite of the early skepticism that had been expressed, to some, the Australian results sounded reasonable enough. Almost immediately the Yale Poliomyelitis Unit decided to try to confirm or at least throw some light on this important observation—even if it had come out of Australia. The plan, however, was to use various poliovirus strains that had been obtained in the United States. One of these (the We strain from Connecticut) had been isolated from a patient with a minor illness during the epidemic of 1931 and had been "established" during the winter of 1931–32, so that it was quite usable and reliable in cross-neutralization tests. Another strain, isolated from a fatal case during that same 1931 epidemic, had been received from Dr. Flexner (the F strain). These two, which were at first inappropriately called "human" strains, were compared with the "standard" MV strain that had come from W. H. Park's laboratory.

The experiments performed by the Yale group were essentially a repetition of those by Burnet and Macnamara, and the results were completely in accord with the Australian findings.[4,5] Thus the experimental disease in the monkey induced by the two so-called human strains failed to immunize animals against subsequent reinfection by the old passage (MV) strain; and the neutralizing power of human convalescent sera taken from patients who had sustained recent infections in the 1931 outbreak differed qualitatively from the neutralizing power possessed by normal human sera when tested against the old MV strain. At least the findings by the Yale group were enough to settle the argument whether the Australian results had been entirely due to an exotic or special Australian virus. The detection of antigenic differences among various strains started the Yale Poliomyelitis Study Unit (YPSU) in a new direction that was to last for some five years. At the onset, these explorations were begun with the premise that the former methods of testing the neutralizing capacity of human sera against various strains of poliovirus, methods which had been in use for some twenty-five years, left something to be desired. What came to light was evidence of the existence of qualitative differences in immune human sera which reflected differences in the strain or strains of poliovirus which were responsible for the individual's immunity. In spite of certain crudities of the neutralization tests performed in those early days, coupled with statistical inadequacies, these experiments told an important story.

In the meantime, in 1934, three years after Burnet and Macnamara had

4. J. R. Paul and J. D. Trask: A comparative study of recently isolated human strains and a passage strain of poliomyelitis virus. *J. exp. Med., 58*: 513–29, 1933.

5. J. R. Paul and J. D. Trask: The neutralization test in poliomyelitis; comparative results with four strains of the virus. *J. exp. Med., 61*: 447–64, 1935.

announced their discovery, a report describing a plurality of polioviruses had come from Erber and Pettit in Paris.[6] The latter, it may be remembered, had for some fifteen years prepared serum in horses for treatment of acute poliomyelitis. These French investigators were among the few who still maintained that immune serum was a useful therapeutic measure in spite of growing evidence which had appeared in the United States and elsewhere that human convalescent serum was ineffectual. In their 1934 paper the Parisian workers compared strains of poliovirus from such widely separated parts of the world as Canada, Czechoslovakia, and France and concluded that the existence of immunologic differences between these strains made it necessary to prepare a polyvalent horse serum for the treatment of the disease. It was a reasonable but belated suggestion.

Another attempt by the Yale Unit to try to bring some sort of order to the classification of polioviruses was reported in 1937.[7] It had taken some two and a half years of work and required the use of hundreds of monkeys before Dr. Trask and his colleagues were able to report the results of these long and complicated experiments which demonstrated clearly that at least two types of poliovirus existed, as Burnet and Macnamara had indicated six years earlier. The differences were shown to be related to the epidemic source of the virus, and they were inherent in the strain. Eleven years later the findings were further amplified by Hammon and Roberts, who used more sophisticated methods.[8]

Six years after Burnet and Macnamara's discovery, Simon Flexner, in the last paper he was ever to write on the subject of poliomyelitis, continued in his skepticism about antigenic differences between strains of poliovirus. This alone is a measure of current unwillingness at that time to accept the new doctrine. Today it may be difficult to imagine the protracted confusion which beset poliovirus workers during the 1920s and 1930s by their failure to recognize the diversity of members of the poliovirus family. The idea expressed by Rivers, who was caught in the same morass, that strains of poliovirus did not seem to immunize satisfactorily, still was based on this same mistake. And, in self-defense, Aycock and others resorted to hypotheses which fitted the facts, as they saw them. Such theories maintained that factors other than specific immunization were responsible for the promotion of immunity. It was only after 1950 that real progress was made, coincident with the recognition of the three distinct serotypes. Before that there were two—the Lansing-like strains, of which there were several ex-

6. B. Erber and A. Pettit: À propos de la pluralité des souches de virus poliomyélitique. *C. R. Soc. Biol. (Paris)*, *117*: 1175, 1934.

7. J. D. Trask, J. R. Paul, W. J. German, and A. R. Beebe: Viruses of poliomyelitis; immunological comparison of 6 strains. *Trans. Ass. Amer. Phycns*, *52*: 306–10, 1937.

8. W. McD. Hammon and E. C. Roberts: Serum neutralizing antibodies to the infecting strain of virus in poliomyelitis patients. *Proc. Soc. exp. Biol. Med. (N.Y.)*, *69*: 256–58, 1948.

amples, and the Brunhilde-like strains, the latter being named after a chimpanzee with certain physical assets which qualified her for that title.

There the situation remained for several years. But with World War II over, it became obvious to many investigators that the problem of the multiplicity of strains had received but a temporary solution. It was high time something solid be done about it. The majority had agreed that until this matter was straightened out there was little use in trying to get anywhere with artificial immunization. To this end, in 1946, a conference on mechanisms of immunity in poliomyelitis was called by the National Foundation for Infantile Paralysis (NFIP), at which, among other topics, the timely matter of multiple strains of poliovirus was aired, particularly in relation to artificial immunization. The meeting was also an early example of the kind of conference which the NFIP was in a peculiar position to promote. The discussion quickly settled down to the question as to whether any one laboratory could accomplish the colossal task of sorting out and classifying strains of poliovirus. It was here that the seeds of cooperative endeavor were sown among National Foundation grantees. The approach was opened with a statement by the chairman:

DR. MAXCY [Johns Hopkins]: Perhaps the opportunity can be developed on a basis of group cooperation.

DR. HAMMON [Univ. of California]: . . . The hope of an effective vaccine still depends to a great degree on how many strains of virus we are going to have to immunize against. We need a great deal more work to find out how complex the antigenicity is, and it may be quite hopeless if we have too many of them.

DR. BODIAN [Johns Hopkins]: It might be possible to relieve the situation regarding virus strains a little if each laboratory took upon itself the responsibility for finding out something about the few strains it uses.

DR. RIVERS [Rockefeller Inst.]: I think workers in this country should decide sooner or later whether poliomyelitis produces an immunity and how good it is. Is it good enough to warrant bothering our heads about, and spending a lot of money on vaccines? I do not believe that we can get far in developing a vaccine until we know the number of different strains of virus operating.[9]

The upshot of the 1946 conference was that after a delay of some fifteen months, the NFIP finally got around to holding another meeting,[10] in

9. Mechanisms of Immunity in Poliomyelitis. A round table conference held under the auspices of the Dept. of Epidemiology, School of Public Health & Hygiene, Johns Hopkins University, Baltimore, Md., Sept. 1946, unpublished, pp. 72–75.

10. "Immunologic Types of Viruses of Poliomyelitis," a conference held in New York City, July 1948.

which plans for action were drawn and a strong committee[11] was appointed to implement the program.

The majority of the committee, having agreed that a large-scale attack on this problem was timely, proceeded to outline a series of standard techniques as to how it would go about the task. Technical details of the comparison of strains of virus will not be given here. Had the program been delayed five or more years (when tissue-culture methods became available) it could have been accomplished far more cheaply and probably more accurately. But in 1948, the initiation of a typing program was not merely urgent—it cried aloud to be done. As Drs. Hammon and Rivers had stated, little progress in poliomyelitis research could be made until this matter had been cleared up, expense or no expense. With regard to the methods used, suffice it to say that the outmoded monkey neutralization test was resurrected. This time with not one or two monkeys per serum, but more lavishly—five monkeys per serum.

Years afterward, a long-time clinical and academic member of the National Foundation's General Advisory Committee said to me that he considered the Typing project was the greatest single piece of developmental research that the NFIP was to accomplish during the years of its existence. The way was opened automatically, as it were, to all subsequent developmental projects.

The Committee on Typing, which began to publish its results three years later, in 1951, started with the premise that:

> prior to 1931, the problem of antigenic variation of poliomyelitis viruses was so little appreciated that most investigations did not mention the sources of viruses used in their published experiments, and as late as 1935, vaccines prepared for the immunization of human beings contained a virus which, although initially a mixture of strains of unknown antigenic composition, had been passaged so extensively in monkeys that it could only have been presumed to consist of a single strain.[12]

The committee started its work on a polyglot collection of about 250 strains of poliovirus of unknown type, which came from different geographical areas and different anatomical sources—oropharynx, stools, and

---

11. Members of the Committee on Typing of Strains were: Drs. Charles Armstrong, Washington; David Bodian, Johns Hopkins; Thomas Francis, Jr., Michigan; Louis P. Gebhardt, Salt Lake City; John F. Kessel, Los Angeles; Albert B. Sabin, Cincinnati; Jonas E. Salk, Pittsburgh; Herbert A. Wenner, Kansas City; and H. M. Weaver, ex-officio (the latter representing the NFIP).

12. The Committee on Typing of the National Foundation for Infantile Paralysis: Immunologic classification of poliomyelitis viruses: I. A Cooperative program for the typing of one hundred strains. *Amer. J. Hyg., 54*: 191–274, 1951. See also subsequent papers: Nos. II–V (1951) and VI–VII (1953).

(in fatal cases) central nervous system. One hundred strains were eventually chosen. Of these, 86 percent came from the United States, the rest from widely distributed areas around the globe. The routine technical work was parceled out among several universities, which included Bodian and Howe's laboratory at Johns Hopkins, Baltimore; Gebhardt's at the University of Utah; Salk's at the University of Pittsburgh; Wenner's at the University of Kansas; and Kessel's at the University of California at Los Angeles. That the bulk of the program was to prove to be dull work, few could deny. Conceivably the whole project could have been better done by a wholesale drug house, hired for the job. But certain members of the NFIP committee were so vitally interested in the Typing Program and so anxious that it be brought to a satisfactory conclusion that they wanted to do this task themselves and would have been willing to expend any amount of effort in furthering the cause. In spite of dire predictions that neither the quota nor the global source of poliovirus strains tested was sufficiently adequate, the mission of the Typing Committee succeeded better than anyone had hoped. A total of seven papers were published, tracing the progress of the testing program. Bodian served in the capacity of chief editor of the first papers that came out under the auspices of this committee; Wenner edited the next series.

One may remember that a major fear had been expressed (particularly by Dr. Hammon) that so many different strains of virus might be turned up by this enterprise as to make any idea of a vaccine which embraced the whole "large" family of polioviruses impractical. Fortunately this did not prove to be the case. The poliovirus family turned out to be surprisingly small—in fact, limited to only three members, or serotypes. The Yale group had predicted at least two serotypes in 1937, and the Johns Hopkins group, in a report published at the start of the Typing Committee's work in 1949 had predicted three. But to have this conclusion confirmed by an investigation that started with 100 strains, and later expanded to 196 collected from far and wide, was not only surprising, but convincing. When tissue-culture methods were added to the techniques then in vogue, the results were even more convincing. A proper search had been made, and in the following years no one had been able to turn up a fourth or fifth type of true poliovirus, using the most foolproof and up-to-date methods.

The final count of the percentage distribution of these three types among the 196 strains is listed in table 5. The percentages, which were reported in 1953 (see n.12), have pretty much held for the distribution of poliovirus types in sporadic cases and epidemics around the world ever since.

The results placed Type I in by far the most prominent position with regard to the prevalence of paralytic poliomyelitis. In spite of the dearth of strains tested from outside the United States in the first series of 100, the concentration of strains from one nation did not prove to be a defect of the Typing Program as several had predicted.

TABLE 5. Distribution of the three types of poliovirus as determined
in 196 strains tested by the NFIP's Committee on Typing

Type	No. of Strains	Percent
I	161	82.1
II	20	10.2
III	15	7.7

See n. 12.

In subsequent correspondence with Dr. Bodian about the work of the committee, he said:

It seems to me in retrospect that the Committee problems were mainly practical ones, such as acquiring a definite assortment of strains, and expanding laboratory facilities to accomplish the huge task of dealing with so many monkeys. The procedures had been tested in practice beforehand, and were generally acceptable.[13]

Bodian adds that in only one of the laboratories were there moderately discrepant results—not a bad record for research by individual groups who were singularly wedded to their own ideas and methods. It was a major triumph for the NFIP to have engineered this cooperative endeavor among a highly individualistic group of research workers, some of whom had hitherto no doubt considered their laboratories to be sacrosanct.

Dr. Wenner's comments were:

Salk served as a spearhead in the venture—but not necessarily the leadership—excepting for the typing by the adjuvant method. Credit must be given Salk however; he wished to discharge the program and was effective in doing so. Weaver played a considerable role in coordinating, expediting (among the four laboratories) and seeing to it that we were financially able to get the job done.

Among other features inherent in Dr. Wenner's statement, it is evident that the degree of skill and efficiency in expediting research programs already shown by Dr. Salk was beginning to be recognized, not only by his colleagues but by leaders of the NFIP as well.

We can leave the Typing Program for the time being to discuss what manner of research workers were engaged in it. Several of them went on to become actively identified with virus work in the poliomyelitis field.

The career of David Bodian already was established; he was to assume a position of continued major prominence in the whole broad field of polio-

13. I am indebted to two members of the NFIP's Committee on Typing for their accounts of this program which were kindly furnished almost 20 years after the project had been initiated. These are Dr. David Bodian, of Johns Hopkins University (letter to the author of December 22, 1967) and Dr. Herbert A. Wenner, of the University of Kansas Medical Center (letter to the author, December 19, 1967).

myelitis. Bodian (see fig. 34) was born in St. Louis, Missouri in 1910 and received the Ph.D. degree at the University of Chicago in 1934 and an M.D. degree from this same university in 1937. After preliminary experience on the faculty of several medical schools in their departments of

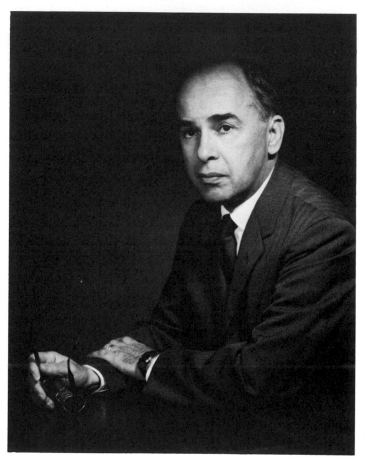

FIG. 34. David Bodian, Ph.D., M.D. Photograph (by Leonard L. Grief, Jr.) in the author's possession.

anatomy, in 1942 he joined the recently organized poliomyelitis team at the Johns Hopkins School of Hygiene and Public Health. This team had already assumed stature under the leadership of Dr. Kenneth F. Maxcy, Frost's successor as professor of epidemiology at Johns Hopkins. Other members of the team consisted of Dr. Howard A. Howe, a neuroanatomist who was to concentrate his talents on experimental and human poliomyelitis and whose work and writings have received constant and well-merited mention in this history, and Dr. Isabel Morgan, whose experiments on the immunization of monkeys we shall hear much of later. In the coming years this team was to play a major role in dealing with the subjects of the neuro-pathology, epidemiology, pathogenesis, and immunology of poliomyelitis.

By 1942, Kenneth Maxcy, the chairman of the Johns Hopkins Poliomye-litis Group; which had received a sizable financial grant from the National Foundation, became the acknowledged leader of the first important unit to be substantially supported by the foundation. When Maxcy was forced to resign in the 1950s due to ill health, Bodian assumed leadership.

The Johns Hopkins laboratory was responsible for the introduction of the chimpanzee as an animal superior to the rhesus and other species of monkeys. Chimpanzees were to prove the nearest to man with respect to susceptibility to poliomyelitis. Their greater sensitivity to the virus became manifest not only by the ease with which alimentary tract infection could be induced by feeding the virus (unlike the rhesus monkey) but also by their ability to acquire inapparent poliovirus infection. So, in spite of their cost, chimpanzees gradually became a necessity rather than a luxury for some few poliomyelitis laboratories. It was a conspicuous step forward in the history of experimental poliomyelitis. Chimpanzees were exploited to such a degree that experimental poliomyelitis emerged with quite a new and efficient, albeit an expensive, look.

Under the leadership of David Bodian, studies by the Hopkins group flourished in the 1950s.[14] The work dealt with the main and timely issues of poliomyelitis research. Although the unit had begun in the field of neu-ropathology and had been a champion of neural pathways along which poliovirus was supposed to travel,[15] when Bodian announced his opinion with regard to the pathogenesis of the infection and the role of the blood-stream invasion by poliovirus in the human disease, it represented a cou-rageous step—almost an about-face—for him.

Particularly in the 1950s and 1960s Bodian assumed a position of author-ity, and somewhat of an arbitrator, during the difficult years when prob-lems about poliovirus vaccines were being debated, occasionally with acri-mony. Here he was vocal and articulate. His talent for seeing clearly what was to be done or said at the moment drew Bodian forcibly into the NFIP's Typing Program, where he was to occupy a position of leadership which he did not relinquish until the NFIP ceased its activity on poliomyelitis.

Another prominent member of the Committee on Typing, but a differ-ent kind of personality, was Dr. Herbert A. Wenner. He was born in a small town in Pennsylvania in 1912 and received his medical degree in 1939 at the University of Rochester School of Medicine. He had planned

14. Bodian meanwhile had found time to accept the editorship of the *American Journal of Hygiene,* which had its headquarters in the Johns Hopkins School of Hygiene and Public Health, a position which he maintained from 1948 until 1957.

15. H. Howe and D. Bodian: *Neural Mechanisms in Poliomyelitis.* New York, Common-wealth Fund, 1942.

to go into pediatrics but had his ambitions in that direction cut short by an attack of tuberculosis, which, fortunate to say, turned out to be mild. As a result he was advised to go into medical rsearch, even though it is a naïve mistake to assume that a successful and effective career in medical research has any less frustration or hard work in it than goes into the practice of medicine. During the years 1942–46 Wenner had held fellowships in the Yale Poliomyelitis Study Unit and with the Johns Hopkins Poliomyelitis Group. In each place he was to endear himself to his colleagues and to demonstrate his ability as an independent worker. In fact, during this brief period of apprenticeship he had several published papers to his credit, on subjects ranging from clinical and statistical epidemiology to field- and benchwork in the poliovirus laboratory.

He joined the faculty of the University of Kansas Medical School in 1946 and became research professor of pediatrics in 1951 with headquarters in the Hixon Memorial Laboratory of this university, a position which he held with distinction up until his recent transfer to the University of Missouri.

Herbert Wenner was to prove an ideal member of the Committee on Typing, and once launched on this type of activity he pursued his interest in taxonomy avidly and productively. It was an example of the right man being chosen for the right job—and of both seeking each other. He was ready to jump into the Typing Program immediately, and he set such an example of quiet industry and meticulous work in sorting the various strains of poliovirus that it was enough to put to shame some previous attempts along these lines.

Herbert Wenner has followed in his subsequent career along channels which have taken him into investigations of other tribes of viruses, some neurotropic and some with different properties. All of them have presented familiar problems, although the agents were endowed with new names when the subfamilies of enteroviruses (which are much larger than the poliovirus family) swarmed onto the scene. Today he is the man to whom one turns when confronted with the bewildering intricacies of the many strains of Coxsackie and echoviruses and what their role might be in the matter of human infections.

Biographical sketches of Drs. Francis, Salk, and Sabin, who were also members of the Committee on Typing, will be taken up when it comes to discussions of their respective roles in the development and testing of poliovirus vaccines. As to the other two members of the committee, Drs. Gebhardt and Kessel, their histories will not be recounted, only because the mainstream of their subsequent interests has flowed in other directions since their early work on polioviruses.

I have dwelt on the Typing Program not only because it produced such a satisfying and definite answer but also because it was a milestone in the field of cooperative "research and development." It represented the first interuniversity venture in poliomyelitis research in which eight members of a committee, who directed four laboratories, pooled their brains and resources in the interest of a common problem. Three types of poliovirus had at last been established on a firm footing. It had taken an unconscionably long time—too long, it would seem—since Burnet and Macnamara had first pointed the way, in 1931.

A more significant feature was the emergence of the idea that other problems in poliomyelitis could be solved in this same manner. Thus the cooperative concept may be said to have been born as a result of the success of the Typing Program. It was felt that too long had the "fate of polio" rested upon individual whims of self-styled authorities. Dr. Harry Weaver, the NFIP's director of research, had no difficulty in deciding that what the "cause of polio" needed was *good direction.* The idea was firmly created that by long-term financial support of some of the major laboratories in the poliomyelitis field in the United States, the National Foundation could now climb into the driver's seat and assume a commanding position. This novel and revolutionary idea, whether good or bad, at least brought the foundation into a position of power to which it had long aspired but had never really achieved. Whatever previous plans the organization might have had, the success of the Typing Program provided a vision of future accomplishments to be implemented through its advisory committees and facilities. A major strategy for leading the fight against infantile paralysis to its ultimate conquest had begun, with Dr. Rivers as a commanding figure.

As a result, the foundation started something in this country: namely, the policy of directed interuniversity "research," an approach which depends mightily for success on at least two or three features: (1) the type of work involved; (2) dominant budgetary control in support of it; and (3) the degree to which universities could submit to it.

If the general principles of (1) *research* and (2) *development* are to be considered separately, and sometimes a division between them is impossible, the second type of activity (development) sometimes has a much better chance of success when farmed out to a group of cooperating laboratories; not so, the former. Exploratory research is one situation in which individual genius should be left to its own devices. These were lessons which the NFIP learned slowly. It might have been at an even slower pace had not Dr. Rivers been on hand to guide the foundation on these delicate points of policy in dealing with various research projects and the investigators who were going to direct them. But now I have anticipated my story.

CHAPTER 23

The Nose as a Portal of Entry?

After the Swedish team of clinical virologists had reported in 1912 that they had successfully isolated poliovirus not only from the throat but, what was more important, from intestinal excreta in a series of paralytic and nonparalytic cases, it would have seemed mandatory for other investigators to have repeated these observations regardless of doubts having been expressed about the validity of some of the results. Prior to this, in 1911, a futile attempt had been made by Rosenau and colleagues to transmit poliomyelitis to monkeys by inoculating them with nasal and pharyngeal secretions from eighteen human cases.[1] It was more than a pity that they were completely unsuccessful. Unfortunately Rosenau was to prove extraordinarily unlucky with his various ventures into clinical virology in the fields of both poliomyelitis and influenza, for his voice would have carried much weight.

It is not known how many similar efforts were made after 1912. At least one attempt at the Rockefeller Institute was reported by Flexner, Clark, and Fraser.[2] These authors stated that in 1913 they had succeeded in only a single instance in isolating poliovirus from the throat of the healthy parent of a child who had recently suffered from paralytic poliomyelitis. The virus that they recovered was active and virulent, and produced characteristic lesions in the monkey. It was a small contribution to the story, although it might have proved that the Swedes had at least been on the right track. However, strange to say, the major part of the Swedish results remained under a cloud for some twenty years, particularly the isolation of the virus from the intestinal tract, which after 1915 was not to be resurrected until the late 1930s. At least this type of clinical virology was not pursued at the Rockefeller Institute in subsequent years in spite of innumerable opportunities during the epidemic of 1916. A few efforts reported from other laboratories include one highly questionable positive result with oropharyngeal washings obtained in Boston in 1913;[3] Sawyer's

---

1. M. J. Rosenau, P. A. E. Sheppard, and H. L. Amoss: Anterior poliomyelitis; attempts to transmit the disease to monkeys by inoculation with the nasal, pharyngeal and buccal secretions of eighteen human cases. *Boston med. surg. J., 164*: 743, 1911.

2. S. Flexner, P. F. Clark, and F. R. Fraser: Epidemic poliomyelitis. Fourteenth note: passive human carriage of the virus of poliomyelitis. *J. Amer. med. Ass., 60*: 201, 1913.

3. W. P. Lucas and R. B. Osgood: Transmission experiments with the virus of poliomyelitis;

recovery of virus from intestinal washings in California in 1915;[4] and Taylor and Amoss' isolation from nasopharyngeal washings in Vermont in 1917.[5]

Reasons for the lack of interest in pursuing the cause of clinical virology at this crucial period in the history of the disease are not at all clear. Probably authorities considered that the case for the nasal portal of entry and for nasal carriers had been well established and henceforth need not be tested or disproved. As for the presence of the agent in intestinal excreta, it could represent virus from the nasopharynx which had been swallowed. And yet information on the conditions under which infective virus could be recovered from both nasopharyngeal and intestinal sites had barely been tapped. Countless timely questions might have been answered had suitable investigations been carried forward in the period between 1912 and 1930. Were the Swedes really in error in the bulk of their observations? What was the duration of the carrier state in convalescence? This point had a vital bearing on the duration of the quarantine period. What was the frequency and age distribution of so-called healthy carriers? Did they occur more frequently in infants? Did they occur more frequently in families in which one child had poliomyelitis or in those in which no one had been ill?

The technical problems involved in isolating virus from clinical specimens were admittedly difficult; but, more than likely, prevailing interpretations, emanating in large part from the Rockefeller Institute, were accepted as the authoritative word on the human disease, and it was a bold man indeed who offered contrary opinions. Several of the institute's staff members had pronounced the Swedish results as inconclusive and not to be taken seriously—and that was that. But fortunately, the small Research Laboratory of the State Board of Health of Vermont recognized the importance of continuing efforts to recover the virus from patients and, as a result, succeeded in outshining the larger, more important laboratories.

On June 1, 1917, poliomyelitis had broken out in Washington County, Vermont, and before the summer was over, 79 cases had occurred in a population of 45,000. The director of the Vermont Department of Health was still Dr. Caverly, who had maintained an active interest in poliomyelitis since the 1894 epidemic in his state. With customary alertness, he had been instrumental in securing the services of Dr. Amoss (from the Rockefeller Institute) with the view of trying to isolate poliovirus from some of the

finding the virus in the nasal secretion of a human carrier four months after the acute stage of a second attack of poliomyelitis. *J. Amer. med. Ass., 60*: 1611, 1913.

4. W. A. Sawyer: An epidemiological study of poliomyelitis. *Amer. J. trop. Dis., 3*: 164, 1915–16.

5. E. Taylor and H. L. Amoss: Carriage of the virus of poliomyelitis, with subsequent development of the infection, *J. exp. Med., 26*: 745–54, 1917.

cases. The opportunity presented itself when, early in the epidemic, a family with four children came under special observation because of a fatal case of paralytic poliomyelitis in the oldest child, aged 16. This boy had died on the fourth day of his disease. On the same day specimens were obtained by nasopharyngeal irrigation from two of the remaining children, Hazel, aged 13, who had remained well, and Everette, aged 10, who had experienced a one-day minor illness at the time of onset of the fatal case. An effort was made to obtain washings from the youngest child, Dwight, aged 7, but he proved refractory to this unpleasant procedure.

The original idea that Amoss and his assistant Taylor had was to detect the virus in the three apparently normal children in a family in which there had been a frank case. If washings from Everette, who had had the abortive attack, were positive, he might be classified as a "convalescent carrier"; while a positive result with specimens from Hazel, who had no sumptoms of illness, would indicate that she was a so-called healthy carrier. What happened was that virus was recovered from both of these children. Furthermore, an unexpected finding was in store for the investigators. Somewhat to their dismay, the child Dwight, from whom they had been unable to obtain washings, came down two days after the attempted nasopharyngeal irrigation with a moderately severe form of paralytic poliomyelitis, from which he recovered and for which he was treated with immune serum. Equally dismaying was that Hazel developed a mild attack five days after the irrigation. Thus the original idea of the tests, which was to determine whether "healthy" carriers existed within a family group, went completely awry when two children who had hitherto escaped significant illness contracted the disease. Taylor and Amoss had made a discovery: children actually harbored poliovirus in the nose and throat passages a few days before the disease appeared in recognizable form, but it was not the kind of discovery they had been looking for, and it was cold comfort to these two investigators.

Years afterward, Dr. Amoss, then a practicing physician in Greenwich, Connecticut, told me that he had been deeply concerned at the outcome of the tests, for when Hazel and Dwight came down with poliomyelitis, not only did it vitiate the avowed purpose of the experiment, but he had been continually haunted by the idea that the nasopharyngeal irrigations might have been instrumental in precipating the attacks of poliomyelitis which followed—attacks which might not have occurred had the irrigations not been done. This idea was based on the then accepted belief that poliovirus entered the human brain via the nose and the olfactory cranial nerves. Perhaps Dr. Amoss' reluctance to continue nasopharyngeal irrigations was subsequently imparted to others, and this may account for the many years which elapsed before the method was tried again. Had Taylor and Amoss known in 1917 that gargle washings and throat swabs were equally good sources of virus, or even better, had they considered using washings from the intestine—the best source—they would have been spared an immense amount of worry and, incidentally, would have made not only one but two discoveries. At the basis of their misinterpretation of the findings was a conviction that the pathway which the virus always followed was up the nose and through the brain into the spinal cord.

Ideas regarding the nasal portal of entry were already firmly entrenched in 1917. As early as 1910, Flexner and Lewis[6] had first suggested that poliovirus gained access to the central nervous system via the nasal mucosa. This was reasonable enough. It was in line with the recently discovered manner in which meningococci were supposed to produce meningococcal meningitis. Also it rested on experimental data on the pathogenesis of the disease in rhesus monkeys that were interpreted as incriminating the rich network of blood vessels, lymph channels, and tiny nerves just below the surface of the nasal mucosa and close to the brain. Further support for this notion was obtained from experiments in monkeys which Flexner and Clark performed in 1912.[7] In these tests, swabs containing poliovirus were introduced into the nose of the monkey and rubbed vigorously over the upper nasal mucous membrane; following this the virus could be detected in the olfactory nerves within 48 hours.[8] These results, which seemed to be convincing evidence, were obtained in highly artificial experiments using neuro-adapted strains. Nevertheless, on such observations Flexner based his interpretation that the virus gained ready access to the human brain from the nose. It was tacitly assumed that in the natural infection in man the virus traveled the same route as in the intranasally inoculated monkey.

Flexner and his associates had also confidently stated their belief that all or most poliovirus strains possessed a very special affinity for nervous tissue, as distinct from other tissues of the body. But they did not take into account that this neurotropism had been aided artificially by laboratory procedures.

The conclusions drawn by Flexner and his colleagues in these early years

6. S. Flexner and P. A. Lewis: Experimental epidemic poliomyelitis in monkeys. *J. exp. Med., 12*: 227, 1910.

In another article, published that same year, Flexner had occasion to say: "We are disposed to the view that the nasal mucosa serves not only as the portal of infection but as the path of elimination of the virus. . . ." S. Flexner: The contribution of experimental to human poliomyelitis. *Trans. Ass. Amer. Phycns, 25*: 108–30, 1910.

7. S. Flexner and P. F. Clark: A note on the mode of infection in epidemic poliomyelitis. *Proc. Soc. exp. Biol. Med. (N.Y.), 10*: 1, 1912–13.

8. The two olfactory nerves represent the first and most anteriorly placed pair of nerves that emanate from the brain. At their peripheral ends they terminate in bulbous swellings known as *olfactory bulbs*, from which delicate and tiny nerve fibrils extend down through a small perforated portion at the base of the skull, the cribriform plate, to terminate in the nasal mucosa.

were regarded as great progress toward an understanding of the pathogenesis of poliomyelitis. A start had been made, although obviously certain obscurities remained. For instance, there was the knotty question of how the lymphatic system could become so extensively involved at the onset

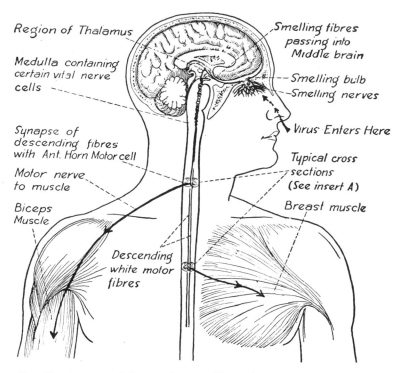

Region of Thalamus

Medulla containing certain vital nerve cells

Smelling fibres passing into Middle brain

Smelling bulb

Smelling nerves

Virus Enters Here

Synapse of descending fibres with Ant. Horn Motor cell

Motor nerve to muscle

Typical cross sections (See insert A)

Breast muscle

Biceps Muscle

Descending white motor fibres

Fig. 35. Anatomical diagram from an illustration by Draper (see n. 9) of the manner whereby the virus was supposed to enter the nose, pass through the "smelling nerves" into the "middle brain," and thence to the spinal cord. Reproduced by permission from Appleton-Century-Crofts, Div. of Meredith Corp.

of the human disease, as was evident from a general enlargement of lymph nodes, if this system had little or nothing to do with the pathogenesis of the infection.

Nevertheless, the views emanating from the Rockefeller Institute seemed so convincing that theory soon hardened into firm belief. Even after some twenty years, as late as 1935, the second edition of Draper's *Infantile Paralysis*[9] contained an illustration depicting a semisagittal section of the upper third of the human body (see fig. 35) indicating how a tuft of small delicate nerve fibers emanating from the olfactory nerves seemed to be ready and eager to absorb poliovirus and conduct it to the midbrain and thence to the spinal cord. So strong was this theory fixed in the minds of

9. G. Draper: *Infantile Paralysis*, 2nd ed. New York, Appleton-Century, 1935.

the medical profession that it imparted the erroneous idea that poliovirus had such an intimate and special tropism for nervous tissue that it became locked away in the cells of the brain and cord almost at once, at the very start of the acute disease, making it difficult of access to any form of therapy directed toward destroying the virus. This affected medical views on treatment as well as prophylaxis. So the theoretical experimentalists, like so many who have immured themselves in their laboratories before and since, drifted further and further away from the human disease in their attempts to use experiments in the monkey for interpretations of the disease in man. But even Draper, the model of an astute and well-trained clinician, had been led astray.

And yet, even before the year 1912, doubts were beginning to be expressed in some places, especially in Europe, that the nose was not the Achilles heel that it was supposed to be. Enough evidence had accumulated to permit the assumption that by the first few days of illness virus somehow had gained access to the body, probably through the oropharynx, and soon became widely distributed throughout the lymphatic system, although the way it got to the central nervous system still remained mysterious. Rissler, Medin, and Wickman all had an inkling of the generalized nature of the infection during its first hours or days.

Wickman had even concluded that the gastrointestinal route of infection was the more probable. And in Germany, Krause, after examining eight victims who had succumbed during an epidemic in Westphalia in 1909, agreed from pathological findings that the intestinal tract was the portal of entry.[10] Römer, in 1911, thought that the virus might enter the body through the nasopharynx or the intestinal tract or both. He believed this varied in different epidemics.

Others had straddled the fence. Although the authors of the monograph from the Hospital of the Rockefeller Institute were not ready to abandon Flexner's view, they called attention at this time (1912) to the swelling of the mesenteric lymph nodes and the spleen, concluding that such a general reaction meant to them that acute poliomyelitis was a *general infection* even though it especially affected the central nervous system. In the "Polio Bible" published in 1932[11] writers gave first priority to the nasal portal of entry but were quick to add that many felt there was evidence that the virus also gained access to the body by way of the digestive tract and pointed to an impressive list of authors, mostly from Scandinavia and other European countries. A late convert to the latter idea was Lawrence Smith of New York. In his series of 134 autopsies performed during the epidemic

10. P. Krause: Zur Kenntniss der westfalischen Epidemie von akuter Kinderlähmung. *Dtsch. med. Wschr., 35*: 1822, 1909.

11. *Poliomyelitis*. International Committee for the Study of Infantile Paralysis, Baltimore, Williams & Wilkins, 1932.

of 1931, he found evidence which prompted him to imply that the gastro-intestinal tract was probably the usual portal of entry of the infection.[12] However, no one except Kling, Levaditi, and associates had been able to contribute any impressive evidence for the presence of the virus in this site.

So in the early 1930s the direct nasal pathway of the virus was still the favored one, although Draper's whole experience and philosophy would seem to negate this idea. It was he who had emphasized the general and systemic nature of the early preparalytic stages of an acute poliomyelitis infection. And it was he who had stressed that the time to administer immune serum was in the preparalytic stage—before the central nervous system had been invaded.

One man who in the early years was definitely unsympathetic with the view that the nasal pathway was the important one was Dr. Montrose Burrows. In 1916, the year of the great epidemic, Burrows was resident pathologist at the Johns Hopkins Hospital, a position which Dr. Flexner had held some twenty-five years earlier. Burrows had spent the summer doing autopsies on fatal cases of poliomyelitis and had accumulated a wealth of data. Although he had had no experience with experimental poliomyelitis, he was convinced that the human disease was primarily a systemic one that involved the lymphatic system. This involvement was manifest by a general enlargement of lymph follicles and nodes, especially those in and adjacent to the intestinal tract, somewhat as Rissler had shown twenty years earlier and as Lawrence Smith was to do in 1931. Burrows claimed that only secondarily or accidentally did the virus penetrate beyond the lymphoid system to the central nervous system. He also recognized the fallacy of making deductions concerning the human disease from experiments in monkeys. He was particularly vehement in expressing his views on the pathogenesis of poliomyelitis to the class of medical students in pathology at the Johns Hopkins Medical School that he taught during the academic year of 1916–17—a class of which I happened to be a member. But his was a voice crying in the wilderness. He never got around to publishing these vigorous but unorthodox views until fifteen years later. If he had not waited so long to explain his theories and the lesions on which they were based, his contribution might have had some effect, and the cause might have been advanced by several years.

However, after this long delay Burrows understated his case about poliomyelitis by saying that "even now there is a tendency to class this disease as one primarily of the central nervous system rather than in the light of its true pathology." But he was still ahead of his time, even in 1931, in voicing the following belated sentiments:

12. Ibid., p. 258.

Too many deductions were being drawn from studies on monkeys in which the virus had been introduced directly into the brain or some site chosen by the operator, rather than from the clinical cases in which the natural routes of infection and spread of the disease could be followed more accurately.[13]

Regardless of whether poliomyelitis was considered to be a generalized systemic infection or not, the haggling over whether the virus got in through the nose or the mouth was not an inconsequential preoccupation. The nasal portal implied that the virus was circulating in the air and was breathed in, perhaps in the form of droplets, similar to the manner in which influenza is spread. The oral portal, on the other hand, carried the idea that the virus was swallowed or found its way into the mouth on children's fingers. In this way the differences had considerable significance, for in prevaccinal days ideas about the prevention of poliomyelitis were firmly based on notions as to how the disease was spread. Indeed, infection by way of the alimentary tract was the ultimate characteristic on which the oral vaccine was based.

As a case in point were the futile attempts to block the nasal route of virus invasion with chemicals applied to the mucous membranes of the nose, a method which had been enthusiastically taken up during the period of 1935–38. The suggestion was first advanced in 1935 by Armstrong and Harrison that monkeys might be protected from experimental poliomyelitis following intranasal instillation of the virus if the nasal passages were first treated with certain chemicals such as alum.[14] Other investigators promptly followed suit using zinc sulfate or picric acid and eventually little doubt remained that this prophylactic measure was effective in the *experimental disease* when the virus was introduced intranasally. It was thus inevitable that this procedure should be proposed as a means of preventing poliomyelitis in man.[15] And by 1937 a nasal spray containing an astringent solution as a prophylactic measure had strong support, notably from Schultz and Gebhardt of California[16] and Dr. Max Peet of the Department of Neurosurgery of the University of Michigan. But no less of an authority than Thomas M. Rivers of the Hospital of the Rockefeller Institute was also behind the idea and is quoted by *Time Magazine* as saying: "If I had a child in an area where poliomyelitis appeared, I would

13. M. T. Burrows: Is poliomyelitis a disease of the lymphatic system? *Arch. intern. Med.,* *48*: 33–50, 1931.

14. C. Armstrong and W. T. Harrison: Prevention of intranasally-inoculated poliomyelitis of monkeys by instillation of alum into the nostrils. *Publ. Hlth Rep. (Wash.),* *50*: 725–30, 1935.

15. C. Armstrong: Experience with the picric acid-alum spray in the prevention of poliomyelitis in Alabama, 1936. *Amer. J. Publ. Hlth,* *27*: 103, 1937.

16. E. W. Schultz and L. P. Gebhardt: Zinc sulphate prophylaxis in poliomyelitis. *J. Amer. med. Ass.,* *108*: 2182, 1937.

take my child to a good otolaryngologist and ask him to apply the spray in the manner set forth by Dr. Peet."[17]

An early opportunity to test the zinc sulfate spray, known as the "Schultz-Peet prophylactic," soon arose when an epidemic of poliomyelitis occurred in 1937 in Toronto, Canada. The nasal spray project, under the auspices of the University of Michigan, was promptly launched in the Toronto epidemic, and as promptly failed.[18] It was another demonstration that the problem of preventing human poliomyelitis was not to be easily solved on the basis of evidence deduced from the experimental disease in the rhesus monkey.

Added to other evidence from several directions, the experience in Toronto aroused uneasiness about the whole hypothesis of a nasal portal of entry in man. Some years before, in 1929, Kling and his colleagues at the Pasteur Institute had claimed that cynomolgus monkeys could be infected by the alimentary route,[19] although their opponents raised the objection that the possibility of nasal contamination had not been adequately excluded. But two years later, in 1931, the same group brought further evidence to bear on this point and definitely succeeded in inducing paralytic poliomyelitis in cynomolgus monkeys by feeding the virus to them, an observation which Saddington in the United States was able to confirm in 1932.[20] Unfortunately, advantage was not taken of this discovery for another six or seven years, perhaps because of Saddington's untimely death. For in spite of the growing evidence pointing to the alimentary tract as a portal of entry, public opinion favoring the nasal route in the human disease was at an all-time high in the early and mid-1930s and proving to be well-nigh irreversible.

By 1936, however, Sabin and Olitsky, working in the laboratories of the Rockefeller Institute, which had heretofore been a stronghold of the opposite camp, had shown that in those monkeys succumbing to poliomyelitis after nasal instillation of the virus, histological lesions in the olfactory apparatus were demonstrable, but these were *not* present when the virus had been administered intracerebrally.[21] The point is graphically illustrated

17. *Time Magazine*. Sept. 6, 1937.

18. F. F. Tisdall, A. Brown, R. D. deFries, M. A. Ross, and A. H. Sellers: Zinc sulphate nasal spray in the prophylaxis of poliomyelitis; observations of a group of 4,713 children age 3–10 years, during an epidemic in Toronto. *Canad. publ. Hlth J.*, *28*: 523, 1937.

19. C. Kling, C. Levaditi, and P. Lépine: La pénétration du virus poliomyélitique à travers la muqueuse du tube digestif chez le singe et sa conservation dans l'eau. *Bull. Acad. Méd. (Paris)*, *102*: 158, 1929.

20. R. S. Saddington: An intravascular lesion in poliomyelitis induced by feeding in *Macacus cynomolgus*. *Proc. Soc. exp. Biol. Med. (N.Y.)*, *29*: 838, 1932.

21. A. B. Sabin and P. K. Olitsky: Influence of pathway of infection on pathology of olfactory bulbs in experimental poliomyelitis. *Proc. Soc. exp. Biol. Med. (N.Y.)*, *35*: 300–01, 1936; ibid., The olfactory bulbs in experimental poliomyelitis. *J. Amer. med. Ass.*, *108*: 21–24, 1937; A. B. Sabin: The olfactory bulbs in human poliomyelitis. *Amer. J. Dis. Child.*, *60*: 1313–18, 1940.

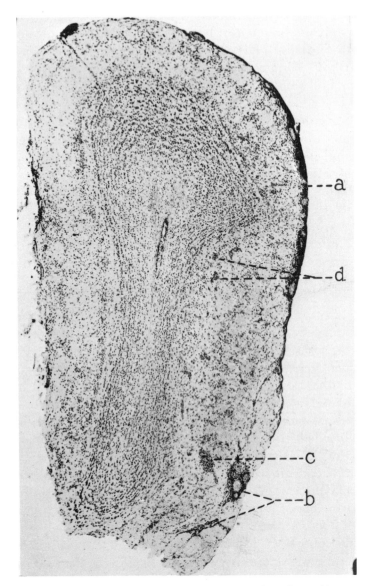

FIG. 36. Low-power photomicrograph of a section of an olfactory bulb from a monkey succumbing 8 days after nasal instillation of poliovirus. Note small lesions at locations a, b, c, and d (from Sabin and Ward, n. 23, by permission).

in figure 36 from a photograph taken from one of Sabin's papers that demonstrates small lesions in the olfactory bulb of a monkey after intra-nasal inoculation of the virus.

Among other pathologists, L. W. Smith, whose extensive autopsy studies performed on human cases during the epidemic of 1931 were mentioned earlier, had already reported on the surprisingly slight involvement of the olfactory apparatus in the human disease.[22] Sabin and Olitsky further emphasized that the presence of lesions in the olfactory bulbs of monkeys was simply a reflection of the intranasal route of inoculation; and in a later study (1940) Sabin raised the question whether absence of lesions in the olfactory bulbs did not indicate absence of virus in these structures. This would be strong evidence against the nasal portal of entry of the virus in man. Sabin promptly answered his own question by demonstrating (in collaboration with Robert Ward) that in six fatal human cases, tests for virus in the olfactory bulbs all proved negative.[23] This was another in the long series of telling observations, begun in his student days in 1931, that Dr. Sabin was to make in the field of poliomyelitis.

By the late 1930s a considerable degree of disenchantment had developed in some quarters with the idea that a similarity existed between the pathogenesis of experimental poliomyelitis induced by intranasal inoculation of the rhesus monkey and the natural disease in man. Added to this was the chance finding by Howe and Bodian of the Johns Hopkins School of Hygiene of a 1935 report by Müller, describing spontaneous poliomyelitis in two chimpanzees in a children's zoo in Cologne, Germany. The observation suggested to them that this primate relative of man might possess a greater susceptibility to the disease than did monkeys of several species. As mentioned previously, in a series of experiments begun in 1939, Howe and Bodian established the much greater ease with which the chimpanzee could be infected by feeding the virus as compared with other primates, even cynomolgus monkeys. And in one of their experiments they not only succeeded in excluding the possibility of contamination of the olfactory portal but also presented added evidence that the clinical and pathological picture after experimental infection by the oral route closely resembled that observed in man.[24]

Thus the concept of infection via the olfactory pathway, vaguely linked to "droplet infection," was at long last severely challenged. An alternate, the oral-alimentary tract portal of entry was not only supported by persuasive experimental data but also, after 1938, by a growing body of circumstantial evidence including the recovery of poliovirus from fecal excreta of patients with the acute and subacute disease.

An explanation of this long and devious path that eventually arrived

22. J. F. Landon and L. W. Smith: *Poliomyelitis; A Handbook for Physicians and Medical Students Based on a Study of the 1931 Epidemic in New York City.* New York, Macmillan, 1934, p. 50.

23. A. B. Sabin and R. Ward: The natural history of human poliomyelitis; I. Distribution of virus in nervous and non-nervous tissues. *J. exp. Med., 73*: 771, 1941.

24. H. A. Howe and D. Bodian: Poliomyelitis in the chimpanzee; a clinical pathological study. *Bull. Johns Hopk. Hosp., 69*: 149–81, 1941.

at the truth involves a number of factors.[25] For one thing, the experimental animal first used extensively was the wrong one, for the rhesus monkey is virtually insusceptible to infection by the alimentary route. This had led experimentalists down the wrong road. Another point was that a conscious and prolonged effort seems to have been made on this side of the Atlantic to repudiate the Scandinavian observations that poliovirus could be found in intestinal washings from children suffering from the acute infection. This was a grievous error, compounded by the tendency to accept dogmatically the voice of authority which emanated from the Rockefeller Institute, regardless of the facts in the case.

It is not to be presumed, however, that an idea of thirty-years standing was relinquished with alacrity. Physicians were especially loathe to reverse themselves on the conviction that poliovirus entered through the nose. It was a view they had been explaining to patients for many years, and it had been taught in medical schools for a generation. However, after years of error the record was finally set straight—for most authorities at least.[26] Actually, the correct interpretation of the pathogenesis of the human disease became the basis of an idea that an effective poliovirus vaccine could be administered orally, an idea born in the 1940s and eventually implemented in the United States in the late 1950s.

25. I am indebted to both Dr. Albert B. Sabin of Cincinnati and David Bodian of Baltimore for their explanations of the long period during which the nasal portal of entry theory prevailed.

26. This comment is made advisedly, for the booklet issued by the American Public Health Ass. on the "Control of Communicable Disease in Man," edition of 1945, contained the statement that the virus enters the body by way of the "nose and mouth."

Also, in a personal conversation held as late as 1946 with Dr. Haven Emerson, a long-time authority on poliomyelitis, I found he was still unconvinced that the nasal portal of entry was not the common one.

CHAPTER 24

Ill-Fated Vaccine Trials of 1935

Almost from the time that acute poliomyelitis was first recognized as a distinct disease it became apparent that one attack was sufficient to confer immunity; second paralytic attacks very seldom occurred. This observation was of little practical value in previral days, but when the virus was discovered the idea of prevention through artificial immunization of some sort was immediately and avidly seized upon. It was *the* logical approach considering the success achieved by similar methods in other human viral diseases such as smallpox and apparently—rabies.

In the first experiments and for the next twenty-five years, attempts were made to stimulate immunity in monkeys by the subcutaneous injection of antigens that consisted of emulsions of ground-up monkey spinal cord containing live, virulent, untreated poliovirus. Infected monkey cord was the only available source of the virus—and parenteral injections the only route of administration which was used. Emulsions containing live virus were given in various dilutions, which were injected (usually into or under the skin) in several small doses over a period lasting a few weeks to a few months. If the animal survived this procedure, its immunity was tested by a drastic challenge in the form of an injection of virulent poliovirus into the brain, using a dose which would ordinarily produce paralysis in a nonimmunized animal. If the monkey remained well and withstood this procedure, it was concluded that immunity had indeed been established.

Flexner and Lewis,[1] in 1910, were the first to induce active immunity[2] in monkeys by this method, but the results were irregular and the technique was risky. Others, in 1911, did not meet with such success, not only because an occasional "immunized" animal succumbed when challenged but also because difficulty was encountered in keeping the monkeys alive during the long period of immunization.

Thomsen in Denmark probably did the most significant early work in this field in 1913–14.[3] He achieved success only by using gradually in-

---

1. S. Flexner and P. A. Lewis: Experimental poliomyelitis in monkeys. Seventh and eighth notes. *J. Amer. med. Ass., 54*: 1780, 1910; and *55*: 662, 1910.

2. *Active immunity* signifies an immunity induced by the host's response to a natural infection or to artificial immunization. Passive immunity, in contrast, refers to the transfer of serum antibody from one host to another for the purpose of transient protection.

3. O. Thomsen: Experimentelle Arbeiten über Poliomyelitis. *Berl. klin. Wschr., 51*: 309, 1914.

creasing doses of virus at intervals of not less than a week and over a period which generally lasted two months. Almost all animals so immunized resisted intracerebral challenge with virulent virus.

Ten years later Flexner and Amoss, working with a strain of poliovirus that as a rule produced a nonfatal form of the experimental disease, found that the recovered monkeys uniformly resisted subsequent inoculations of a more virulent strain. However, immunization of monkeys using any live poliovirus proved too risky, especially when administered in the usual manner—parenteral injections into the muscles or under the skin. Had another species of monkey, *Macaca cynomolgus*, been considered in the 1920s and had the poliovirus been administered orally instead of parenterally, the story might have been very different.

During the period 1910–14, Römer, Flexner and Lewis, Leiner and von Wiesner, and Levaditi, finding their trials with live poliovirus to be unsuccessful, turned attention to the use of inactivated or partially inactivated virus to see what luck they might have with this technique. Since it had already been discovered that completely killed poliovirus had no immunizing power whatsoever, virus which had been only partially killed (inactivated by physical or chemical methods) was tried. Such antigens had been successfully employed in immunization against bacterial infections and therefore seemed to be the ones with the most promise. First on the list was the use of heat, applied at a temperature of 56° C for 30 minutes or an hour, a treatment which had proven sufficient to destroy the virulence of typhoid bacilli without at the same time destroying antigenicity and therefore immunizing power.

So, taking a leaf from the bacteriologist's book, virologists began to use this method with poliovirus as early as 1910. Unfortunately, although such heat-inactivated virus proved harmless enough when injected into monkeys, it was relatively ineffective in producing immunity. This was a disappointment to several teams of workers, among them Flexner and Lewis, and Landsteiner and Levaditi.

In the same year Römer and Joseph found that poliovirus which had been subjected to heat of a lower degree (45°C) did have immunizing power when given subcutaneously but unfortunately was still unsafe to use, for several of the monkeys developed paralysis during the process of immunization.[4] Levaditi and Landsteiner soon confirmed these results. They split the difference between 45° and 55° and settled on 50° C as the correct temperature but still had only partial success. They felt that the modification of the virus induced by heat was probably quantitative in its effect rather than qualitative. In any event the heat inactivation of poliovirus was given up.

4. P. H. Römer and K. Joseph: Noch einige Experimente zur Poliomyelitis-frage. *Münch. med. Wschr.,* *57*: 2685, 1910.

The use of poliovirus weakened by chemical rather than physical means was also tried in those early days. Kraus in Germany used virus which had been treated with small concentrations of phenol (carbolic acid) and achieved some success, although he worked with a very small number of monkeys.[5] He also made the bold suggestion that this method might be used for prophylactic vaccination in man! Fortunately, due to the outbreak of World War I, Kraus was unable to carry out this suggestion. It was twenty years later, in 1930–31, before he took up his investigations again, and this time he was much more cautious in his pronouncements. In 1927 Aycock and Kagan had also tried phenolized vaccines in monkeys and found them wanting.

Inactivation of the virus by formalin was attempted for the first time by Römer in Germany as early as 1911, but without success.[6] A number of other chemicals was tried, including aluminum hydroxide and a combination of virus plus immune serum. Similar efforts were continued spasmodically in the ensuing twenty years, by Aycock, Rhoads, Olitsky, Cox, and others, but all of these attempts, using crude techniques, turned out to be disappointing. Immunization against poliomyelitis, after enjoying an initial burst of enthusiasm, appeared to require an infinite amount of experimentation, time, expense, and labor. Through it all, however, the principle still held that the ideal way to attack poliomyelitis was prevention through vaccination. It was to take long years for the dream to become a reality.

In the early 1930s two new personalities arrived on the scene, and there was a sudden reawakening of interest not only in experimental immunization against poliomyelitis but even in vaccine trials in man. The first of these men was Dr. Maurice Brodie. He had started his experiments on monkeys in Montreal, shortly after he had graduated from medical school. He first used subinfective doses of live virus, but finding this method unsuccessful, as others had before him, he turned to other practices, such as mixing live poliovirus with hyperimmune serum as a method of inactivation without destroying antigenicity. Rhoads at the Rockefeller Institute had tried this approach the year before, but although it had been used successfully in toxin-antitoxin injections which could immunize man against diphtheria, it did not work for poliomyelitis. So Brodie began to experiment with such inactivating agents as phenol and formalin.[7] His early reports had the distinction of being accepted for publication by the

5. R. Kraus: Ueber das Virus der Poliomyelitis acuta, zugleich ein Beitrag zur Frage der Schutzimpfung. *Wien. klin. Wschr., 23*: 233, 1910.

6. P. H. Römer: *Die epidemische Kinderlähmung (Heine-Medinsche Krankheit)*. Berlin, Springer, 1911, p. 49.

7. M. Brodie and A. Goldbloom: Active immunization against poliomyelitis in monkeys. *J. exp. Med., 53*: 885, 1931; M. Brodie: Active immunization against poliomyelitis. *J. exp. Med., 56*: 493, 1932.

Journal of Experimental Medicine in 1931, which was tantamount to scientific approval of the investigations. Shortly thereafter Brodie moved from Montreal to New York City, where he became associated with the staff of Dr. W. H. Park's City Health Laboratory and with New York University and the Bellevue Hospital Medical School.

The antigen that Dr. Brodie used in his animal experiments consisted of a 10 percent emulsion of infected monkey spinal cord.[8] He eventually arrived, through a process of trial and error, at formalin as the optimal inactivating agent, a method which had been given up by Römer some twenty years previously as unsuccessful. Brodie succeeded where others had failed. He reported on the successful immunization of two groups of rhesus monkeys (numbering 12 and 8) with either one or two intracutaneous inoculations of formalinized vaccine. He maintained that his results constituted sufficient evidence that "definite immunity could be developed against the virus of poliomyelitis using virus rendered non-infective by formalin."[9] This statement, as it turned out in later years, was to be of major significance and not far off the beam. But Brodie acted on it far too precipitously by rushing into human vaccination too soon. His haste was attributable in part to his desire to be ahead of his competitor in the field, Dr. John A. Kolmer of Philadelphia, who was also championing a poliovirus vaccine at the time. Otherwise Brodie would not have taken the risks which he did by barging into a program involving the immunization of 3,000 children, using a vaccine which had been tried on only 20 monkeys. Nevertheless in his next paper,[10] which was published six months later, he described how after trying out his immunizing methods on adult volunteers, who must have sustained very little risk as they no doubt already possessed specific antibodies and were therefore immune, he proceeded to inoculate 12 children between the ages of 1 and 6 with either one or two intracutaneous doses of his vaccine. To his delight all the children showed a rise of neutralizing antibody. Eight months later Brodie and Park were able to report that "formalin inactivated virus is probably a perfectly safe vaccine inasmuch as no harmful effects have developed after more than 3,000 inoculations."[11] This was a brash statement. Brodie had no doubt been driven by a fierce competitive urge to give his vaccine what

8. Up to this time and for many years thereafter the only source of poliovirus consisted of an emulsion of the spinal cords of monkeys that had succumbed or had been sacrificed during an experimental infection.

9. M. Brodie: Active immunization in monkeys against poliomyelitis with germicidally inactivated virus. *Science*, 79: 594–95, 1934. Brodie's investigations were supported by the New York Foundation and the Rockefeller Foundation.

10. M. Brodie: Active immunization of children against poliomyelitis with formalin inactivated virus suspension. *Proc. Soc. exp. Biol. Med. (N.Y.)*, 32: 300–02, 1934.

11. M. Brodie and W. H. Park: Active immunization against poliomyelitis, *N.Y. St. J. Med.*, 35: 815, 1935; *J. Amer. med. Ass.*, 105: 10: 9, 1935.

was considered as "good" a trial as possible, but on the other hand he may have been egged on by Dr. Park, who was never one to let grass grow under his feet, especially when either a therapeutic or prophylactic measure was involved. In any event, it has always been difficult for me to ascertain exactly what happened during the Brodie-Park vaccine trials of 1935. But something went wrong—and Brodie's vaccine was never used again.

Immediately after this episode, Dr. Rivers of the Rockefeller Institute addressed two meetings of the American Public Health Association, the first in Milwaukee in October and the second one in St. Louis in November. Rivers was apt to speak up at meetings in a forthright manner, and his voice carried a great deal of weight. He took both Brodie and Kolmer to task in his presentations. He mentioned that in the Brodie trial it was more than likely that there had been postvaccinal (vaccine-induced) cases of poliomyelitis. And yet he said that actually no case of vaccine-induced poliomyelitis had as yet been identified, nor could he find "any evidence for or against the efficiency of [the] vaccine."[12] Years later, Rivers quoted Norman Topping (who had been in California at the time the vaccine trial was conducted there) as saying that "some of the children who received the Park-Brodie vaccine could have come down with polio as a result of the vaccine."[13] Also, in 1935 Rivers did not happen to have a particularly high opinion of formalin as a method for inactivating poliovirus, saying that others had used this method "before Brodie and had found results so discouraging that the matter was not pursued." He went on: "There is one fact that must be held in mind. It is that the virus of poliomyelitis, either active or inactive acts as though it was a poor antigen." (See n. 12.) Rivers was distinctly in error here on this "one fact." Within a year, poliovirus inactivated by formalin was being used in monkeys, not only to induce solid immunity but also for the production of a supply of hyperimmune serum. And eventually, formalin inactivation of poliovirus did prove to be the method of choice for a killed vaccine. So Rivers had been wrong in his altogether too sweeping condemnation of the Brodie-Park vaccine.

The Kolmer vaccine, which had been widely used in that same summer (1935), was a different matter. Dr. John A. Kolmer of Philadelphia was a quiet, unassuming, earnest, little man who preferred to spend his energies less on theory than in recording the results of his efforts at the laboratory bench.[14] He was particularly interested in practical bacteriologic problems

12. T. M. Rivers: Immunity in virus diseases with particular reference to poliomyelitis. *Amer. J. publ. Hlth, 26*: 136–42, 1936.

13. S. Benison: *Tom Rivers; Reflections on a Life in Medicine and Science.* Cambridge, Mass., MIT Press, 1967, pp. 186 and 190.

14. As a member of a small professional club composed largely of laboratory directors of Philadelphia hospitals in the 1920s, I got to know Dr. Kolmer quite well, long before he had any ambitions as a champion of a poliovirus vaccine. He recounted to me with great serious-

and immunological techniques such as the complement-fixation test for syphilis, generally known as the Wassermann test. Soon after graduating from the Medical School of the University of Pennsylvania in 1908, Kolmer became the pathologist to the Philadelphia Hospital for Contagious Diseases and shortly afterward joined the staff of a private laboratory in Philadelphia known as the Dermatological Research Laboratory. In 1939 this became part of the Medical School of Temple University with Dr. Kolmer as professor of medicine and director of the institute, which subsequently was named the Institute of Public Health and Preventive Medicine.[15] During his entire professional life John Kolmer displayed an amazing capacity for continued and prolonged activity, not only in the laboratory but as a prolific writer. He turned out more than 600 articles and wrote numerous successful textbooks, largely on laboratory techniques, which went through repeated editions.

Philadelphia had suffered a severe epidemic of poliomyelitis in 1932, and it was at this point that Kolmer began his work in an effort to deal chemotherapeutically with the acute disease. He also tried to infect small animals such as rabbits, guinea pigs, and mice with poliovirus. In these two ventures he was unsuccessful, but his appetite had been whetted, and in the following year he tried his luck at immunization. Starting out with ideas different from Brodie's, his view was that a killed virus vaccine was less likely to be effective in producing immunity than one containing living virus. He therefore decided to use live but slightly attenuated virus. In fact, he was the first to apply the term *attenuated* in connection with poliomyelitis vaccines in the sense in which it was to come into general use subsequently. But his method of attenuation was distinctly novel. In the first place he had convinced himself that strains of poliovirus then in common use in experimental work had become materially altered by having been continuously passed in monkeys. As a result, or so he claimed, they had become "of greatly reduced infectivity for human beings." But he also compromised in the preparation of his *live* vaccine by exposing a 4 percent emulsion of infected monkey spinal cord to a 1 percent concentration of sodium ricineolate, a soaplike substance that he claimed pro-

---

ness that during the revision of his numerous textbooks on clinical laboratory methods he was accustomed, night after night, to awaken at half-past three in the morning, never later than four o'clock, and work through until breakfast time. Then he would go through the normal day's work at the laboratory. Apparently, long hours of work never bothered him.

15. This laboratory, founded shortly before World War I, had a curious history. During the war the supply of the chemotherapeutic drug developed by Ehrlich for the treatment of syphilis, "606" (or Salvarsan), had been cut off, and the drug became unavailable in the United States. So the Dermatological Research Laboratories of Philadelphia as part of the Institute of Cutaneous Medicine took over the task of preparing Salvarsan and soon became the sole source of its supply, not only for the U.S. armed forces but also for the civilian population. This saved the government considerable sums of money. Profits from the sale of the drug, together with some other funds, were used to keep the Institute of Cutaneous Medicine running.

vided slight inactivation of the virus. In addition the emulsion was subjected to various other technical procedures. Anyway the race was on between Brodie and Kolmer as to which of their respective vaccines was to prove superior. Competition in this matter should not have been a factor which played a vital role; nevertheless it usually is and certainly was in this particular instance.

The experimental information which Kolmer and his associate, Miss A. Rule, amassed was published in a long series of papers that was summarized in one submitted for publication early in 1935. The immunizing procedure had been tried first on 42 monkeys, then on 2 adults including himself, then on his 2 children, aged 11 and 15, and following this on 22 other children. Presently, he was able to state:

> I believe, therefore, that sterile vaccine carrying 4 percent of very finely divided remote monkey passage spinal cord is safe by subcutaneous injection for both monkeys and human beings after treatment with 50 percent glycerol for one week and 1 percent sodium ricinoleate and 1:80,000 phenyl mercury nitrate at 37°C. for twenty-four hours followed by from ten to fourteen days in a refrigerator at 12° to 16°C.[16]

This vaccine, which some said was a veritable witch's brew, administered in 3 doses at stated intervals, was the preparation which Kolmer felt safe in distributing to the medical profession during the summer of 1935.

In a footnote obviously written after the paper had been submitted for publication and before it was set up in final proof, Dr. Kolmer stated that since January of 1935 some thousands of children had been given the vaccine.[17] It was also mentioned in a footnote that there had been 10 instances of poliomyelitis developing shortly after administration of one or two doses. This suggested a rate of vaccine-associated poliomyelitis cases which may have been as high as 1 per 1,000. Considering that paralytic poliomyelitis was not epidemic in any of the localities at the time the vaccine was given, this was an ominous sign. The day of reckoning for Kolmer and Brodie and their premature vaccine trials was bound to come, and it came swiftly.

At the meeting of the Southern Branch of the American Public Health Association held in St. Louis in November 1935, Rivers and Leake went out to discuss the safety of the Kolmer and Park-Brodie vaccines, prepared

---

16. J. A. Kolmer: Susceptibility and immunity in relation to vaccination in acute anterior poliomyelitis. *J. Amer. med. Ass., 105*: 1956–62, 1935.

17. During the first half or so of 1935, Dr. Kolmer's institute had distributed 12,812 doses of the vaccine in amounts of 0.5 cc each to 582 physicians in 36 states; and the William S. Merrell Company of Cincinnati had distributed 8,910 cc to 137 physicians. Altogether it might seem that many thousands of children received the vaccine.

to do battle. This time, Dr. Rivers, with all of his bluntness and honesty, was not above indulging in certain pyrotechnics. He took Dr. Kolmer to task for basing his claim for the safety of his vaccine on the fact that it had been prepared from a strain of *remote monkey passage* poliomyelitis virus that had been partially inactivated by the chemicals mentioned above. And he went on to state that in view of the resulting cases of poliomyelitis, some of them fatal, which had apparently been due to the vaccine, it was essential that Kolmer show definitely that his vaccine was safe (see n. 12).

Also at this meeting Dr. James P. Leake of the U.S. Public Health Service is recorded as having made severely critical statements directed against Kolmer. The published version of his remarks is presumably watered down. After mentioning 12 cases, 6 of them fatal, Dr. Leake went on to say:

> Paralytic poliomyelitis was not epidemic in any of the localities at the time of the occurrence of these cases. . . . The likelihood of whole series of cases having occurred through natural causes is extremely small. Although any one of these cases may have been entirely unconnected with the vaccine the implication of the series as a whole is clear.[18]

This criticism and these admonitions were enough to call a halt on both vaccines. Enthusiasm quickly drained away, and the disastrous results of these early efforts were sufficient to dampen any further attempts to immunize man for a dozen or more years. At the time, this episode was believed to be a tragedy of the first magnitude, yet in the light of subsequent experiences it would appear that the Brodie-Park results had been blown up out of all proportion. Despite an unfortunate outcome, the roots of Brodie's ideas at least had some truth in them. True, the mistakes made by the two investigators were numerous. The crude, nonquantitative methods used in virus inactivation might be described as "kitchen chemistry." The substrate monkey spinal cord was far from ideal, and in fact it was subsequently shown that the continued injection of such material is a dangerous procedure that occasionally results in a characteristic type of encephalitis. One of the most glaring errors committed by both investigators was the total disregard of any antigenic differences between strains of polioviruses, although by 1934–35 there was plenty of evidence on this score, beginning with the observations of Burnet and Macnamara in 1931. Finally, to rush into human trials on the basis of results in so few monkeys (Brodie, 20; Kolmer, 42) was completely unwarranted. The impact of the whole episode on the scientific world was such that as a result

18. J. P. Leake: Poliomyelitis following vaccination against this disease. *J. Amer. med. Ass.,* *105*: 2152, 1935.

a wave of revulsion against human vaccination attempts in poliomyelitis took place that lasted many years. As one of those who bore the brunt of this wave, Kolmer is quoted (see n.13) as having said at the meeting in St. Louis in November 1935, "Gentlemen, this is one time I wish the floor would open up and swallow me."

Thus the pressures of scientific rivalry, "the strife of science" as Pasteur put it, plus a sense of urgency to produce a vaccine which would prevent a crippling disease and save lives combined to drive two scientists into premature human trials of methods based on inadequate experimental data. Yet when human vaccination was taken up once again some twenty years later, when far more was known about the subject, even then unfortunate accidents occurred. Indeed such accidents are very prone to happen. In the case of the Salk-type vaccine, which also contained poliovirus inactivated by formalin (as Brodie had tried to use), "the Cutter incident" that followed was of many times the magnitude of the accident which occurred as a result of the Brodie and Kolmer trials. But in the case of Salk-type vaccine, the circumstances were different. The Brodie-Park and Kolmer vaccines had been launched with a degree of ignorance which was unwarranted; the Salk-type vaccine program had been undertaken when there had been infinitely more knowledge about the problem. Furthermore, the Salk-type vaccine had been licensed by the Public Health Service, and powerful groups including a vaccine committee made up of prominent scientists, public health workers, and a benevolent organization, the National Foundation for Infantile Paralysis, were backing the show, so in this instance hostile words and castigations against guilty individuals were less in order. Still later, in the case of the Sabin attenuated vaccine, the occasional vaccine-associated cases of poliomyelitis, although extremely rare, were enough to exert quite a sobering effect upon the committees charged with the responsibility of guaranteeing the safety of this product. But in 1935 a vaccine did not have to undergo the lengthy process of being approved and licensed by the U.S. Public Health Service. The individual promoters of any such preparations were the only ones who had to bear full responsibility for the safety of their product for human use.

Fortunately, in the aftermath of the ill-fated vaccine trials of 1935, Dr. Kolmer weathered the storm and took up the threads of his usual work. Apparently the episode did not seriously interfere with either his career or the flow of articles which emanated from his laboratory, some of them on poliomyelitis. Nevertheless in 1938, in describing the present status of methods for the prevention of poliomyelitis, he intimated that vaccines containing active virus were too dangerous for human beings. Actually, in an obituary note on Dr. Kolmer in 1964[19] his biographer even wrote that

19. L. Tuft: Memoir to John Albert Kolmer, 1886–1962. *Trans. Coll. Phycns Philad., 32:* 49–51, 1964.

he was far ahead of his time in anticipating Dr. Sabin in the latter's attempts to produce attenuated strains of poliovirus!

To poor Brodie, on the other hand, failure was a crushing blow. During the early days of his experimental work on immunization everything had seemed to be going well. He had received many flattering offers from universities as well as opportunities to serve on the staffs of prominent drug houses. But after 1935 such offers ceased abruptly, and Brodie was hard put to find a place to work. Eventually he accepted a minor position in Michigan. He died shortly after accepting this post. It is alleged that he took his own life—a tragic end for one who had started out with such high hopes. After all, he had almost succeeded in a good cause and was at least on the right track in choosing formalin to inactivate the virus. His work on adapting poliovirus to mice seemed equally hopeful.[20] In fact, had he lived, he would have seen himself partially vindicated on two counts. The story of poliomyelitis has no dearth of tragic episodes of this nature.

The events of 1935 cut more deeply into progress in the immunization of man against poliomyelitis than most people realized at the time. It put an immediate stop to human vaccine trials that was to last for more than fifteen years—so dramatically and traumatically had the research programs of a whole generation of investigators on the immunization problem been jolted. True, World War II intervened, and this interrupted many investigations both in the United States and Europe, but the subject of human vaccination had received such a blow that attempts to reopen it in the decade following 1935 would have been regarded with horror. Even after eleven years, immunologists had hardly yet recovered from their phobia of vaccine trials in man. At a meeting held in September 1946, called at the instigation of the National Foundation for Infantile Paralysis to discuss mechanisms of immunity in poliomyelitis, a report was given by Isabel Morgan of the Johns Hopkins School of Hygiene on a progress in orthodox methods of immunizing monkeys. This was received with acclaim. Yet one of the participants at the meeting said:

> The time has come to find out what happens in man; to study his immune reactions, and to get on with new attempts to produce artificial evidence of immunity in man.[21]

At this, a veritable shudder went round the room—and the subject was im-

20. Among other failings that these two vaccines had was the practically insoluble problem of how to procure an adequate supply of monkey spinal cord material. If the demand were to be great, it would have required a colossal number of monkeys, which would soon have exhausted the world market. Brodie, however, had made the effort before his death to switch from the use of monkey supply to mice (see chap. 26).

21. Proceedings of a conference on mechanisms of immunity in poliomyelitis. This meeting was held at Baltimore under the auspices of the Department of Epidemiology, School of Public Health, Johns Hopkins University. Unpublished report, Sept. 17–18, 1946, p. 75.

mediately changed. But it was becoming obvious to many of the participants that although the basic principles of artificial immunization against poliomyelitis might be worked out in primates, the final test would *have* to be made in man. No amount of vaccination of rhesus monkeys, particularly when the intracerebral challenge was used, would ever be sufficient as *the* crucial test.

CHAPTER 25

Mouse Encephalomyelitis
Classifications of Polioviruses

Nature has seen fit that certain members of the animal kingdom shall be subject to the same general types of infections that cause human disease, or perhaps it should be stated the other way around, considering that animals were here long before man. Thus tuberculosis affects both cattle and man, although the two diseases are usually caused by slightly different varieties of tubercle bacilli. Among viral infections, smallpox virus differs somewhat from the agent that causes cowpox. Other examples are porcine and human strains of influenza virus. Perhaps such families of bacteria and viruses have been derived from a single ancestral strain which, through thousands of years of evolution affecting both host and parasite, has gradually produced variants and achieved a degree of mutual specific adaptation. These are matters that involve too much speculation for our concern at the moment, but a more pertinent point is that polio-like diseases of animals do exist. Furthermore the commoner of the polio-like viral agents, although somewhat similar to poliovirus in some respects, are different in antigenicity. It was due to the discovery of one such virus that research in experimental poliomyelitis was deflected into new channels.

This discovery was made in 1934 in the laboratory of Dr. Max Theiler (see fig. 37), who was then working at the Rockefeller Institute on problems connected with yellow fever vaccine.[1, 2] On Dr. Theiler's laboratory staff there was an alert technician named George Martin, who had noticed among the normal mouse colony, one mouse with flaccid paralysis of the hind legs. This animal was promptly killed, and portions of its brain and spinal cord were inoculated intracerebrally into other mice, which resulted in the reproduction of the paralytic disease. It was found that the infection could be maintained indefinitely by serial mouse passage. The type of paralysis, which was for a time given the name of "George's disease" (G.D.), was a perfect replica of human poliomyelitis. Thus, following an incubation period of varied length, mice suffered from flaccid pa-

1. I am indebted to Dr. Max Theiler for an account of how he chanced to detect this virus disease of mice and of events in the subsequent years in which he engaged in work on the subject.

2. M. Theiler: Spontaneous encephalomyelitis of mice—a new virus disease. *Science, 80*: 122, 1934.

ralysis. Histopathologically, the chief lesions were in the anterior horn cells of the spinal cord, and according to the British neuropathologist E. Weston Hurst they resembled almost exactly those of human poliomyelitis. However, the murine virus differed in that it was not pathogenic for

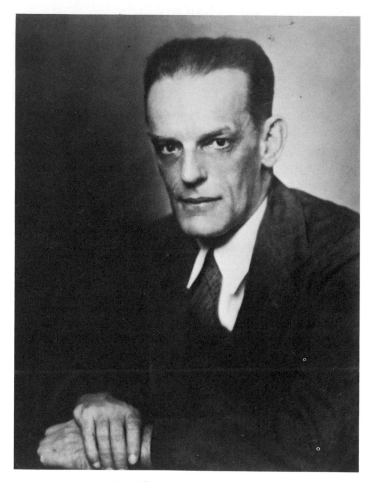

FIG. 37.   Max Theiler, M.D.

rhesus monkeys; nor did it have any *immunological* relationship with human poliovirus. But "George's disease" nonetheless became *mouse poliomyelitis,* and, for a time, *spontaneous encephalomyelitis* of *mice.* The incidence of such paralysis among a colony of normal mice was low indeed, being only of the order of four or five per year, although many thousands of mice were under observation annually in Dr. Theiler's animal quarters. For the time being it was uncertain as to how the mice became infected.

In 1939, a few years after Theiler's discovery, Olitsky,[3] also working at

3. P. K. Olitsky: Viral effect produced by intestinal contents of normal mice and of those having spontaneous encephalomyelitis. *Proc. Soc. exp. Biol. Med. (N.Y.), 41*: 434, 1939.

the Rockefeller Institute, made an observation which shed light on this point. He found that from the intestinal contents of apparently normal mice a viral agent could be recovered which in all respects resembled the virus of "George's disease"; by cross-immunity tests he was able to show that the two agents were the same. Olitsky proposed furthermore that the name of the virus be changed to TO virus (Theiler's original virus).

These findings suggested a new approach to the study of the epidemiology of the murine disease; the thinking about human poliomyelitis had by this time veered around to a belief that it too might, after all, turn out to be an intestinal disease. In Sweden, Kling immediately spotted the implications of Olitsky's new discovery and dispatched one of his young assistants, Dr. Sven Gard, to the United States with instructions that he spend a few months with Dr. Theiler at the Rockefeller Institute in New York and a few months with the Yale Poliomyelitis Study Unit at New Haven, Connecticut, where investigators were hot on the trail of human poliomyelitis as an intestinal disease. With Dr. Gard as the initial emissary, this marked the vigorous reentry of Sweden into the field of poliomyelitis research after a twenty-five-year period of lessened activity.

To Theiler and Gard[4] it soon appeared reasonable that both Theiler's and Olitsky's viruses were the same and that in all probability an intestinal carrier state with TO virus existed in most mouse colonies. Evidence for this was that almost all mice became infected and immune before they were 30 days of age, although they seldom developed signs of central nervous system disease; i.e. the infections were largely inapparent. In this respect also, TO infection of mice was a replica of human poliomyelitis.

To many, mouse encephalomyelitis (TO virus infection) was just another example of an animal disease caused by a neurotropic virus, but to the few whose interest was in the epidemiology of poliomyelitis the new discovery offered something more. It suggested a model for the study of their favorite disease, not only from the standpoint of pathogenesis but experimental epidemiology as well. With luck, the results could even uncover leads as to how the human disease might be controlled.

It was somewhat unfortunate that the investigation of "mouse poliomyelitis" was not immediately pursued to the limit in the United States, Scandinavia, and elsewhere. But with the outbreak of World War II the activities of the various groups were of necessity diverted elsewhere. Dr. Gard returned to Sweden where he continued to work periodically on the murine disease for at least a few years,[5] but after this, other interests intervened, and communications were interrupted until the end of the war.

Dr. Theiler reviewed his studies on TO virus infection in an excellent

4. M. Theiler and S. Gard: Encephalomyelitis of mice. I. Characteristics and pathogenesis of virus. *J. exp. Med., 72:* 49–70, 1940; Ibid., III. Epidemiology. 72: 79–90, 1940.
5. S. Gard: *Purification of Poliomyelitis Viruses. Experiments on Murine and Human Strains.* Uppsala, Almqvist & Wiksells, 1943.

summary paper published in 1941 in which he pointed out that it could be a model for studies on human poliomyelitis.[6] Shortly after this the United States became embroiled in hostilities, and apart from sporadic activities maintained by Olitsky and to a lesser extent by Jungeblut, interest in mouse poliomyelitis waned. Indeed there seemed to be few if any master plans to guide the direction of poliomyelitis research at this time. Other groups, which should have been intensely interested, had become so involved with human poliomyelitis as an intestinal infection and with the problems that poliomyelitis posed as a *military* disease that other interests were dropped for the time being. The course of events was typical of the crablike manner of progression that has characterized the whole poliomyelitis story.

Nevertheless, the subject was not abandoned completely, for beginning during the war years, Dr. Herdis von Magnus of the State Serum Institute in Copenhagen, Denmark concentrated her efforts on TO virus infection in mice.[7] It was a period when Denmark had been cut off from the majority of the scientific world. Monkeys were unavailable, but mice were plentiful, and Dr. von Magnus seized the opportunity to make a complete study of spontaneous encephalomyelitis of mice, comparing its pertinent features with those of human poliomyelitis.

The significance of Dr. von Magnus' contributions, which have been largely overlooked, was that she found that nearly all laboratory mouse colonies were naturally and constantly infected with TO virus, and, as a result, the great majority of mice acquired immunity to the infection at an early age. But by taking newborn mice from their mothers and having them suckled by rats, she was able to build up a mouse colony that was free of TO virus. Such animals proved to be 10–250 times more susceptible to the virus than the young mice in the ordinary colony. Here was abundant food for thought, if one can switch from mice to men. To substitute the human scene at the dawn of the sanitary age, perhaps the resistance of certain human populations to polioviruses at this time had been similarly decreased by eliminating early exposure and infection in an era when the slogan "cleanliness is next to godliness" was beginning to be accepted. If one can go a step further, such a train of events could have been the reason for the sharp increase in incidence of human poliomyelitis in the developed countries where improvements in sanitary methods had occurred at about the turn of the century. It was therefore unnecessary to postulate an enhancement in virulence of poliovirus as an explanation, but rather a shift in human resistance brought on by man's changing habits. Thus the

6. M. Theiler: Studies on poliomyelitis. *Medicine, 20*: 443–62, 1941.

7. H. von Magnus: Studies on mouse encephalomyelitis virus (TO strain). Acta pathologica I, 27: 605–10; II, 611–24, 1950; III, *28*: 234–49, 244–50, 251–57, 1951; Ibid., Studies on mouse encephalomyelitis virus (TO strain). *Observations on the Oral route of Infection and on the Epidemiology of the Disease.* Copenhagen, State Serum Institute, 1952.

principles that had accompanied the introduction of sanitary methods at the turn of the century might have provided the sort of improvements that resulted indirectly in increasing man's susceptibility to poliovirus, much as was the case in von Magnus' TO-free colonies of mice. Of these hypotheses we shall hear more in chapter 34.

Besides elucidating epidemiologic, pathogenetic, and immunologic aspects of the problem, Dr. von Magnus' observations also illustrated the point that investigators had been concentrating their attention heretofore too much on the use of a few highly neurotropic strains of poliovirus in experiments on the monkey. It was high time that scientists should shift their perspective to see how a model of their favorite disease acted in another species, and under various environmental conditions.

Actually in the early 1930s, or about the same time that Theiler discovered the poliomyelitis-like disease of mice, a similar spontaneous infection of pigs was found to be caused by a neurotropic virus. This disease had been known in eastern Europe as Teschen disease, named for the city in Czechoslovakia where it was originally observed. Reference to the first experimental transmission of the virus in 1930 by the Czech scientist Klobouk was included in a review of the European literature published in English in 1948,[8] in which similiarities between Teschen disease and human poliomyelitis were stressed. Investigations of Teschen·disease proved considerably more expensive and less convenient than those of the murine infection, for one pig is unfortunately more difficult to handle in the laboratory than one mouse. But Teschen disease eventually came to be regarded as still another type of poliomyelitis-like infection, caused by an immunologically distinct agent spread by the alimentary route.

No doubt there are other animal species that have their own special kinds of poliomyelitis. In fact, in the 1940s, with Theiler's "mouse poliomyelitis" and Teschen disease being dubbed "pig polio," the question arose whether there was not perhaps a whole tribe of neurotropic viruses, quite apart from the encephalitic viruses described in chapter 17 that had a predilection for the spinal cord of both man and animals. Jungeblut and Sanders considered that their Columbia Sk (Col-Sk), which eventually turned out to be a virus that caused natural infection of several wild rodents, should be included.[9] There were also the related EMC (encephalomyocarditis) viruses. These had been isolated in Africa from mosquitoes

8. M. M. Kaplan and D. R. Meranze: Porcine virus encephalomyelitis and its possible biological relationship to human poliomyelitis. *Vet. Med., 43*: 330–41, 1948.

9. The current interpretation is that the Col-Sk virus was picked up as a native virus of cotton rats, the rodents that had been used in the process of adaptation to mice. Another and similar agent, the MM strain, had been recovered by Jungeblut and Dalldorf from the brain of a hamster that had died 19 days after inoculation with central nervous system material derived from a fatal human case of poliomyelitis. The several strains (Col-Sk, MM, and EMC) were eventually shown to be related, but antigenically distinct from the Lansing strain of poliovirus.

and also from a physician ill with encephalitis. The same infection cropped up at odd places around the world.

It was Mollaret in France in 1950 who proposed that the above viruses all be included in one large family and that those agents which were not true (human) poliomyelitis viruses be designated as parapoliomyelitis or pseudopoliomyelitis viruses. His suggestion, fortunately, won only limited support. Another totally unacceptable proposal, put forth in 1948, grouped poliomyelitis virus together with a number of completely unrelated agents under the genus *Legio*.[10] Obviously things were getting out of hand, and the time had arrived for an international body to tackle the problem, which was done in 1948.[11]

It might be mentioned that although foreseen and unforeseen problems inherent in the classification of any biologic species have existed since the days of Linnaeus, the main reason for laboring the point here is that the manner in which a given entity is classified usually reflects contemporary ideas concerning it and as such has a certain amount of historical value.[12]

After vigorous debate the international committees of 1947–48, which met prior to the time that the three serotypes of poliomyelitis viruses had become established, came to the conclusion that such viruses as TO, Col-Sk, MM, EMC,

> which produce paralysis and neuronal lesions in the anterior horns of the spinal cord in experimental animals, but which do not otherwise satisfy the criteria set down for poliomyelitis virus, should not be called "poliomyelitis virus," "mouse poliomyelitis virus," or "poliomyelitis-like virus."

This action temporarily closed a chapter that had been characterized by a certain amount of loose thinking about the limits of the term poliomyelitis virus.

Between 1948 and 1955, Mollaret in France, Jungeblut and Koprowski in the United States, and Rhodes in Canada aired their respective views as to how poliomyelitis viruses should be classified. Also, Sir Christopher Andrewes of London entered the arena. To him it was obvious that such matters should be decided by an international group, and as a result another committee was appointed with the assignment to get on with the task of defining polioviruses and assigning them a proper place in the general microbiological scheme of things.

10. R. S. Breed, E. G. D. Murray, and A. P. Hitchens: *Bergey's Manual of Determinative Bacteriology*, 6th ed., Baltimore, Williams & Wilkins, 1948, p. 1257.

11. Committee on Nomenclature of the National Foundation for Infantile Paralysis: A proposed provisional definition of poliomyelitis virus. *Science, 108*: 701–05, 1948.

12. Typical of the way ideas of classification change is the present-day fashion of dividing viruses according to whether they contain DNA or RNA; according to this scheme it may be doubtful whether viruses should be regarded as microbes at all.

This newest committee submitted a brief report in 1955[13] that carried the suggestion, made originally by Dr. Burnet of Australia, that the name poliomyelitis viruses should be shortened so as to have some uniformity with the provisional names arrived at by other nomenclature groups. Thus the term *poliovirus* was coined, in line with already accepted terms such as *poxvirus, herpesvirus,* and *myxovirus*. In retrospect, the only lasting feature of this committee's suggestions was that the name *poliovirus* became universally adopted.

For within two years the family of polioviruses was embraced by a far larger group. What was more extraordinary was that the uniqueness of polioviruses in inducing characteristic lesions in the central nervous system was given up. Now it was the intestinal tract with which taxonomists were concerned. Viruses that had similar physical and chemical properties, i.e. small size and resistance to ether, and behaved in a similar fashion biologically with regard to the human intestinal tract as their special, though transient, habitat were all placed together in a new category regardless as to whether or not they affected the central nervous system. Thus the large family of *enteroviruses* was created as a subgroup of the newly designated *picornaviruses*. TO, Teschen, and other similar agents were classified as *picornaviruses* of lower animals.[14] Included besides polioviruses in the human enterovirus group were the Coxsackie and echoviruses, of which we shall hear much in a subsequent chapter. This complete change in the image of polioviruses coincided with the general decline in the incidence of paralytic poliomyelitis. As vaccination became more and more effective the tragic paralytic results of the disease began to fade, and the virus acquired the more earthy name of its main anatomical site of predilection, which had so long been denied it. Polioviruses thus became members of the enterovirus family, incredible as this would have sounded to past generations of investigators. Dr. Flexner must surely have turned in his grave at the thought.

13. The group of three, appointed by the Virus Subcommittee of the International Nomenclature Committee, were: H. von Magnus of Denmark, J. H. S. Gear of South Africa, and J. R. Paul of the U.S.A. For their report, see: A recent definition of poliomyelitis viruses. *Virology, 1*: 185–89, 1955.

This committee reversed the decision made in 1948 and admitted Theiler's (TO) virus into the fold, although none of the other murine viruses were taken back. This action was prompted by the demonstration that this disease in mice had proved to be such a striking model for human poliomyelitis, not only from the standpoint of pathology and pathogenesis but also in its epidemiology. It was decided that the *Poliovirus Family* should include two major divisions: *Poliovirus hominis,* which embraced the three established human serotypes; and *Poliovirus muris,* which included only Theiler's (TO) virus.

14. Committee on Enteroviruses. Classification of Human Enteroviruses. *Virology, 16*: 501, 1962; and International Enterovirus Study Group. Picornavirus group. *Virology, 19*: 114–16, 1963. The term *picornavirus* was derived from *pico,* implying small size, and *RNA,* which refers to the type of nucleic acid which these viruses contain.

CHAPTER 26

Adaptation of the Lansing Strain to Rodents

During the thirty years or so following the discovery of the virus of polio-myelitis, repeated, almost desperate attempts had been made to infect lab-oratory animals other than primates. The usual animals tested were rab-bits, guinea pigs, and mice; others, including dogs, cats, pigs, lambs, and calves, had been tried, all with equally discouraging, negative results. As monkeys were not only expensive but also difficult to handle, it would have been a godsend to investigators if some smaller, cheaper animal could have been shown to be susceptible. The result was that progress had been slowed more or less to a snail's pace in the 1920s and early 1930s. The field was dominated by a relatively few individuals or small groups, who con-tinued to occupy the stage for a long time, because it was thought that they were the only ones who could afford the luxury of a primate colony. This was to the detriment of new ideas.

By the year 1930, a review of the literature and a summary of the various attempts to infect animals other than primates were made by Harmon, Shaughnessy, and Gordon.[1] Their report left little doubt that the only ani-mals susceptible to poliovirus infection were primates, a dictum which became so fixed that it held for another eight or ten years.[2] But during the late 1930s, things began to happen.

Early in 1935 Maurice Brodie, the same Brodie of the ill-fated vaccine, had made repeated efforts to infect rabbits, guinea pigs, rats, and mice—all of them unsuccessful.[3] And yet, despite these early failures, he and his collaborators continued and decided to concentrate on mice as the most suitable laboratory host. They went further than usual in their experi-ments and employed a number of approaches aimed at reducing the re-sistance of refractory animals; finally they succeeded.

Actually what they did was to expose a series of mice to repeated small

1. P. H. Harmon, H. J. Shaughnessy, and F. B. Gordon: The effects upon animals of inocu-lation with the virus of poliomyelitis. I. Rabbits. II. Dogs, cats, guinea pigs and other animals. *J. prev. Med., 4*: 59, 89, 1930.

2. J. A. Toomey: Experimental poliomyelitis in animals other than the monkey; review of literature. *J. Pediat., 16*: 519–27, 1940.

3. M. Brodie: Attempts to produce poliomyelitis in refractory laboratory animals. *Proc. Soc. exp. Biol. Med. (N.Y.), 32*: 832, 1935.

doses of x-rays and then inoculate them with virus both intracerebrally and intraperitoneally.[4] On the 11th postinoculation day, one series of mice so treated showed signs of weakness of the hind legs. A suspension of the brains of these animals, when passed to other, nonirradiated mice and a monkey, failed to produce any reaction. This must have been a discouraging blow, and one which might very well have ended their efforts.

Undaunted, Brodie and his colleagues made a second try. This time some of the second passage mice were successfully infected and developed paralysis. One monkey that received infected mouse brain material responded with nothing more than a rise in temperature, but this was enough to arouse a faint flicker of hope. After continued transfer through 17 serial mouse passages, they began to get much more definite results, due probably to progressive adaptation and higher concentrations of virus. A monkey inoculated with 17th passage mouse brain actually ran the typical course of experimental poliomyelitis and showed characteristic histological lesions in the spinal cord. At long last they seemed to be in business! The pathologic features in mice differed from the picture in primates in that the lesions occurred mainly in the brain and meninges; the virus thus induced a meningoencephalomyelitis rather than having a predilection for the spinal cord, as in man.

This was a revolutionary finding. It came just at the time (March 1935) when Brodie was doing all sorts of remarkable things with his formalin-inactivated poliovirus vaccine, including the immunization of monkeys and children. In fact, Brodie's work with mice had been motivated with a practical objective in view: he knew that should the demand for his vaccine become as enormous as he hoped, it was inevitable that the supply of monkeys would soon be exhausted. If the mouse experiments were successful, it would enable him to switch from monkey spinal cords to mouse brains, which might make his vaccine project vastly more feasible.

But the scientific world was decidedly skeptical over this new and startling development coming along at the height of the Brodie success story. How had he been able to succeed in so many fields where others repeatedly had failed? One important authority, in speaking of the mouse venture, made the pronouncement that "if indeed, Brodie has done what he has claimed, he has turned a mighty neat trick, but if he has not, he has dug himself a mighty deep grave."

As it happened, the repudiation of Brodie's vaccine did not help his reputation as a scientific worker in other projects, particularly his claim to have given poliomyelitis to mice. Shortly after the failure of his vaccine,

---

4. M. Brodie, S. A. Goldberg, and P. Stanley: Transmission of the virus of poliomyelitis to mice. *Science, 81:* 319, 1935.

he had left New York City's Public Health Laboratory, where it was maintained afterwards that the vaccine had been "made in the most incredible sloppy manner."[5]

This was enough to cast a cloud over all of Brodie's efforts in the field of poliomyelitis, and there is no record of his having published anything further about the adaptation of poliovirus to mice. It was a pity, because if he had really succeeded (and it is likely that he had) and if he had continued to follow up this lead, it would have been a tremendous step forward. At least he would have been four years in advance of other successful efforts in the same direction. And yet poor Brodie, who was to die within a short time, had been right about a number of things. In the opinion of the author of this book, he deserves more recognition than history has allowed him to date. He had succeeded in showing (Dr. Rivers to the contrary) that formalin could be used effectively to inactivate poliovirus and provide an antigen or vaccine that was capable of inducing protective neutralizing antibodies—even immunity—in both monkeys and man. But even though the vaccine was not to live up to expectations, if Brodie and his group had actually been the first to get poliovirus going in mice, they would indeed "have turned a mighty neat trick."

The next episode in the adaptation of the virus to rodents involved Dr. Charles Armstrong of the U.S. Public Health Service. He succeeded in such a convincing manner that his results gave an entirely new direction to research on poliomyelitis and polioviruses in general.

Charles Armstrong (see fig. 38), a native of Alliance, Ohio, was born in 1887.[6] He received a B.S. degree from Mt. Union College there in 1910, and then went on to pursue his medical education at Johns Hopkins. After two years of internship at the New Haven Hospital he suddenly decided, as a result of notices posted on the hospital bulletin board, to join the Public Health Service—just in time to serve, during World War I, on a Coast Guard cutter in European waters.

The war over, he was assigned to work with Dr. Frost at the Johns Hopkins School of Hygiene, an experience that contributed to his education and took him on field projects having to do with diverse subjects including epidemic influenza, and even an outbreak of botulism due to canned ripe olives. His subsequent career as a research scientist began in 1921 in the old Hygienic Laboratory of the Public Health Service. This was the predecessor of the present National Institutes of Health (NIH), where he was eventually to become chief of its Division of Infectious Diseases.

One of the unique qualities of Charles Armstrong was his versatility

5. S. Benison: *Tom Rivers; Reflections on a Life in Medicine and Science.* Cambridge, Mass., M.I.T. Press, 1967, p. 185.

6. I am indebted to Dr. Armstrong's daughter, Miss Mary Emma Armstrong of Washington, D.C., for much helpful information about her father's career. See also *N.I.H. Report* (July 1967).

and competence in many fields, but especially in the new and rapidly developing field of virology. A list of the subjects that he tackled would be entirely too long to include here; it certainly was a mixed bag. Among his accomplishments was the discovery of the causative virus of a disease

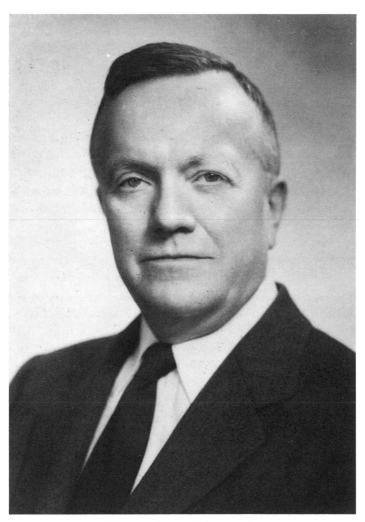

Fig. 38. Charles Armstrong (1887–1967). Kindness of his daughter, Miss Mary Emma Armstrong of Washington, D.C.

known as *lymphocytic choriomeningitis* (LCM) that often involves the central nervous system. He did considerable work while at the NIH on *psittacosis*, better known as "parrot fever," and he also was a pioneer worker on neurotropic arthropod-borne virus diseases such as St. Louis encephalitis.

As a result of experience with various viral and other infections Armstrong developed, one might say, a fundamental philosophy about infectious disease. True, he was to stray occasionally up a few blind alleys, such as his continued, dogged pursuit of the nasal spray as a prophylactic measure in poliomyelitis long after other people had given up the whole idea. But what inquisitive and industrious research worker has not been guilty of following up blind alleys? Charles Armstrong was able to rectify his mistakes better than most.

From the time of the establishment of the National Foundation for Infantile Paralysis he served constantly in an advisory capacity to that organization. Indeed, from the first meeting of Rivers' Committee on Scientific Research, which was formed as early as July 1938, the foundation constantly looked to him for counsel.

In August of the previous year, 1937, Dr. Armstrong had received a strain of poliovirus from Dr. Max Peet of the University of Michigan, soon to be a fellow member of Rivers' NFIP Committee on Scientific Research. The particular strain supplied by Dr. Peet had been isolated from a fatal case of bulbar poliomyelitis that had occurred at Lansing, Michigan; hence the name *Lansing strain.*

I have many times tried to extract the reasons from the late Charles Armstrong which prompted him to attempt to adapt poliovirus to cotton rats instead of to mice. Rats would seem to have been a singularly unfavorable species of rodent, particularly since many a trial had shown that they are quite resistant to the commoner viral infections that attack man. Furthermore Brodie's work had indicated that as far as intracerebral passage was concerned, the rat maintained viable poliovirus in its brain only up to the 16th passage, whereas in the mouse it persisted up to the 45th passage.

The only satisfactory answer I could ever obtain from Dr. Armstrong was that there was currently at the NIH a colony of various species of rats being used in investigations on Weil's disease, a spirochaetal infection transmitted to man by rats. Apparently an excess supply of these rodents, including a specimen of the cotton rat (*Sigmodon hispidus hispidus*), was turned over to Dr. Armstrong, who promptly tested its susceptibility to the Lansing strain of poliovirus.

Armstrong's first experiments were begun in November 1937. Luck was with him on two counts: in his choice of the particular species of rat as the test animal; and in his choice of the Lansing strain, eventually identified as belonging to Type II poliovirus, which, as it turned out later, was the type most amenable to this sort of adaptation. He began by inoculating the 19th monkey passage of Lansing virus into several species of rodents, including one cotton rat. This lone animal remained well until the 25th day, when it developed a disease resembling experimental poliomyelitis, and, lo and behold, when it was sacrificed the pathological report confirmed the diagnosis. During the winter the experiment was repeated, but this time only 1 out of 11 of the injected cotton rats developed signs of the disease, and all attempts to pass the virus to other animals proved negative. So the investigations were abandoned for a time in the belief that the early success had been just a fluke.

There was a lapse of about eighteen months before these experiments were repeated, and it is to Dr. Armstrong's infinite credit that he took them up again. This time he was able to produce experimental poliomyelitis in a series of cotton rats. The findings enabled him to make the following report:

> Efforts were again made, however, during the poliomyelitis season of 1939, and up to the time of this report the Lansing strain of virus has been carried in series through 7 cotton rat transfers and animals of the eighth transfer are developing symptoms.[7]

It was only a matter of a few short months before Armstrong was able to make the much easier adaptation from cotton rats to mice. Three months after his first paper on the subject, he announced that

> The Lansing strain of poliomyelitis virus after adaptation to the eastern cotton rat has been successfully transmitted through twelve generations in white mice.[8]

This discovery, soon confirmed by others, meant that at last a strain of poliovirus was available that could be used to study the experimental disease in a far cheaper animal than the monkey. It meant neutralization tests could be done by using this strain with a sufficient number of animals to yield statistically significant results. Infinitely more important, instead of there being only a few laboratories which could afford to work with polioviruses, many could now join in the attack. In fact, Armstrong's discovery turned out to be one of those tremendously significant ones that have occasionally punctuated the history of poliomyelitis and turned it in a new direction. It suddenly accelerated progress that had only been inching along during the previous decade. A new era had begun.

When Armstrong began to think about the epidemiological implications of his discovery, his thoughts turned on the suggestion as to whether it meant that rats could serve as a reservoir of polioviruses, as they were for the spirochetes in Weil's disease and for the infected ectoparasites that carried murine typhus. It happened that during the summer of 1939 a severe epidemic of poliomyelitis was in progress in and about the city of Charleston, South Carolina, and to follow up this lead, Armstrong dis-

7. C. Armstrong: The experimental transmission of poliomyelitis to the Eastern cotton rat, *Sigmodon hispidus hispidus. Publ. Hlth Rep. (Wash.), 54*: 1719–21, 1939.

8. C. Armstrong: Successful transfer of the Lansing strain of poliomyelitis virus from the cotton rat to the white mouse. *Publ. Hlth Rep. (Wash.), 54*: 2302–05, 1939.

patched Dr. Gilliam of the Public Health Service to make a survey of the rat population in the affected area with orders to bring the rats back alive to the National Institute of Health without delay. But nothing came of this investigation. There was no evidence of the existence of a reservoir of poliovirus infection in wild rodents, and the cotton rat story proved to be a matter of laboratory manipulation without apparent epidemiological implications.

Naturally, immediate efforts were made to repeat Armstrong's results with many different strains of poliovirus. Dr. John Toomey used 9 strains unsuccessfully. It was little wonder that he had difficulty since more than half of them in all probability were Type I. Kessel and Stimpert also came up with negative results in similar attempts. Their account ended with the statement:

> At least insofar as practical application to poliomyelitis research is concerned, it appears that adaptation of a poliomyelitis virus to the rodent is so rare that such animals cannot be utilized for routine experimental work in the isolation and comparisons of strains of virus.[9]

These last two authors obviously had a special kind of practical poliomyelitis research in mind, namely the direct isolation of virus from patients. Their pronouncement was another example of the confusion that existed because of a lack of awareness that the poliovirus family was composed of three serotypes, which differed in antigenicity and in biologic properties. Within a few years, however, investigators began to appreciate that there was a Lansing-like group of strains of poliovirus, many of which possessed a special tendency for mouse adaptability. The next strain to be recognized through its ability to infect mice *directly* was the MEF-1 strain from Egypt, which we will hear about in chapter 33; others followed—the Sk from New Haven and the Wallingford from Los Angeles. All of these strains later turned out to be members of Type II. Other serotypes, including the important Type I, were eventually adapted to mice;[10] but by the time these successes occurred they had little impact because by then the three serotypes of poliovirus had been found to be readily propagated in tissue culture, and the urgency of adapting them to small animals had faded into the background.

And yet Charles Armstrong's discovery in 1939 suddenly shed a completely new light on the behavior of poliovirus, with implications which neither he nor anyone else had appreciated or even contemplated. Not only could mice replace monkeys as the test animal in many studies of

9. J. F. Kessel and F. D. Stimpert: Attempts to transmit poliomyelitis virus to rodents. *Proc. Soc. exp. Biol. Med. (N.Y.)*, *45*: 665–67, 1940.

10. C. P. Li and M. Schaeffer: Adaptation of Type I poliomyelitis virus to mice. *Proc. Soc. exp. Biol. Med. (N.Y.)*, *82*: 477, 1953.

experimental poliomyelitis, but investigators could start considering the possibility that they might, after all, manipulate strains of poliovirus so as to change their virulence for humans without altering their antigenicity. As a result, such strains might be used as immunizing agents in man.

It may be remembered that Dr. Kolmer had conceived of this hypothesis five years before and had erroneously claimed that his vaccine strain of poliovirus had been so altered by continuous passage from monkey to monkey that it had lost its pathogenicity for man. This turned out not to be true, for the alteration in the properties of Kolmer's virus was too slight. But through adaptation to rodents, the Lansing strain had undergone a far greater change, and this did provide a more hopeful situation, at least one which could be put to the test. It remained for Dr. Max Theiler to pick up and casually report on the idea in 1946. He had been recently working in the laboratories of the Rockefeller Foundation on a similar problem, an attenuated strain of yellow fever virus that could be used as an immunizing agent against that disease. As might be imagined, he was alert to the potential usefulness of biological attenuation of viruses and had a very special interest in this approach to immunization. So, in due time (World War II having intervened), at a conference held under the auspices of the National Foundation for Infantile Paralysis, he reported as follows:

> Some years ago through the courtesy of Dr. Armstrong, I obtained the Lansing strain of poliomyelitis virus. The material received from Dr. Armstrong was an infected cotton rat brain representing the 34th passage in this rodent. On receipt the virus was inoculated intracerebrally into monkeys, cotton rats and mice. Serial passages were made in both cotton rats and mice.
>
> After 52 serial passages in mice, the virulence was tested by intracerebral inoculation of three rhesus monkeys. All remained well. This was the first indication that the Lansing virus, by serial passage in mice, was losing its pathogenicity for monkeys.[11]

Theiler's experiments (see table 6) indicated that after 150 mouse passages the Lansing strain could be used with impunity as an immunizing agent, at least for rhesus monkeys! After 100 passages, vaccines composed of 2–6 doses of such live poliovirus protected 95 percent of the monkeys, whereas an injection of the original, virulent Lansing virus would have induced paralysis in 100 percent of the animals. Theiler's investigations marked the first series of studies that traced the actual course of the process of attenuation of virulence for the monkey. The results produced a

11. M. Theiler: A mutant strain of the Lansing virus. Unpublished report given at a conference, "Mechanisms of Immunity in Poliomyelitis," Baltimore, Md., Sept. 17–18, 1946, pp. 29–36.

TABLE 6.   Intracerebral inoculation of monkeys with mouse-adapted
Lansing poliovirus

No. of Passages in Mice	No. of Monkeys Inoculated	Monkeys that Developed Paralysis	
		Number	Percent
1–50	12	7	58
51–100	21	3	14
101–150	24	1	4
150+	18	0	0

ray of hope that one could so manipulate virulent poliovirus as to render it progressively less virulent without injuring its antigenic composition. In retrospect it seems reasonable to expect that this lead would have been either taken up by members of Rivers' NFIP Committee on Scientific Research or farmed out to other investigators. But in 1946, the scientific world was not ready for these findings; at least not ready for them to be put to any practical use. The family of polioviruses had not yet been separated into its three component types, and in view of the tragic failure of the Kolmer vaccine, 1946 was hardly the year to contemplate any renewal of vaccine trials.

As Theiler's interest meanwhile had been diverted along other lines, he did not pursue this series of experiments further. He preferred instead to let "polio experts" do what they could with his finding. Unfortunately they did nothing. Nevertheless his observation deserves a high place in the history of poliomyelitis. He had pointed the way in a direction that eventually led to the development of the live, attenuated poliovirus vaccine that is used today.

CHAPTER 27

The Revival of Poliomyelitis as an Intestinal Disease

By 1937 more than twenty-five years had elapsed since Kling, Pettersson, and Wernstedt[1] had first reported the isolation of poliovirus from human excreta. They had recovered the virus from the intestinal contents of fatal cases (see table 3), from specimens obtained from patients in the acute phase of the disease, and from patients during convalescence. The following year (1913) this success was repeated by Kling and Levaditi,[2] who demonstrated the agent in the intestinal tract of a single fatal case; in the United States another lone positive result with fecal material from an ill patient was described by Sawyer in 1915.[3] Shortly thereafter, however, such attempts were discontinued. The significance of the presence of poliovirus in the intestinal tract sank into oblivion in spite of spasmodic efforts on the part of Kling and his colleagues to revive interest in the subject. Progress in poliomyelitis research did not recover from this setback for almost a generation.

Indeed, as mentioned earlier, in the years following 1915 concerted efforts were made in some quarters in the United States to downgrade the Swedish findings of 1912, with the claim that unreliable criteria had been used in evaluating the virus isolation results. By the 1920s and 1930s it had become fashionable to say that no one paid attention anymore to the discredited work of old Kling and his team—or words to that effect. Growing support for belief in the nasal portal of entry and the olfactory pathway to the central nervous system had so completely overshadowed all other considerations of pathogenesis during this period that the possible role of the intestinal tract was thought to be simply not worth bothering about. Doubters maintained that maybe the virus was excreted now and again in the stools, but this only meant that its original source had been the pharynx and the swallowed virus had somehow survived the long passage through the alimentary tract.

But from 1931, with the rebirth of *clinical* virological investigations, isolations of the virus from nasopharyngeal secretions of patients once

1. C. Kling, A. Pettersson, and W. Wernstedt: The presence of the microbe of infantile paralysis in human beings. *Communications Inst. med., État.* Stockholm. *3*: 5, 1912.

2. C. Kling and C. Levaditi: Études sur la poliomyélite aigüe épidémique. *Ann. Inst. Pasteur. 27*: 718–839, 1913.

3. W. A. Sawyer: An epidemiological study of poliomyelitis. *Amer. J. trop. Dis., 3*: 164, 1915.

again began to be reported, and one wondered whether Kling and his team had been so wrong after all.

A jolt came in 1937 when Harmon of Chicago made casual mention in a paper dealing with quite another subject[4] that he had been successful in isolating the virus from intestinal washings from 5 of 17 patients, 2 of them fatal cases. This *was* news. It immediately stirred the Yale Poliomyelitis Unit into action to have another look at the human intestinal tract. It may be recalled that this unit had tried unsuccessfully to isolate the virus from intestinal washings collected during an epidemic in Philadelphia in 1932 (see chap. 20), and in the face of disastrous results had practically decided to abandon such attempts. But five years later, in the fall of 1937, upon receipt of Harmon's report, the search for virus in fecal specimens was renewed. An opportunity came during a small outbreak of poliomyelitis in New Haven and Meriden, Connecticut. Twenty-two patients from these cities furnished specimens; 3 of 9 nasopharyngeal washings yielded poliovirus, and 3 of 13 fecal specimens were also positive!

Clinical circumstances under which the three isolations from fecal material were obtained are worth recording and best presented in a family chart which follows the same pattern as that illustrated in a previous chapter. The situation in family Sk is portrayed in figure 39. This family had three children. The oldest child, Teddy, had contracted severe paralytic poliomyelitis early in October, and the youngest, Daniel, whom we visited at home on October 18, was suffering from what appeared to be a mild, nonparalytic attack, with fever, listlessness, and slight stiffness of the back but with no evidence of muscular weakness. Nasopharyngeal washings and a stool specimen were obtained from all three children. The rest of this eventful story is graphically illustrated in figure 39 as well as being documented in two publications.[5]

The finding of poliovirus in the stools of Daniel Sk came to the laboratory of the Yale Poliomyelitis Unit by pure chance. We happened at the time to have a *cercopithecus* monkey in the laboratory named Bosco by our animal caretaker, Tony Coppola. Bosco was indeed a beautiful animal and was Tony's special pet. But Bosco seemed to be serving no good purpose in the laboratory. Actually he had been eating into our none too generous budget for many months. And yet no one had the heart to use him in an experiment that might cause paralysis and perhaps death. Besides, Tony's good will was at stake. That was worth more than many monkeys. But at the suggestion of Dr. Alfred J. Vignec, the extract of fecal

4. P. H. Harmon: The use of chemicals as nasal sprays in the prophylaxis of poliomyelitis in man. *J. Amer. med. Ass., 109*: 1061, 1937.

5. J. D. Trask, A. J. Vignec, and J. R. Paul: Isolation of poliomyelitis virus from human stools. *Proc. Soc. exp. Biol. med. (N.Y.), 38*: 147–49, 1938; Ibid., Poliomyelitis virus in human stools. *J. Amer. med. Ass., 111*: 6–11, 1938.

material obtained on October 18 from the infant Daniel Sk was inoculated *intraperitoneally* into Bosco. Both Drs. Trask and Paul believed that he would safely survive this procedure. But in spite of our predictions, Bosco was paralyzed in all four limbs within a few days of inoculation and suc-

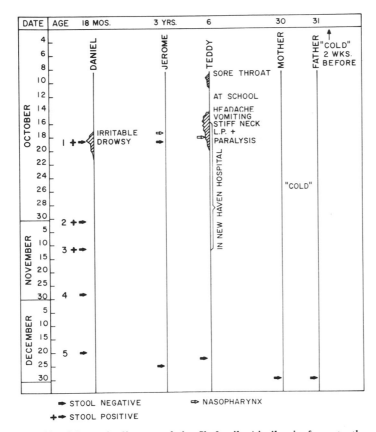

FIG. 39. Schematic diagram of the Sk family (similar in form to the one shown in fig. 32). But here, both nasopharyngeal washings and stool specimens were collected.

cumbed quite rapidly. Sad as his death was, it certainly shed new light on the pathogenesis of poliomyelitis that was quickly exploited. The mistake we and almost everyone else had been making all along was to insist on following the technique of inoculating small amounts of treated fecal extracts into the brains of monkeys, a procedure which that delicate organ could not withstand, considering the crude methods which were used to make the inoculum bacteria-free. If others, including ourselves, had followed the initial Swedish technique of using intraperitoneal, instead of intracerebral, injection, the pathogenesis of poliomyelitis would have been resolved years earlier.

It will be seen from the diagram in figure 39 that not only had Daniel

Sk's first stool specimen yielded the virus, but his second and third specimens, which had been obtained on the 11th and 24th days of his disease respectively, were also positive. It soon became apparent that it was easier to detect the virus of poliomyelitis in the feces during the acute infection and first weeks thereafter than to find it in the nasopharynx. The reason was that not only was the quantity of virus present in feces much larger, but excretion continued for a far longer time, in contrast to the brief period of its presence in the nasopharynx. The results implied that virus had not been merely swallowed but that multiplication in the alimentary tract continued for at least several weeks. This was strong evidence that intestinal wastes might be a potential source of periodic community virus distribution.

The change in point of view came suddenly and was indeed unacceptable to all but those few members of the Kling school of thought. In America the reaction was more or less one of disbelief by the rank and file of microbiologists and epidemiologists. Prior to 1937, apart from the ideas which Kling, Levaditi, and Lépine had expressed in 1929, the notion that poliomyelitis was "an intestinal disease" was to all intents and purposes dead. One lone champion of this cause in the United States had been Dr. John A. Toomey, a pediatrician with headquarters in the Municipal Hospital in Cleveland, who had long held out for the alimentary portal of entry of the virus. During the 1930s he had tried to substantiate his claims by the use of a highly artificial experimental technique in which he traumatized a loop of intestine and inoculated poliovirus directly into it. The animals developed paralytic poliomyelitis. Toomey's theory had been right, but his method of proving his point left much to be desired.

To give some idea of how unpopular the idea was that the alimentary tract had anything to do with the pathogenesis of poliomyelitis in 1938, it may not be amiss to recount a highly personal incident. The occasion was the 1938 meeting of the American Epidemiological Society, which was held in Baltimore in April. At this meeting I gave an account of events of the previous October that have been illustrated in figure 39. My report ended with the statement that poliomyelitis just might, after all, "deserve to be considered as an intestinal disease." This pronouncement was greeted with a chilling silence. In the audience were several men that had had considerably longer experience with poliomyelitis than the speaker. To them this was old and outmoded heresy. Such men included Haven Emerson, Lloyd Aycock, and James Leake, among others. One member of the Public Health Service at length arose and said, "For some years now we have been following the good work that the Yale unit has been doing, but now, although I am loath to say it, they have apparently gone off the deep end."

Yet, in spite of this reaction, this position was soon joined by others, who went on to exploit the new finding. In a paper published in July 1938, we had occasion to say:

That the stools in these mild and generally unrecognized cases (which may outnumber the paralytic cases eight times) may be infectious over a period of three weeks places these patients almost in the status of "healthy carriers." Furthermore, that the virus may survive in vitro in the stools for ten weeks suggests that during an epidemic a high degree of pollution of sewage with poliomyelitis virus could readily occur. In fact, one could almost term this hypothetic degree of sewage pollution as "massive."

As stated, the immediate reaction, particularly of the public health profession, to the announcement that poliovirus not only was present in human stools but was commonly found in such excreta was one of militant disbelief. Reasons for such skepticism were eminently logical as far as they went. Not only did this finding contradict the favorite theory that the nasal mucosa was *the* portal of entry, but it also carried the suggestion that poliomyelitis might be a waterborne disease, comparable to typhoid fever and some of the bacterial dysenteries. This was in conflict with all past experience. All available data testified that poliomyelitis was very different from typhoid fever in its epidemiology. Epidemics did not occur in relation to grossly contaminated water supplies, and to this' day it is unlikely that water has any significant role in its transmission.[6] For a brief period only, the Yale Unit believed that watercourses polluted with polioviruses were instrumental in the spread of poliomyelitis. But our adherence to this view was short lived.

The entire story of viral diseases considered to be associated with the human intestinal tract had not even begun to be written by the late 1930s. What most of the members of the public health profession missed was that the mere presence of virus in the stools did not necessarily signify a disease that behaved like typhoid fever. When carriers, either convalescent or long-term ones, like "Typhoid Mary" excreted typhoid bacilli into an already polluted water supply, these organisms, if given the proper conditions of temperature, protein content, and other organic materials, could actually multiply. No matter how heavily the water supply might be contaminated with polioviruses, there was little reason to believe that multiplication could occur in this medium because, as with other viruses,

6. J. W. Mosely: "Transmission of viral diseases by drinking water," in *Transmission of Viruses by the Water Route*, ed. I. Berg. John Wiley, 1966, pp. 7–11.

With the much larger family of enteroviruses now on the scene, including the Coxsackie and echoviruses, which share many of the epidemiologic features of poliomyelitis, it seems unlikely that there have been any true waterborne epidemics. On the other hand, it is uncertain whether any really serious attempts have been made to detect them.

growth is possible only in the presence of living cells. Had the proponents of poliomyelitis as an intestinal disease been more specific or explained some of these points to their public health colleagues from the start, they might have saved themselves an infinite amount of controversy.

Dr. Rivers is quoted by Benison in this connection:

> let me say that the initial impact of the discovery of poliovirus in the feces of abortive and paralytic cases of polio by Dr. Trask and Dr. Paul made them focus their attention on sewage as the likely agency in the spread of polio. I would like to add that they got quite an argument when they published such views. I personally didn't think much of that particular idea, because polio epidemics hit good sanitary environments and clean healthy kids with more force than it did slums, where the kids might have been scrawny and dirty, and certainly not as well fed. One of the important corollaries of the sewage idea was that polio epidemics might be water-borne, and Dr. Paul and Dr. Trask pursued that notion very carefully. In this way they went back to an idea of old papa Kling, the Swedish epidemiologist, who pointed out that some of the early polio epidemics in Sweden followed streams. Well again they could find no hard proof that water was actually related to the spread of polio epidemics. I opposed them on these ideas but I don't know that I wouldn't have done the same had I been in their shoes.[7]

On the other hand, confirmation of intestinal excretion came quickly. The first support was from a team headed by Kramer, Aycock's former partner, and composed of members of the Long Island College of Medicine and the Jewish Hospital of Brooklyn, New York. These investigators succeeded in isolating poliovirus from the feces of a patient a few days after the onset of illness. This finding, they said,

> further suggests that improper disposal of feces from patients with poliomyelitis may leave serious public health consequences, particularly in smaller communities where inadequate sewage disposal may result in the contamination of surrounding beaches or even local water systems.[8]

But Kramer went considerably further in his explorations of this aspect of poliomyelitis. A few months later, in the summer of 1939, Detroit experienced a large epidemic. Kramer had recently joined the Michigan Department of Health, and along with A. G. Gilliam, of the U.S. Public

7. S. Benison: *Tom Rivers; Reflections on a Life in Medicine and Science.* Cambridge, Mass., M.I.T. Press, 1967, p. 266.

8. S. D. Kramer, B. Hoskwith, and L. H. Grossman: Detection of the virus of poliomyelitis in the nose and throat and gastrointestinal tract of human beings and monkeys. *J. exp. Med.,* *69*: 49–67, 1939.

Health Service, and a member of the local municipal health department, J. D. Molner,[9] he investigated a sharp outbreak in a children's home in that city. In one wing of the institution which housed only 20 children 2 to 5 years of age, 5 had come down with frank poliomyelitis, a remarkably high incidence. Fecal specimens were collected from all of the children and from 8 of their nurses. Poliovirus was recovered from 3 of 12 children who had remained well and from 2 of 3 who had experienced brief febrile episodes lasting 24 to 48 hours. From 2 of these, virus was again recovered from stools collected 19 days after the first isolations. One of 8 asymptomatic nurses was also found to be excreting poliovirus. These observations, besides representing a remarkable technical accomplishment, had a more far-reaching significance. Not only did they confirm by laboratory test the carrier theory, which Wickman and, later, Wernstedt had been at such pains to document a generation earlier, but the demonstration also pointed to preschool children as being in all likelihood a major reservoir of infection, which could easily serve as a source of spread, whereas prior to this time the youngest age group had been regarded as innocents in this connection. Kramer and his team seem not to have been aware of the implications of this finding at the time. At least they were content to settle with the statement "that the virus of poliomyelitis is usually spread throughout the general population by the agency of healthy carriers.[10] Amplification of these views came promptly.

Years later Dr. Sven Gard of the Karolinska Institute in Stockholm reemphasized the point that *infants* could be regarded as specially "dangerous carriers." He reported in 1960, as a result of a study carried out with more sophisticated methods, that children between the ages of 6 and 18 months, who were not yet toilet trained, were the main virus disseminators and were a far greater menace to susceptible young parents, or to nursemaids, or any other members of the household, than were older children.[11]

Recognition of the importance of inapparent infection in infants and others received a further boost a few years after the Detroit study, in 1942, as a result of a field observation made during an epidemic in the area of Buffalo, New York by Alexander D. Langmuir, then a member of the New York State Department of Health.[12] In the course of this investi-

9. Dr. Molner became commissioner of health of Detroit after this investigation and in subsequent years attained prominence as the author of a syndicated newspaper column dealing with health matters.

10. S. D. Kramer, A. G. Gilliam, and J. G. Molner: Recovery of the virus of poliomyelitis from the stools of healthy contacts in an institutional outbreak. *Publ. Hlth Rep. (Wash.)*, *54*: 1914–22, 1939.

11. S. Gard: *Second International Conference on Live Poliovirus Vaccines.* Washington, D.C., Pan American Sanitary Bureau, 1960, p. 187.

12. A. D. Langmuir: Carriers and abortive cases in a rural poliomyelitis outbreak. *Amer. J. publ. Hlth, 32*: 275, 1942.

gation he observed a cluster of 5 paralytic cases which occurred under circumstances that pointed strongly to their having been infected by contact with healthy persons carrying the virus. Unlike Wickman and Wernstedt, he was able to document this by laboratory means—i.e. by virus isolation. Langmuir and McClure examined stool specimens from 27 intimate contacts of patients and recovered virus from 20 of them, whereas no virus was isolated from 4 individuals that had sustained attacks of poliomyelitis in the past.[13] This work unfortunately was somewhat clouded by the interpretations of the pathologist of the team, McClure, who had employed considerably broader pathological criteria as to what was to be regarded as positive evidence of poliomyelitis in the monkey than had been used by other investigators. Be that as it may, certainly some of the 20 isolations, perhaps the majority of them, were acceptable according to the usual orthodox standards of interpretation. The results constituted the first intimation that during a *rural* epidemic the proven poliovirus carrier rate might be infinitely higher than had been suspected.

Besides this, a more important new finding now emerged, viz. that the carrier rate seemed to follow the same age distribution as the frank paralytic cases. This meant that inapparent carriers were more common in infants and preschool children than in those of school age, and infinitely less common in adults. Thus, in addition to a growing awareness that a great deal of poliovirus infection lay completely below the surface, the idea now emerged that in epidemics a huge reservoir of virus might be in infants and young children who were actually suffering from acute asymptomatic infections.

Meanwhile the Yale Poliomyelitis Unit had gone off on another tack. As a follow-up of its prediction made in 1938 that poliovirus might be found in urban sewage, the unit was the first to succeed in demonstrating that this was indeed the case by recovering it from the sewage of Charleston, South Carolina during the large epidemic in that city in 1939; also in other epidemics, in Buffalo, New York (1939) and in Detroit, Michigan (1940).[14]

For a brief period the discovery that poliovirus was easily recoverable from sewage induced our Study Unit to reconsider Dr. Kling's *theorie hydrique*. When almost the only cases that occurred in the western part of Connecticut in 1939 were sequentially grouped about a heavily polluted river, this was thought to be supporting evidence.

But after one or two years the Yale group had begun to talk more cau-

13. G. Y. McClure and A. D. Langmuir: Search for carriers in an outbreak of acute anterior poliomyelitis in a rural community. *Amer. J. Hyg., 35*: 285, 1942.

14. J. R. Paul, J. D. Trask, and C. S. Culotta: Poliomyelitic virus in sewage. *Science, 90*: 258–59, 1939; J. R. Paul, J. D. Trask, and S. Gard: Poliomyelitic virus in urban sewage. *J. exp. Med., 71*: 765–77, 1940.

tiously about the role of sewage in the *transmission of poliomyelitis*. The following view was expressed in 1941:

> It is not evident . . . whether [the virus'] presence in sewage is a direct or even an indirect link in the chain which leads this potentially infectious agent from one patient to another in this disease. Our observations merely call attention to the fact that the virus is there during epidemics.[15]

The question was soon raised whether poliomyelitis virus might not be a normal or constantly replenished inhabitant of urban sewage, similar to the situation with tubercle bacilli. The mere finding of tubercle bacilli in sewage obviously told little about the epidemiology of human tuberculosis. Of particular interest in this connection was an experiment made during both epidemic and interepidemic periods to determine whether or not poliovirus might be universally present in urban sewage winter and summer, or only occasionally, i.e. during the epidemic season. If it were present all the time, this would have been in keeping with Aycock's theory; namely, that the population was constantly exposed to the virus, and only when profound alterations occurred in the human host did the clinical disease come to the surface. To answer this question the Yale Poliomyelitis Unit began a six-year study in which we tested samples of sewage collected monthly from one of the larger sewer effluents of New York City, which discharged into the East River.

These tests were continued, largely by Dr. Melnick, from 1940 until 1945.[16] The frequent negative but occasionally positive tests told an interesting story. In a given year when cases of poliomyelitis reached a peak during the summer within that particular urban district of New York City (drained by the East River sewer), poliovirus began to appear in the sewage. On the contrary, during interepidemic times the frequent tests for polioviruses were all negative. These findings lent no support to Aycock's theories. In fact they spoke loudly in favor of the idea that polioviruses circulate widely in the population and the environment only during epidemic seasons; in line with this thought, infection is acquired in the same manner as in measles, i.e. by exposure of a susceptible child to an infected person during a period when measles virus is existent in the community. But that infection was waterborne was not implied.

Another feature of Melnick's work was that it marked the beginning of a method of *sewage assay* for viruses that was to be widely used in subse-

15. J. R. Paul and J. D. Trask: The virus of poliomyelitis in stools and sewage. *J. Amer. med. Ass., 116*: 493–97, 1941.

16. J. R. Paul: Clinical epidemiology of poliomyelitis. *Medicine, 20*: 495–520, 1941; J. L. Melnick: Poliomyelitis virus in urban sewage in epidemic and nonepidemic times. *Amer. J. Hyg., 45*: 240–53, 1947.

quent years. Gradually the idea dawned that one could, by this means, detect the presence of polioviruses in a particular city and map its distribution at a given time within the area. Eventually, when other enteroviruses came on the scene, these too could be traced in similar fashion; and when attenuated poliovirus vaccines were introduced into the general population, virus isolation surveys from samples of sewage collected in different parts of the city could understandably be put to use in a variety of ways. Thus, in the few years following 1937 not only had a new leaf been turned, but concepts of the nature of poliomyelitis had undergone a metamorphosis. Most of all, examination of stool specimens had become the method of choice for tracing clinical poliovirus infections.

In looking back, it is remarkable that this change had been so long in coming. Kling and his colleagues had been on the right track as early as 1912; following this lead, in 1929 Kling, Levaditi, and Lépine had shown that cynomolgus monkeys could be infected via the oral route. As a matter of fact, Levaditi, one of Landsteiner's original collaborators and a most enthusiastic supporter of Kling's, also deserves credit for keeping this concept precariously alive. He it was who, with Kling, had confirmed the presence of virus in the intestinal tract in 1913; he had steadfastly championed this finding through the dark and relatively unproductive period of World War I and in the 1920s. For this alone, a brief sketch of his life is indicated here.

Constantin Levaditi (see fig. 40), who spent almost his entire career at the Pasteur Institute in Paris, has not been given the place that he deserves in the history of poliovirus research. His was the only career besides that of Landsteiner that spanned the age of Pasteur and modern times. Pierre Lépine of the Pasteur Institute has stated that Levaditi's work covered a range of subjects that today would be considered prodigious.[17] He was almost the first, and for a long time the only person in France, to study viruses systematically. As such he occupied a position in virology in France which Rivers was to hold later in the United States.

But Levaditi was familiar with viruses long before Rivers, so when the discovery of the etiologic agent of poliomyelitis by Landsteiner and Popper was announced in 1908, he was ready. His eagerness and enthusiasm led to a quick collaboration with Landsteiner in some of his earliest investigations. But, differing from Landsteiner, Levaditi never relinquished his interest in poliovirus research.

I had the good fortune to meet Levaditi during the winter of 1928–29 on one of his visits to the United States and was immediately struck by the enthusiasm which seemed so much a part of him. Though I was many years his junior, our encounter started a steady flow of correspondence

17. P. Lépine: C. Levaditi, 1874–1953. *Ann. Inst. Pasteur, 85*: 535–40, 1953.

that was kept up for years. When the Yale Poliomyelitis Commission, with Dr. Trask at the helm, started its clinical virological investigations during the U.S. epidemic of 1931, although separated from us by an ocean much wider than it is today, Levaditi proved an enthusiastic supporter

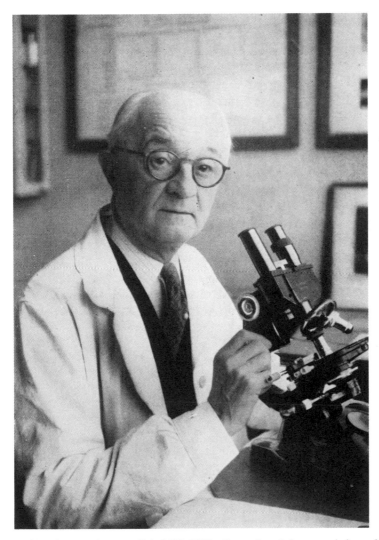

Fig. 40. Constantin Levaditi (1874–1953). Reproduced by permission of Annals of L'Institute Pasteur (see n. 17).

of our work. In fact, in the early 1930s the Pasteur Institute sent an emissary, in the form of Dr. Harry Plotz, bearing Levaditi's urgent and special message that our publications in the United States on "la theorie des infections inapparents" was to be exploited in America as being the whole key to the epidemiology of poliomyelitis.

Constantin Levaditi was born in France in 1874; having lost both parents early in life, he was brought up by an aunt who lived in Bucharest, Romania, where he obtained his medical education. Shortly after his internship he became, in 1899, a demonstrator at the Bacteriological Institute at Bucharest. After a brief interval of training under Paul Ehrlich in Germany, he returned to spend the rest of his life in Paris.

Here, by a stroke of good fortune, he was able to obtain a position in Elie Metchnikoff's laboratory at the Pasteur Institute. Dr. Emile Roux, then director, soon gave him the chance of establishing an independent laboratory at the institute. He retained his position as head of that laboratory until the time of his retirement in 1940. Levaditi has been characterized as bridging the gap between nineteenth-century pathology and twentieth-century immunology. He exercised an immense influence on both of these sciences; there was scarcely a microbiological laboratory in Europe that did not boast of at least one worker who had been trained in Paris by Levaditi.

In the words of Lépine, Levaditi shed a radiance upon the "House of Pasteur" which will long be remembered with emotion. He kept this light constantly burning until his death in 1953. It was a pity that he did not live two more years to witness the conquest of poliomyelitis achieved through the science of which he had so long been a champion, namely immunology. But he lived to see his work with Kling and Lépine vindicated, and that was, to say the least, no small triumph.

CHAPTER 28

Insects and Their Potential in the Spread of Poliomyelitis

From the beginning of the twentieth century, perhaps before, the idea that poliomyelitis was spread by insects seemed to be particularly appealing. For one thing, this would account for its striking summer incidence in temperate climates. Yellow fever, another summer disease, had at the turn of the century been discovered to be carried by the mosquito, and this had led to all sorts of speculations about the nefarious and universal role of insects in the spread of disease. As far as poliomyelitis was concerned, the idea had received a sudden but short-lived burst of enthusiasm in the excitement over the stable fly in 1912. The following year, and for some years thereafter, Frost had included in his epidemiological investigations any data that could possibly implicate insects as potential vectors; in the great epidemic of 1916, Haven Emerson had continued these observations, but found them unproductive.

The excitement over the stable fly did not represent the first attempt to test the capacity of flies to carry the virus, for in 1911 Flexner and his colleagues at the Rockefeller Institute had succeeded in inducing experimental poliomyelitis through the agency of nonbiting common house flies, *Musca domestica*.[1] In these experiments, a suspension of ground-up flies that had been allowed to come in contact with a thick emulsion of spinal cord from a fatal case of poliomyelitis was injected into the brains of monkeys. It was a highly artificial experiment to say the least, and it was not surprising that it produced a positive result; virus was recovered from the flies for a brief time (48 hours), but whether from the surface of the fly or from an internal site was not clear.

It was at Harvard a year later that Dr. Milton J. Rosenau, at that time the professor of preventive medicine in the Medical School, and the entomologist C. T. Brues began their work on the biting stable fly (*Stomoxys calcitrans*), using rhesus monkeys (*Macaca mulatta*) as test animals.[2] They allowed thousands of flies to feed first upon a monkey in the acute stage

1. S. Flexner and P. F. Clark: Contamination of the fly with poliomyelitis virus. Tenth note. *J. Amer. med. Ass., 56*: 1717, 1911.

2. M. J. Rosenau and C. T. Brues: Some experimental observations upon monkeys concerning the transmission of poliomyelitis through the agency of *Stomoxys calcitrans*. A preliminary note. *Mass. St. Bd. Hlth, M. Bull.*, n.s. 7: 317, 1912; Trans. XV Int. Cong. Hyg. Demog., Washington, *1*: 616, 1913.

of poliomyelitis, and immediately afterwards, upon a normal monkey. On the basis of their results in such experiments, the stable fly was heralded as the answer to the mechanism of spread of poliomyelitis. The implication was that stable flies transmitted the disease in much the same way that anopheles mosquitoes transmit malaria and biting sand flies transmit sand-fly fever. In 1912 this seemed a highly reasonable suggestion. It could explain why the virus was so much more widespread in summer than in winter, and it could account for its worldwide distribution; for what could be more universal than biting flies? But enthusiasm for this theory lasted only a few months.

Immediately following Rosenau and Brues' announcement, Anderson and Frost, working at the Hygienic Laboratory of the Public Health Service in Washington, also reported success in the transmission of poliomyelitis by stomoxys flies; but their experiments must have been hastily designed, for within a year they retracted their published results after examining possible loopholes. Others were also unable to confirm Rosenau and Brues' findings, notably Howard and Clark, the latter having shared in one of Flexner's original 1911 investigations on the common housefly and poliovirus. Later Brues himself said, in 1916; "But these experiments have failed of further confirmation, and cannot now be regarded as free from possible error."[3] Thus the idea that a biting fly was the explanation for the dissemination of poliomyelitis, which had been so enthusiastically received at first, was discredited almost as quickly as it had come on the scene.

To digress a bit and consider other biting insects: Japanese workers, in subsequent years, raised the interesting possibility from time to time that mosquitoes might play a part in the spread of poliomyelitis. Their work on the subject has been intermittent and never attracted sufficient enthusiasm to warrant a serious attempt to repeat it. Other biting insects, such as lice, bedbugs, biting midges, and sand flies, have also been suspected of playing some role, but no one has considered this possibility of sufficient importance to set up the elaborate experiments that would be necessary to prove the point, particularly as other explanations seemed to be so much more plausible.

If a biting fly did not satisfy all criteria, however, it was thought that nonbiting flies might do as well, since it was entirely conceivable that a fly, contaminated within or without by one means or another, might transfer the infection from a sick to a well child. The sudden upsurge of interest in the intestinal aspects of poliomyelitis in 1938, together with the recent isolation of the agent under natural conditions from privies

3. C. T. Brues: "Insects as carriers of infection. An entomological study of the 1916 epidemic," in *A Monograph on the Epidemic of Poliomyelitis (Infantile Paralysis) in New York City in 1916.* Dept. of Health, New York City, 1917, p. 137.

and from urban sewage, was enough to bring nonbiting flies back into the picture. If infected infants and children shed the virus in their stools, it was easy to see how they might contaminate their immediate environment and provide an opportunity for flies to pick up the virus. Furthermore, this line of reasoning led to the suspicion that flies, particularly of the feces-eating variety, might even be a ready source for contamination of certain varieties of food.

It was not remarkable therefore that, through the use of various vastly improved methods, three American laboratories reported almost simultaneously, within the short space of a few weeks, the detection of poliovirus in samples of flies collected in rural and urban areas where the disease was epidemic during the summer and fall of 1941. The investigators included those of the Yale Poliomyelitis Unit,[4] Sabin and Ward of the Children's Hospital Research Foundation in Cincinnati,[5] and Toomey, Takacs, and Tischer of the Department of Pediatrics at the Cleveland Municipal Hospital.[6] All were successful in isolating the agent from feces-eating flies including common blowflies (*Phormia* and *Protophormia*), green bottle flies (*Phaenicia sericata*), and various other members of the *Phaenicia* family.

The next chapter in this story dealing with practical studies on the dissemination of poliovirus by flies is an unhappy one for those who had had their hopes aroused by the news that poliomyelitis might indeed be a fly-borne disease and that fly-abatement measures might serve as a useful means of prevention. Within a few years, however, this matter was settled as far as the United States was concerned—in the negative, as had been the case with many another onetime hopeful means of prophylaxis. Luckily the question did not drag along in an undecided state for long.

Within two years of the time that flies captured under natural conditions had been incriminated as possible mechanical vectors of polioviruses, the chemical insecticide originally known as *neocid* (1943), and later as DDT, was introduced. At first it was a restricted product with priorities especially for the armed forces in the mosquito-infested malarious areas of the South Pacific islands and other strategic locations. The almost miraculous results achieved in the control of mosquitoes led to delirious hopes that all insect pests could be controlled by small doses of this powerful chemical. In fact, one high-ranking medical officer from the Preventive Medical Division in the surgeon general's office in the U.S. Army went

4. J. R. Paul, J. D. Trask, M. B. Bishop, J. L. Melnick, and A. E. Casey: The detection of poliomyelitis virus in flies. *Science, 94*: 395–96, 1941.

5. A. B. Sabin and R. Ward: Flies as carriers in human poliomyelitis virus. *Science, 94*: 590, 1941.

6. J. A. Toomey, W. S. Takacs, and L. A. Tischer: Poliomyelitis virus from flies. *Proc. Soc. exp. Biol. Med. (N.Y.), 48*: 637, 1941.

so far as to publish an article in a popular magazine ascribing almost magical qualities to DDT.

Coincidentally, in the winter of 1943–44, questions were being raised as to whether this new pesticide, which had proved so effective in eradicating the mosquito vectors of malaria in the South Pacific and had apparently succeeded in suppressing epidemic, louse-borne typhus in Naples, Italy, could not be used with the same effectiveness for diseases spread through the possible agency of flies, notably bacterial dysenteries, and perhaps even poliomyelitis. The idea that flies *spread* this last mentioned infection was only hypothetical, but it was also high time that the question be looked into from the theoretical as well as the practical aspects.

The incrimination of the fly as an actual contaminator of food was soon demonstrated by a single ingenious experiment undertaken by the Yale Poliomyelitis Unit and reported in 1945.[7] Dr. Robert Ward (Sabin's former partner) had joined the unit earlier, and he and fellow members of the team proceeded to expose food (sliced bananas with sugar and water) to flies, which were flying about outside the homes of poliomyelitis patients during an epidemic in North Carolina. The food which the flies had contaminated was collected after 24 hours, frozen, and transported to the laboratory in New Haven. There it was subsequently fed to a series of chimpanzees. The investigators did not have long to wait, for several of the test animals promptly developed subclinical infections, as demonstrated by prolonged excretion of poliovirus in their stools. This result indicated that it was theoretically possible that flies might deposit poliovirus on food and so indirectly induce the infection in children.

Hence it seemed logical to try fly control as a measure to suppress poliomyelitis epidemics, particularly since Public Health Service teams working in Texas had reported that the new insecticide had proved successful in fly-abatement programs; not only was the fly population in selected areas reduced markedly, but a significant reduction in diarrheal disease had followed close upon the heels of DDT application.

It had immediately become apparent however that the fly was far more resistant to DDT than the mosquito, thus making the task much more difficult than had been anticipated. Obviously, only when a disease such as bacterial dysentery was highly prevalent, as it was in Hidalgo County, Texas in 1946–47, would an experimental fly-control program be likely to give significant results. As far as poliomyelitis was concerned, it would be necessary to choose a site where the disease was approaching epidemic proportions for a similar experiment to provide meaningful data. Needless to say, because of these practical problems, setting up valid experi-

7. R. Ward, J. L. Melnick, and D. M. Horstmann: Poliomyelitis virus in fly-contaminated food collected at an epidemic. *Science, 101*: 491–93, 1945.

ments to assess the importance of flies in poliomyelitis proved extremely difficult.

In 1945, even before the USPHS trial in Hidalgo County was published,[8] the Yale Poliomyelitis Unit had started to carry out some exploratory programs of fly control during poliomyelitis epidemics. In this endeavor we were aided by two entomologists from the Public Health Service and, as it was wartime, by a faithful group of conscientious objectors, who proved to be true to the first part of their title. Plans were drawn with the advice and close cooperation of the Public Health Service. At that time there were premature predictions that the miraculous new insecticides might completely eradicate the fly population within cities. So it was proposed that the use of DDT be confined to urban areas. It was further proposed that application of the insecticide be limited to outdoor areas and that the project be carried out as a *controlled* experiment in which certain areas of a city would be treated with DDT and others left untouched. An effort was to be made to select as favorable an urban site as was possible and certainly to start work as early in the course of an epidemic of poliomyelitis as feasible.

Early in the summer of 1945 a preliminary trial was carried out in Savannah, Georgia, which was not an epidemic area, to see whether such fly-abatement procedures could be conducted successfully within an urban area. As this trial went off without incident, it was decided to undertake experiments in epidemic areas, provided favorable opportunities presented themselves.

The first of these came in the form of a small epidemic that had built up in the early summer of 1945 in Paterson, New Jersey, where an area of four square miles (half the total area) was treated by teams working with hand sprayers, and the rest of the city was left untreated. Definite fly reduction, which lasted only a few days, was achieved in all treated wards, and moreover it was estimated that it was possible to maintain the fly population at about 25 percent of its usual summer level. But no reduction in poliomyelitis cases was shown in the treated area.[9] However, only 62 cases were reported for the city of Paterson in the entire epidemic. This was clearly too few on which to base definite conclusions.

A much more difficult and more painful experience was encountered in Rockford, Illinois, where a severe epidemic of sizable proportions occurred during that same summer. When it was finally over, a total of 321 cases had been reported in the city and county surrounding Rockford, which together had a population of about 85,000. Here we had not reck-

8. J. Watt and D. R. Lindsay: Diarrheal disease control studies. I. Effect of fly control in a high morbidity area. *Publ. Hlth Rep.* (*Wash.*), *63*: 1319–34, 1948.

9. J. L. Melnick, R. Ward, D. R. Lindsay, and F. E. Lyman: Fly-abatement studies in urban poliomyelitis epidemics during 1945. *Publ. Hlth Rep.* (*Wash.*), *62*: 910–22, 1947.

oned sufficiently on the sociological or psycho-social aspects of the problem and had labored under the delusion that we could carry out a carefully controlled experiment that could conform to our own plans. We were much mistaken.

One of the members of the Yale group had been dispatched to Rockford in July to determine whether the epidemic seemed to be progressing or regressing, and whether the area was at all suited to fly-abatement procedures. He was asked to report his findings at a presumably closed meeting of the Board of Health of the City of Rockford. The report which he submitted indicated that the epidemic seemed to be building up and that the city was a likely place for a controlled trial of fly abatement. It was further suggested that perhaps spraying from an airplane might be used, but nothing could be decided until the entire situation had been further checked and investigated. Unbeknownst to the speaker, not only one but several newspapermen were present at this meeting, and they quickly spread the word that the one thing that could save Rockford was to spray it from the air with insecticide. At this unfavorable turn of events the Yale group was inclined to pull in its horns, but it was too late. The situation had got out of hand; in retrospect, we had practically asked for it. Things moved swiftly from then on. The current U.S. senator from Illinois, Mr. Scott Lucas, had been in touch with the Public Health Service and was quoted as saying that efforts were being made to block the spraying of the city at a time when the people of Rockford were seeking desperately for relief. At the time of my first arrival, on August 17, the city was in an uproar. The situation was an oft-repeated example of how all elements of an urban population would unite: Democrats and Republicans, municipal politicians, management and labor, and, most of all, the parents of young children, whatever their race, creed, or color, joined in an almost hysterical common interest over the disaster of a severe poliomyelitis epidemic. Meantime the Public Health Service had communicated with me, saying that all reasonable and necessary steps should be taken to carry out the spraying of the city of Rockford with insecticide at the earliest possible time.

To say the least, it was not the sort of atmosphere in which to carry out a carefully controlled experiment. But decidedly the public had a right to know what was going on, even though, of necessity, the plans so hastily conceived had little chance of success. "Try something—do anything!" was the cry. Local health authorities were satisfied because at least there were outward manifestations that something was being done—wheels were being set in motion to stop the epidemic.

The situation being what it was, prompt arrangements were made under the Armed Forces Epidemiological Board to have a single army plane from nearby Truax Field in Wisconsin undertake the spraying of DDT in a designated area of the city. On the day following my arrival I was greeted by headlines in the local newspapers, with type two inches high, saying: "Professor Expected to Board Mercy Plane at Noon Today"; and "Preventive Spraying for Polio as Important to Rockford as the Atomic Bomb" (which had been dropped on Hiroshima only a few days before).

In the meantime we had distributed sensitive markers around certain areas of the city to enable us to determine whether the insecticide had been laid down in sufficient concentration. Almost immediately it was learned that this objective had not been achieved, so we had to repeat the spraying on the ground, by hand, and by this time we had lost two precious weeks. Eleven men, who worked day and night applying the 5 percent DDT emulsion at a concentration of 1.5 pounds per acre, were required for this six-day project. This maneuver resulted in a temporary reduction of flies, but, as in Paterson, it had no effect on the progress of the polio-myelitis epidemic. Suffice it to say, the Yale Poliomyelitis Unit made no further attempts after 1945 to carry on with this type of experimentation, yet the unsavory reputation that the group had gained in relation to fly abatement as a prophylactic measure during epidemics of poliomyelitis remained for many years. It also became evident during subsequent years that a far more likely, although a more difficult, method of fly control than spraying with DDT was to destroy the breeding places of these insects in advance of the epidemic season.

A final decision in the matter came when the Public Health Service, aided by workers from Johns Hopkins University, administered the coup de grace. By a lucky break it happened that in the same county in southern Texas where experiments in fly control had previously been carried out in connection with diarrheal diseases, numerous cases of poliomyelitis had begun to crop up. This seemed an excellent opportunity to measure the effect of the suppression of flies upon the incidence of poliomyelitis. Eventually the Johns Hopkins group reported, in 1953,[10] that whereas fly abatement had been instituted before and continued during an outbreak of poliomyelitis, it had failed to affect the course of the epidemic. The trial was a thorough testing, and with such a final judgment, this form of prophylaxis was abandoned. Fly control by the emergency use of insecticide was to go the way of the nasal spray and the prophylactic use of convalescent serum. In the light of further and more modern appreciation of the dangerous ecological effects of the indiscriminate and heavy use of insecticides, it would seem that the failure of DDT to check poliomyelitis epi-

10. R. S. Paffenbarger and J. Watt: Poliomyelitis in Hidalgo County, Texas, 1948. Epidemiologic observations. *Amer. J. Hyg., 58*: 269–87, 1953.

demics may have been a blessing in disguise. For inevitably, if there had been a suggestion of success, insecticides would have been universally applied with an overzealous hand and in quantities far exceeding the prescribed amounts.

In brief, Wickman's original contention that poliomyelitis is a disease spread by personal contact still held. Not only was fly abatement unsuccessful in controlling epidemics, but the results seemed to prove that flies did not play a major part in spreading the virus throughout the usual North American environment, in communities where sanitary facilities were mostly adequate. And yet the basic idea that in some fly-ridden cities and villages in the Middle East, India, and North and South Africa, where the eyelids and lips of infants seem to be constantly covered with flies and where flies play a part in the endemic spread of not only diarrheal diseases but also of bacterial and viral eye infections such as staphylococcal and gonococcal infections and trachoma, these same insects could theoretically act as an accessory means of dissemination of poliomyelitis.[11] In fact this would seem highly likely.

Quite apart from the practical implications of fly abatement in the control of poliomyelitis, there is also a biological side of the question. In 1941, feces-eating flies had been incriminated as the only extrahuman or extraprimate host that could act as a vector for polioviruses. Later, in 1942, Syverton et al.[12] discovered that cockroaches had the same unpleasant property. At some future date, it is not unlikely that other insects besides these two species will be shown to harbor polioviruses.

The possible involvement of flies in the epidemiology of poliomyelitis continued to intrigue investigators for some years. In an oft repeated series of carefully controlled and quantitative experiments, poliovirus was shown to survive in the gut of feces-eating flies for about two weeks. During this period the fly may act as a mechanical vector, but there even is evidence to suggest that the virus may undergo a brief temporary period of multiplication.[13] Cockroaches have been demonstrated to harbor poliovirus for 51 days, but there has been no intimation that the virus multiplies in these insects.[14] Indeed the carriage of poliovirus by insects in no way com-

---

11. J. H. S. Gear: "The extra human sources of poliomyelitis," in *Poliomyelitis; Papers and Discussions presented at the Second International Poliomyelitis Conference,* Phila., Lippincott, 1952, pp. 343–54.

12. J. T. Syverton, R. G. Fischer, S. A. Smith, R. P. Dow, and H. F. Shoof: *Fed. Proc. 11:* 483, 1952.

13. M. Gudnadotter: Studies of the fate of Type I poliovirus in flies. *J. exp. Med., 113:* 159–76, 1961.

14. K. H. Dave and R. C. Wallis: Survival of Type 1 and 3 polio vaccine viruses in blow flies (*Phaenicia sericata*) at 40°C. *Proc. Soc. exp. Biol. Med. (N.Y.), 119:* 121–24; Ibid., Preliminary communication on the survival, the sites harboring virus and genetic stability of polioviruses in cockroaches, 119: 124–26, 1965.

pares in significance to the situation in yellow fever, in which the agent undergoes multiplication in the appropriate mosquito and hence merits the name of an arthropod-borne virus.

In the two foregoing chapters it has been said in essence that for a few years during the period from 1941 to 1945, the story of poliomyelitis had temporarily sunk into a slough of feces and flies. And yet it recovered in due time, to go on to more salutory features.

CHAPTER 29

Early Philanthropic and Granting Agencies

After World War I it became increasingly evident in a number of countries that paralytic poliomyelitis was one of those diseases that desperately needed financial help; in fact cried out for aid. Not only would immense subsidy for patient care be required if individuals crippled by extensive paralyses were to be salvaged, but funds were also essential to enable scientists to investigate the intricacies of the disease—its nature, treatment, and prevention. Such research was far more costly than most laboratories could afford. Landsteiner had recognized this as early as 1912, and it accounted in part for his decision to abandon work on poliomyelitis. The great majority of universities and private research institutions were unable to furnish the expensive facilities, technical assistance, and the supply of monkeys which were so necessary at that time for poliomyelitis research.

First and foremost, however, came the appeal that assistance for long-term care was needed for those unfortunate children and young adults that had been struck down and disabled by the cruel affliction. In the latter half of the nineteenth century and before, the numbers of paralytic poliomyelitis cases had been small in relation to other forms of chronic disease and disability, but during the years from 1900 to 1930 the problem of infantile paralysis had grown so as to make it mandatory that something be done. Several countries reached that conclusion simultaneously. One was Australia, where an ardent advocate and organizer of private donations for poliomyelitis emerged in the form of Dr. (later Dame) Jean Macnamara. Whether such support was wholly channeled in the direction of patient care or whether it also provided funds for research is not clear, but · the latter probably was not included, at least at first.

Other countries followed suit. In Sweden, for instance, it had long been the custom to set up national funds donated by the public on the even birthdays of the king. The king then dedicated this money for a particular purpose. King Gustaf V's eighty-year fund in 1938 was dedicated for the support of research in the field of disabling diseases with priorities going to poliomyelitis and rheumatism. From this kind of support, which went along for years, the present Swedish National Association against Poliomyelitis evolved in the late 1940s, and it continues to this day. Various countries subsequently developed their own special patterns of philanthropy, setting up foundations or associations to combat poliomyelitis.

In the United States during the 1920s and early 1930s, when aid for a worthy research project on poliomyelitis was urgently needed, grants were usually obtainable either from private sources or from such agencies as the Rockefeller Foundation or the National Research Council. Such grants, usually made on an annual basis, were not large; indeed to the research worker most of them were painfully small and woefully short term.

A granting agency entirely restricted to an individual disease was rare. In the United States in the early 1920s, as far as can be ascertained, there was only one—The National Tuberculosis Association (NTA). It was a pioneering organization that had come into being in 1904—faced with a huge task. Fortunately it did not have to provide for the care of patients because the state saw to that. But its program did include appropriations for ancillary expenses dealing with various matters in the control of this extremely prevalent disease—then known as the great white plague. The NTA derived its income from contributions from individuals, commercial companies, foundations, and, after 1920, from the sale of Christmas seals. It was run by a group of individuals thoroughly familiar with both medical and administrative problems in tuberculosis, and familiar too with priorities in that field. Among the NTA's officers at the start were physicians of high scientific caliber, and such devoted public servants as Edward L. Trudeau, Charles J. Hatfield, Theobald Smith, E. R. Baldwin, and E. L. Opie, who held the reins more or less tightly. To the association's credit, it was the first of its type to recognize (in 1915) the importance of making its funds available for research. In 1921 its Committee on Medical Research distributed grants for investigation of tuberculosis, to assist only such research fields as had already given promise of success rather than to attempt to create new fields.[1] The association had little of the atmosphere of big business and went about its fund-raising efforts through the sale of Christmas seals with a minimum of fanfare.

But by the 1920s and 1930s, the worldwide and particularly the American incidence of poliomyelitis epidemics had risen so strikingly that the disease came to have an appeal for the public that outweighed that of tuberculosis. Something had to be done about the mounting backlog of patients left with paralytic effects of this devastating disease.

In the United States, perhaps the earliest public support dealing with crippling aspects of poliomyelitis came in 1927, when Franklin D. Roosevelt, having sustained a disastrous attack of paralytic poliomyelitis in the early 1920s, established the Georgia Warm Springs Foundation located at Warm Springs in western Georgia. It is said that in the days before he became president, during his early visits to this watering spot, he took great

---

1. V. Cameron and E. R. Long: *Tuberculosis Medical Research; National Tuberculosis Association, 1904–1955.* New York, Nat. Tuberculosis Assn., 1959, p. 5.

pleasure in splashing about in the crowded swimming pool, cheerfully encouraging, even helping, fellow patients undergoing similar hydrotherapy, most of them less crippled than he, to exert themselves to the best of
their limited abilities. Such was his friendly enthusiasm for this kind of active effort in behalf of other victims of poliomyelitis that it is alleged that
two-thirds of his personal fortune went to the cause of the Warm Springs
Foundation. Its purpose was twofold:

> *First,* to give direct aid to patients through the skill of an able, care-
> fully selected professional staff, in a place with agreeable surround-
> ings and natural warm water; and
>
> *Second,* to pass on to hospitals and the medical profession of the
> country any useful observations or special methods of proved merit
> resulting from this specialized work which might be suitable for prac-
> tical application elsewhere.[2]

Warm Springs, Georgia soon became the leading place in the country
for rehabilitation and physical therapy for patients suffering from the late
effects of paralytic poliomyelitis. Since 1921, when Mr. Roosevelt had
been stricken with the disease, he continued to go there year after year and
even built a house on the premises, which, after he became president of
the United States, was known as the Little White House. Thus this foundation and the place it represented became a symbol to the American people of the *aftercare* of poliomyelitis patients. It has remained so to this
day.

Investigation of the *acute* disease was not included in the program of
the Georgia Warm Springs Foundation, but support for research on this
aspect of poliomyelitis followed shortly. It came about through the efforts
of Mr. Jeremiah Milbank, a philanthropist of New York City. He knew
little about poliomyelitis, but he recognized the havoc it caused and
sought the advice of acknowledged experts in the field as to how one dealt
with a situation of this kind. The men he turned to included Dr. W. H.
Park, the director of New York City's Health Department Laboratories;
three from Columbia University's College of Physicians and Surgeons—
Dr. Joseph A. Blake, a distinguished New York surgeon; Dr. F. P. Gay,
a microbiologist; and Dr. F. Tilney, a neurologist; and Dr. M. J. Rosenau,
professor of preventive medicine at Harvard. This group was chosen as
a steering committee charged with the duty of organizing studies to be undertaken by those best qualified to carry on and direct such work in laboratories that already were active in poliomyelitis research.

The committee was promptly enlarged during the first year of its exist-

2. Georgia Warm Springs Foundation: *Annual Report for year ended on Sept. 30, 1946,*
Warm Springs, Georgia, p. 8.

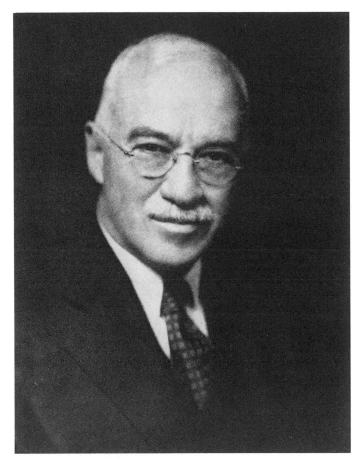

FIG. 41. William Hallock Park, M.D. (1863–1939). Figure reproduced by permission of E. P. Dutton & Co., Inc.

ence, in 1929, and one member was recruited from the Lister Institute of London, England, ostensibly to provide an international flavor. On this tenuous basis it was called the International Committee for the Study of Infantile Paralysis. The committee was given $250,000 and for three years operated by awarding grants from this budget. The original amount was subsequently increased by $30,000 to support the publication of an encyclopedic book containing the most extensive information and opinions about poliomyelitis that had ever been collected in one volume.[3] Dr. Park (see fig. 41) had assumed a position of leadership in the poliomyelitis field, and the new responsibilities bestowed upon him by the Milbank committee gave him a degree of confidence about the disease almost equal to that of Dr. Flexner.

3. *Poliomyelitis.* International Committee for the Study of Infantile Paralysis, Baltimore, Williams & Wilkins, 1932.

Had Park's committee done nothing else, the publication of this volume in itself was an outstanding achievement. One of the best and most enduring parts of the book is its extensive, 45-page "Bibliography of Poliomyelitis," covering the period from the late eighteenth century until 1932.[4] On this, Dr. Park's editorial staff must have spent an enormous amount of time and labor.

In the mid-1930s, however, both the public and the medical profession suffered some disillusionment with poliomyelitis research; Dr. Park himself underwent a certain amount of deflation as the result of the ill-fated Brodie-Park and Kolmer vaccines of which we have heard much. But this setback was short lived, and the cause bounced back with renewed vigor in the late 1930s.

For one thing, the all-around worthiness of the appeal of poliomyelitis was bound to gather strength and could not be suppressed for long. The cause aroused a universal compassionate response—as indeed it should have. It was more than a terrifying epidemic scourge; it was a national affliction, one which had special meaning for the American people. The spectacle of a brave but paralyzed little child, boldy attempting his first steps with steel braces attached to his legs, was well-nigh irresistible; it figured subsequently on posters in many a fund-raising campaign, and the outpouring of money amounted to an exhibition of almost religious fervor.

In March 1933 Franklin Delano Roosevelt had taken office as president of the United States. Not only was he a national political figure, but through his struggle in surmounting, by sheer willpower, great physical disability due to paralysis of both legs, he immediately became the symbol of hope and courage of an almost unbelievable kind. There is no denying that his election to the presidency gave a tremendous boost to the cause of poliomyelitis. The fervent expectation at the time was that the president would lead this nation out of the financial depression that had engulfed it. Added to this, for the majority of American voters, he became overnight a courageous national hero.

Dr. Fishbein subsequently documented this sentiment in the dedication of his *Bibliography of Infantile Paralysis* to Mr. Roosevelt:

> Who, by his triumph over the most dreaded of crippling diseases, which could not conquer him, gave inspiration and courage to thousands of children, men and women similarly afflicted.[5]

4. Ibid., pp. 485–528.

5. *A Bibliography of Infantile Paralysis; 1789–1949,* ed. by M. Fishbein and E. M. Salmonsen, with Ludvig Hektoen, 2nd ed. Philadelphia, Lippincott, 1951. This book was published under the auspices of the National Foundation for Infantile Paralysis. The bibliography mentioned in n. 4 proved of inestimable value to Dr. Fishbein who brought it up to date, as of the year 1949.

Needless to say, fund raisers who were interested in helping the good cause of poliomyelitis were quick to take advantage of the double appeal. Soon after Mr. Roosevelt's election they chose the date of his birthday (January 30) as a fitting one on which to hold a nationwide subscription ball. According to one account,

> The first Birthday Ball to raise funds for Georgia Warm Springs Foundation was held January 30, 1934. Subsequently, from 1935 to 1938, this nationwide celebration of the President's birthday became the principal method of raising money to fight infantile paralysis. On December 15, 1934, a special Birthday Ball Commission of fifteen prominent people was organized to administer the funds raised by the birthday balls. To aid the commission in its work, a special scientific advisory committee was formed early in 1935 and began making grants to medical investigators on May 28, 1935. The first sixteen grants made totalled $241,000.[6]

If any organization in the United States can be said to have seen the light in the matter of obtaining support for poliomyelitis, it was the President's Birthday Ball Commission (PBBC). The National Foundation for Infantile Paralysis, which succeeded the PBBC within a few years, capitalized on this situation to the nth degree; but if priorities are in order, the PBBC deserves the credit. Much to the dismay of some of its organizers, this charity ball become popularly known under the singularly inappropriate name of a "Paralysis Dance."

Although the PBBC was a small organization and its scientific committees largely run by one man, namely Paul de Kruif of science-writing fame, it did its job remarkably well. De Kruif had been an adviser to Sinclair Lewis in the writing of the novel *Arrowsmith* and had himself been author of two provocative books, *Microbe Hunters* and *Hunger Fighters*. Although not exactly knowledgeable about poliomyelitis in 1935, he knew infinitely more about the glamour of medical research and how to turn this on. Thus began a period when the stage was set in America for the promotion of the cause of poliomyelitis by popular and highly important figures in public life.

Considering the relative limitation of the financial resources of the PBBC it accomplished a great deal as far as supporting research was concerned. The committee in charge of planning the research program had distinguished people on it besides de Kruif: Dr. Donald Armstrong, vice-president of the Metropolitan Life Insurance Company, Dr. Max Peet of the University of Michigan, Dr. George McCoy of the Hygienic Labora-

6. S. Benison: *Tom Rivers; Reflections on a Life in Medicine and Science.* Cambridge, Mass., M.I.T. Press, 1967, footnote, p. 179.

tory in Washington, and, later, Dr. Thomas Rivers of the Hospital of the Rockefeller Institute. Paul de Kruif literally ran the show, if anybody can be said to have run a show with Dr. Rivers as one of the committee members.

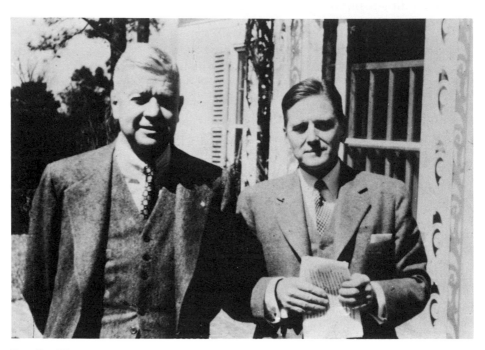

FIG. 42.   Thomas M. Rivers (left) with the author. Picture taken in 1947 at Warm Springs, Georgia.

Although Rivers (see fig. 42) has been quoted as saying that the grants-in-aid made by the President's Birthday Ball Commission were essentially ineffective, here I think he erred. He said: "If you take the good things they did, and substract the bad things that they did, you get a minus. It doesn't mean that everything they did was rotten or useless."[7] Yet in the three short years of its existence this small organization, which operated on a limited budget, was able to support a surprising number of meritorious research projects. However ill fated the Brodie-Park vaccine may have been, the rest of the undertakings represented for the most part quite substantial efforts, and a few of these were *real* contributions. Grants given by the PBBC during its short life included those made to Howard Howe of Johns Hopkins, Joseph Stokes of the University of Pennsylvania, Lloyd Aycock of the Harvard Infantile Paralysis Commission, and the Yale Poliomyelitis Unit. Ten papers supported by PBBC funds were published by

7. Ibid., p. 193.

the Yale group alone. These dealt with the separation of poliovirus into at least two antigenic types; and the rediscovery of the importance of the alimentary tract in the pathogenesis of human poliomyelitis. It was at least another few years before the National Foundation for Infantile Paralysis, successor to the PBBC, could claim to have supported investigations of any such importance.

The PBBC closed up shop in 1938 and was replaced by the National Foundation for Infantile Paralysis (NFIP), which came into being immediately thereafter with Mr. Basil O'Connor, a former law partner of President Roosevelt, as its president. The succeeding organization at least profited from the experience of the earlier one in fund raising on a national basis. It also profited to a certain extent by inheriting members of the PBBC committees. This was to prove of enormous benefit.

CHAPTER 30

The National Foundation for Infantile Paralysis

From the start the National Foundation for Infantile Paralysis (NFIP) deviated from the early example set by the National Tuberculosis Association. The only resemblances between the two were that both directed their efforts against a *single* disease and both were supported as private philanthropies. But the National Tuberculosis Association was a far smaller organization run by men who had labored in that vineyard for a long time and thus were intimately associated with problems of tuberculosis in the United States. Perhaps they were too close to their subject. When Mr. Basil O'Connor took over the presidency of the National Foundation for Infantile Paralysis it was obvious that things began to happen, for with a man of such ability and breadth of vision at its head, one who could recruit many prominent figures for his board of trustees and consulting committees, the organization was bound to move ahead in a big way. After all, with the president of the United States as its spiritual sponsor, it could hardly have done otherwise. It was not as if the foundation had sprung fully formed from the head of Athena, committees and all, and yet this was to some extent the idea of bigness linked to importance that this agency gave at first.

As for Basil O'Connor himself, this remarkable man, besides possessing unusual legal capabilities, was a forceful, able, and imaginative administrator. Not content with limiting himself to activities in downtown New York, he emerged as a leader of good causes. His was a broad outlook of national dimensions. He espoused not only good causes, but great causes.

Born in Taunton, Massachusetts in 1892, he was educated at Dartmouth College and the Harvard Law School. He graduated from the latter in 1915 and practiced law for a while both in Boston and New York. After some years he entered into a law partnership in New York City with Franklin D. Roosevelt in a firm known as Roosevelt and O'Connor. This was in 1924, just three years after Mr. Roosevelt had been stricken with poliomyelitis, which had left him with a severe degree of disability. Their professional association continued during the period of Mr. Roosevelt's governorship of New York State and right up until his election to the presidency of the United States.

Among causes in which Mr. O'Connor exhibited his talent for leadership besides the National Foundation for Infantile Paralysis was the American Red Cross (during the years of World War II), and, later, the National Citizen's Committee for the World Health Organization, to mention but a few. To these tasks he brought an unerring sense of where the public's interest lay—what it would and, even of more importance, what it would not support. He also had that loyalty for the good cause which goes with militant magnanimity. It was inevitable that the NFIP would prosper under his guidance. But through it all he was a tough opponent to face on the witness stand or, for that matter, in committees or anywhere else.

In the earliest days of this organization, most members of its administrative staff were unfamiliar with poliomyelitis except as a dreadful paralytic affliction that ought to be put down at all costs. Although the foundation was quick to learn about this disease, it is fair to say that in its initial years the central office seemed to have placed more emphasis on promoting the specter of paralytic poliomyelitis and on fund-raising activities than on anything else. The keynote seemed to be: Money first, ideas about polio afterward. This concept it regarded as preferable to waiting for the unpredictable pace of medical science, which was bound to move forward, however spasmodically, wherever and whenever well-meaning inquisitive physicians and investigators were allowed to function in a propitious atmosphere. But since the foundation was a private organization that depended upon charitable donations for its existence, the lesson that medical scientists were supposed to learn quickly was that in order for the NFIP to succeed or even to exist, a certain amount of flamboyant publicity was absolutely necessary and they must go along with it. It was plain to see that this caused uneasiness among those who felt that Madison Avenue methods did not mix with anything but pseudoscience.

A source of real dismay especially in the 1930s was the eroding influence of publicity which sometimes forced the hands of investigators with its constant claims that "breakthroughs were just around the corner." This attitude was excused by its supporters on the grounds that the end justifies the means. Charitable agencies nearly always were dependent for their very existence on orthodox methods of promotion—on periodic drives for funds. Nevertheless the NFIP approach gave the appearance that its various functions had been wrapped up in a single package, and scientists and administrators alike were asked to make propaganda speeches hinting year after year that victory was almost imminent. It was like a large company that had a tight grip on both advertising and research departments but above all was intent on the sale of its *own* wares. Perhaps this was a small price to pay, considering how successful the foundation was in the end; and yet, was it?

I will not try to describe the policies that guided the NFIP in its first years (or later), nor could I. Rather, I will attempt to report on what the early impact of this new organization was on those investigators who had thrown in their lots with efforts to solve the poliomyelitis problem.

True to its name the organization soon became national in scope. Within five years it had assembled about forty well-known, prominent figures in American life on its board of trustees and had appointed an experienced group of professional experts and prominent figures in medicine to its various committees: a General Advisory Committee, a Virus Research Committee, another for Research on the Prevention and Treatment of After-Effects, and a Committee on Epidemics and Public Health.[1]

When funds started pouring into the coffers, the next objective was to set up a program to deal with individual aspects of the disease. With this kind of coverage, the NFIP left no doubt of its earnest determination to move into a position of leadership, even dominance, in the fight against infantile paralysis.

By 1940 the public picture of "polio" whether by design or accident, had been transformed from its predominantly medical and public health image to one that had more sentimental—or psychosocial—appeal. At a gala dinner held under the auspices of the National Foundation at the Waldorf-Astoria Hotel in New York in November 1940, several of the more than 130 invited guests sensed the direction that the fight against the disease would take. Whatever one might say, it was definitely a new approach.

Within ten years (1948) the NFIP came out with the following comments on policies and points of view:

> *From these beginnings has evolved the most intensive and comprehensive attack on a single disease ever launched by a private agency anywhere in the world.*
>
> To be sure, we have not found the final answer to any of the many problems. Scientific knowledge can't be purchased over the counter, like groceries. The bits and pieces of information must be gathered in many places in a laborious and sometimes heartbreakingly slow manner.[2]

This statement, intended for public consumption, is nonetheless revealing as to what policies were already being shaped. The casual and early use of the word "we" is significant. It was indeed an essential part of the technique.

To understand the size and the nationwide scope that the foundation

1. See *Annual Report of the National Foundation for Infantile Paralysis, 1943.* New York, Publication No. 47.

2. *A Decade of Doing; The Story of the National Foundation for Infantile Paralysis, 1938–1948.* New York, The National Foundation for Infantile Paralysis, 1948, pp. 7, 8, and 12.

had set for itself, it is important to realize that most of the 3,070 counties in the United States were represented by some sort of branch organization. The plan was that 50 percent of the money raised should remain in the local chapters to provide for hospitalization and the care of patients suffering from the paralytic disease, in fact from any form of poliomyelitis.[3] It was implicit also that efforts be made by each chapter to arouse popular interest in the struggle that the foundation was waging to combat the disease, and to raise money to assist the staggering numbers of individuals crippled by it. This most worthy cause became almost overnight part of the American scene. The aims here have been described by Sills:

1. Making sure that no polio patient—man, woman or child—shall go without the best available medical care for lack of funds.
2. Informing the public about the disease, methods of dealing with it and of the activities and goals of the National Foundation.
3. Raising sufficient funds through the March of Dimes to finance adequately the National Foundation's program of research, professional education, patient care, and polio prevention.[4]

If this account is to deal truthfully with the initial impact which the NFIP made upon that minuscule number of established workers in the field of poliomyelitis, it would be hypocritical not to say that it amounted to the sudden appearance of a fairy godmother of quite mammoth proportions who thrived on publicity. That a certain amount of advertising goes along with fund raising to support agencies for medical research is today regarded not only as essential, but routine; yet, not so in the late 1930s or early 1940s. The part which the NFIP played contributed in no small way to the evolution of present attitudes, which almost ended up with the assumption that any potentially worthy research project should be automatically funded at public expense. Although this is an extreme view, it has a modicum of truth in it. In any event the whole field of medicine gained enormously and materially by the changing approach to research. But it lost an indefinable something too—which was probably inevitable. The NFIP can hardly be blamed for that.

One of the achievements brought about by the effective use of propaganda techniques was the creation of public interest in poliomyelitis research as a *holy* quest. The image of the disease as an evil thing that must be conquered and banished forevermore took hold. The idea that a financial contribution to support research was a legitimate way to achieve such

---

3. Advantage was sometimes taken of this provision of care by unscrupulous doctors who felt that they were doing their patients a kindness by labeling any case with suggestive symptoms, as poliomyelitis. In this way it was thought that the NFIP might foot the bill for hospitalization and treatment.

4. D. L. Sills: *The Volunteers.* Glencoe, Illinois, *The Free Press,* 1957, p. 25.

a goal was a decided innovation—soon to be copied by many another foundation. Much as our grandparents gave to missionary societies of old, in the mid-twentieth century, especially in the 1940s and 1950s, such contributions now went to the March of Dimes. Year after year the public was exhorted to contribute freely to a cause that amounted in some ways to a crusade. But to the credit of the American people it can be said that they never lost heart during the twenty years in which the NFIP existed.

I shall not attempt to trace the growth of the foundation as it gathered strength and incidentally garnered more and more dimes and dollars. I can well remember Dr. Gudakunst, the first medical director, announcing at a public meeting in 1940, just two short years after the organization had come into existence, that the NFIP might look forward to collecting as much as $20 million a year! At that time, with the war on in Europe, this seemed an astronomical and practically unobtainable amount. And yet:

> Between 1938 and 1962, the Foundation's annual income was something like $25 million, or roughly $630 million over the whole period —59 percent of that income was spent on a gigantic Medical-care programme which included hospital support and patients' expenses, 8 percent was devoted to educational programmes, and a most important 11 percent or 69 million, was set aside for research. Fund raising which included advertising and promotional campaigns, proved an expensive item and accounted for $80 million or 13 percent of the total.[5]

By 1940 most of the administrative officers of the NFIP had become familiar with the multifarious problems that the disease presented. Few of them assumed that they were omniscient and that money would solve everything; most recognized the essential need for further carefully planned research. And yet in the early 1940s an uneasy feeling prevailed among clinical investigators that the home and the fountainhead of this disease had somehow been moved to chromium-plated headquarters at 120 Broadway in downtown New York City, quite remote from the hospital wards with all their worries and activities, not to speak of the background grinding noise of respirators known then as iron lungs, which were a constant source of sweat and tears.

Almost from the start, however, the NFIP relied mightily on advisory committees. Indeed, if it was to get on with its task, this was essential. Among de Kruif's scientific advisers of the PBBC who were asked to assume similar positions on the foundation's newly formed Committee on Scientific Research was T. M. Rivers, who was chosen as chairman. He

5. P. J. Fisher: *The Polio Story*. London, Heinemann, 1967, p. 66.

was to be constantly associated in various capacities with many of the foundation's policies and committees until the time of his death in 1962, at the age of seventy-three. He acted as a leading scientific spirit, and his services were to prove absolutely indispensable.

Interesting speculations have been posed as to what the NFIP would have done without Dr. Rivers to guide its destiny from the very start. It is fair to say that without him it would never have gained anything like the support from the academic medical profession that it was soon to enlist. Rivers acted as an interpreter of science for the administrative officers of the foundation; he was there to explain the queer and eccentric ways of medical science, which often consisted of exasperating delays, checks, and double checks. In brief, his contribution was in public relations and consisted of employing his special talent of interpreting in a forthright manner the current story of poliomyelitis, as he knew it, to committee members, science writers, and administrators and, last but far from least, fund raisers.

Although Rivers knew the field of virology intimately and all the personalities who were currently prominent in it, he was not so familiar with clinical poliomyelitis—or even the behavior of poliovirus. He was essentially an arbitrator of scientific questions and by 1940, a powerful and courageous figure representative of science in general. He realized that Mr. O'Connor was out "to conquer polio" according to his own methods and it was up to him to create a fundamental bulwark of solid science to back up these efforts.

I am fortunate to have had the privilege of knowing Tom Rivers from medical school days. In addition to my personal recollections of him I have frequently referred to Dr. Saul Benison's biography.[6] Overall, this book gives the picture of an articulate, formidable man of great courage, who in Benison's own words was a curmudgeon—but he had many other attributes besides.

Thomas M. Rivers came from a Georgia farm background. He achieved brilliant success at college (Emory University) and started out in 1908 to study medicine at the Johns Hopkins Medical School only to have his course rudely interrupted by being told that he had an incurable degenerative neurological disease and had better return home to his native Georgia. But Tom Rivers soon tired of waiting around to die. He even refused to get worse and with customary boldness spent the next eighteen months as a medical technician in a Latin American hospital in Panama City, Panama. He returned to Baltimore none the worse, and probably the

6. S. Benison: *Tom Rivers; Reflections on a Life in Medicine, and Science.* Boston, M.I.T. Press, 1967.

better, for this experience. Not only was he able to complete his medical
studies but also served two years of internship at the Johns Hopkins Hospital. He got out just in time to join the medical department of the U.S.
Army during World War I. It was there in 1918 that he worked on "the
Pneumonia Board," which dealt with pressing wartime problems among
recruits in training camps who suffered disastrous epidemics of pneumonia that had followed close upon the heels of measles and influenza.
Both of these latter highly infectious diseases were eventually proved (although not by Rivers) to be caused by viruses. This army experience gave
Rivers his start in a field in which he became for a time not only preemi-
nent but *the* recognized authority in America.

After the war, through a lucky break, Tom Rivers was fortunate in landing in the Hospital of the Rockefeller Institute, where facilities existed
which enabled him not only to pursue his investigations on viruses under
ideal conditions but also to benefit from a stimulating interchange with,
and a wealth of good advice from, elder colleagues. They in turn were not
long in recognizing his worth.

So it was that Rivers rapidly became the mentor of the expanding science
of virology. He remained at the institute for some thirty-three years, the
major part of this time as director of the hospital. In addition to becoming recognized as a leading expert on viruses, he was for a time the man
to whom many a young scientist in the United States with an ambition
to become a virologist turned. He was not only a tower of strength in his
own particular field but in a variety of other fields as well. He was singularly generous and effective in imparting advice. He took a certain degree of satisfaction from this endeavor. It was here indeed that his strength
lay.

Tom Rivers was not one to hide his light under a bushel. Early in his
career, in 1928, he edited a small book on viruses and virus diseases that
contained more information on this timely subject than had ever been assembled—in the United States at least.[7] This venture gave him the confidence that comes with success. When he became a long-time member of
the Board of Health of New York City his articulateness must have been
irresistible to his fellow board members, not to speak of the effect he had
on some of his colleagues on the various NFIP committees on which he
served. In time, after he had left the Hospital of the Rockefeller Institute,
he became vice-president for medical affairs of the National Foundation,
where he continued to make himself indispensable. And yet in his later
years the accuracy of his statements did not always keep pace with the
forthright manner in which his pronouncements were delivered. He was
formidable enough when he was in the wrong, irresistible when he was

7. *Filterable Viruses,* ed. by T. M. Rivers. Baltimore, Williams & Wilkins, 1928.

right, and sometimes not above the use of pyrotechnics—particularly at meetings.

Benison quotes one of Rivers' intimate friends and a long-time associate, Dr. Richard S. Shope of the Rockefeller Institute, who wrote soon after Dr. Rivers' death:

> Although Dr. Rivers was by nature a friendly person, he had the capacity of being irascible and pugnacious. He was a difficult and formidable person to oppose and could be stubbornly inflexible in maintaining a position. His discussion at scientific meetings of findings with which he disagreed could on occasion be so stinging that the audience, even though realizing the correctness of Rivers' position, often had their personal sympathies entirely with Rivers' opponent.[8]

This outspoken man, so wise in the ways of his world, who was not afraid to express himself on all kinds of occasions, went through life creating many admirers, hosts of friends, and, inevitably, not a few enemies. He was undoubtedly one of the great figureheads of American medical science who lived in the golden age of clinical investigation of infectious diseases—and many other kinds of diseases. As such, the story of his career provides an important chapter here.

Of this period in medical history (from 1920 to 1950) Sir Macfarlane Burnet recently spoke in his *Boyer Lectures.* He said:

> The harvest that Pasteur had sown began to be reaped in full. . . . Over the years since (1920) I have been able to watch the logical unfolding of Pasteur's method, till infectious disease in the civilized world has lost almost all its terrors.[9]

Regardless of how one looks at it, the NFIP was extraordinarily lucky to have entered the arena at just the right time and to have enlisted from the start the talents of just the right man—Tom Rivers.

According to Rivers, the first meeting of his NFIP Committee on Scientific Research was held early in July 1938 and was "very important," even though some of its members do not seem to have done their homework very well; at least it would seem that they had not kept up with the latest literature in the field.[10] The meeting was given over to discussions of

---

8. See n. 6, footnote pp. x, xi.

9. F. M. Burnet: *Biology and Appreciation of Life; The Boyer Lectures,* 1966. Australian Broadcasting Commission, Ambassador Press, pp. 11–12, 34.

10. Membership on this committee included such men as Charles Armstrong of cotton-rat fame, G. W. McCoy of the Hygienic Laboratory in Washington, and Karl F. Meyer of the G. W. Hooper Foundation at the University of California. It was truly an excellent group.

the principal unsolved problems of poliomyelitis, problems which are listed in a series of notes from the minutes:

> Some of these problems agreed to by all present to be important and fundamental, were: (1) What is poliomyelitis? Is the disease a clearly defined entity? Is there more than one form of the virus? If so, are these forms clearly separable and identifiable? (2) Is the pathology of the disease in humans adequately worked out? No. (Much more knowledge is needed of monkey disease pathology.) (3) Is the portal of entry known certainly for humans? Not certainly. But for major epidemics, it is still presumptive that the portal of entry is by way of the olfactory area. But work should continue. (4) Axonal transmission? [via nerves] This appears highly probable. But is it propagated in the body by this route? Should be settled if possible. Work should continue. (5) Chemical blockade? This is certainly the most promising of known methods of prophylaxis, which may be tried in the field. Work in this field should certainly continue, in an effort to find chemicals as effective as zinc sulphate, but less irritating. (6) Basic research should continue on attempts to alter the virus with the hope of making a vaccine. There are precedents for this. Yellow fever, horse encephalomyelitis, etc. (7) The relation of polio to constitution [i.e. body types, etc.] . . . (8) Nature of the virus. Bearing in mind the crystallization of [tobacco] mosaic viruses, and the new physical methods of concentrating and separating viruses, effort should be concentrated on developing this inquiry on multiple fronts. . . . (9) The possibility of setting up a travelling fellowship was discussed. (10) Chemotherapy of the acute disease. This should be pushed. (11) Collection of strains of viruses during epidemic emergency. Grantees should be contacted to find out if they would serve in the field in this capacity.[11]

These eleven items constituted the committee's evaluation of priorities. In spite of being a first draft, the minutes are of singular value in reflecting opinions held in 1938 by a representative group of distinguished virologists. Some of the men were apparently unaware that a substantial amount of work on the separation of poliovirus strains had already been done, dividing the family into at least two types.[12] The foundation could have saved itself an immense amount of labor and money had this information been brought out. Members of the committee also clung to the outmoded theory of the nasal portal of entry of the virus in the human disease and to the nasal spray as a means of prevention. The report of the

11. See n. 6, pp. 229–30.
12. See Burnet's findings in 1931, Chap. 22.

Toronto epidemic in 1937 would seem to have settled that issue once and for all; and if that was not enough, there was the work of Lawrence Smith in the early 1930s on the dearth of lesions in the olfactory bulbs in the human infection; and also of Sabin and Olitsky's observations in 1936, on the olfactory bulbs in experimental as well as in fatal human poliomyelitis. But some of the more skeptical NFIP committee members favored the usual cautious admonition that "more work should be done." Intestinal aspects of poliomyelitis (see chap. 37) received no consideration, whatsoever. One of the items mentioned, however, is of singular interest. Had those present realized the potential of item 6, which carried the suggestion that a live attenuated poliovirus vaccine be tried, a solution of the poliomyelitis immunization problem might have been reached considerably earlier than 1960. Yet in those days (1938), the time was decidedly not ripe for research on live poliovirus vaccines. It is of significance, nonetheless, that the experts had been alerted along these lines.

In a way this first meeting of the NFIP's Committee on Scientific Research set the pace for the next ten or fifteen years. For besides the enumeration of subjects that were considered of highest priority there was something else in the nature of policy making; the seeds had been sown of the concept of a master plan in the field of poliomyelitis research, and, incidentally, of keeping the public well informed about its progress.

The impression I have given so far may be that most established workers in the field of research on poliomyelitis were inclined at first to regard the foundation with a certain degree of uneasiness and more or less as a gift horse. But whether this was true or not, the American people entertained no such reaction. Their response was wholehearted, as it should have been. To the public, the foundation was an organization equipped and ready to lead the fight against this terrible disease and willing and able to provide financial assistance where needed, in patient care, scientific research, education—anything which would help the cause of polio.

The dozen years between 1938 and 1950 represented a period of burgeoning growth for the NFIP. After 1950 this organization assumed a much more aggressive, and I may say much more triumphant, role. This was the period of the controversies that waged over both poliovirus vaccines (the Salk- and the Sabin-type), particularly the former, which will be taken up in the chapters dealing with the years between 1952 and 1962.

In considering what effect the foundation actually had on the disease itself, if the 29 preceding chapters have conveyed any message at all, it is clear that the whole subject of the prevention of poliomyelitis had been relentlessly but unsuccessfully pursued since the discovery of the virus, long before any formal organization entered the picture. Zealous efforts to solve the problem had been pursued since 1910—although they still had a long way to go. But in retrospect, one feature—perhaps the main feature—which contributed to the success of the National Foundation was that it chanced to come on the subject at a time when the omens were favorable and the tide was running with ever-increasing strength in its favor. It would be more than naïve to maintain that the brilliant discoveries made between 1938 and 1953 that furthered the cause of vaccines for poliomyelitis were made as a direct result of the foundation's financial support—as some have vociferously claimed. True, both artists and scientists have thrived on patronage; this is the climate in which genius flourishes. But to claim that certain advances—the discoveries of John Enders and his colleagues, or even of Koprowski and Sabin with their concept of live poliovirus vaccines—were not the result of individual genius, but rather of financial backing, is ingenuous. The NFIP can take credit and pride in what it accomplished in leadership and the manner in which it smoothed the path when it came to organization and exploitation. No doubt these developments could not have come about so promptly—and, it might be added, so hastily—without the foundation's help.

A striking example was the cooperative Typing Program, whose success resulted in the separation once and for all of the family of polioviruses into three antigenic members or types. This cooperative program between laboratories could not have been executed so expeditiously under circumstances other than those that were generously provided by the NFIP (or that might have been provided by some similarly richly endowed agency or institution). But this was not exploration; rather, it was the application of established methods to solve a specific problem. In the planning and implementation of this type of medical "research and development," the foundation was at its best.

Nevertheless it was to the credit of the National Foundation for Infantile Paralysis that from the first meeting of its Scientific Committee it was able to embark on the task of pulling together certain diverse lines of applied research and, with this as an introduction, set up a concerted plan of action—with Rivers as the guiding spirit. Whatever wrong turns were taken, the main overall course was in the right direction. Heretofore the grand strategy of poliomyelitis research had been subject to the whims of individuals, i.e. self-styled authorities. This does not necessarily mean that the individual judgment of these authorities was inferior to the opinions of committee members who had been assembled for an annual one- or two-day meeting. But the latter plan had the advantage sometimes of group continuity and a knowledge of what could be attempted or even accomplished with the assets then available.

During its years of growth, in spite of World War II and in spite (or because) of the increasing incidence of poliomyelitis in the United States, the National Foundation continued to promote and radiate enthusiasm for its cause. Some idea of the extent of this enthusiasm and of the confidence which characterized its middle years may be gained from a series of news releases during 1944. Mr. Basil O'Connor commented on the intentions and generosity of the American people by saying that:

The increase in donations in 1943 and 1944, which probably was due in part to the high incidence of the disease, assured the National Foundation that the public wished it to intensify its activities and to widen its entire field of operations.[13]

He also added:

Some idea of the scope and extent of the National Foundation's program of scientific research is shown by the fact that, since it was organized only six years ago, it has made 298 grants to 74 institutions involving 114 groups of workers, in one of the greatest scientific attacks against any disease.

In another, earlier release, which contains excerpts of a letter to President Roosevelt, Mr. O'Connor said that "unremitting research will provide the key which will unlock the door to victory over infantile paralysis."[14]

In his reply, written in the closing year of World War II, just four short months before his death, President Roosevelt staunchly backed up this policy. In a final paragraph, his timely words were:

"We face formidable enemies at home and abroad," wrote the President. "Victory is achieved only at great cost—but victory is imperative on all fronts. Not until we have removed the shadow of the Crippler from the future of every child can we furl the flags of battle and still the trumpets of attack. The fight against infantile paralysis is a fight to the finish, and the terms are unconditional surrender.[15]

As the foundation gained in experience and grew in size it began to perceive more clearly the directions in which its real talents lay. It was not long before it began to take on the functions of a bureau of health education; it supplied badly needed public and professional information as to what to do "When Polio Strikes." It provided courses in professional education for physical therapists and distributed important information to physicians, pediatricians, and orthopedic surgeons on the use of respirators and special orthopedic techniques.

13. *American People give 30 Million Dollars in 11-year Fight on Polio.* News release for the National Foundation for Infantile Paralysis, Sept. 11, 1944.

14. Letter from Basil O'Connor to President Franklin D. Roosevelt, Nov. 27, 1944, quoted in a National Foundation news release, Dec. 8, 1944.

15. President Roosevelt's reply to Mr. O'Connor, Dec. 1, 1944. See n. 14.

Mr. O'Connor had occasion to write to me a form letter in February 1944, saying:

> You may be interested to see the recently issued folder, "Publications," which lists, with annotations, each of the National Foundation publications now being furnished in response to requests.
>
>   The demand for some of these is astonishing:—

Use of the Respirator in Poliomyelitis	79,974	in 4 years
Respirators—Locations and Owners	185,387	in 4 years
Nursing Care of Patients with Infantile Paralysis	77,933	in 3 years
Doctor . . . What can I do?	238,482	in 2 years
The Importance of Research	18,321	in 1 year[16]

These statistics are a tribute to the truly remarkable administrative ability of Mr. O'Connor in getting his messages across to the public.

Also the NFIP was active in the promotion of other, more serious educational activities. A special and successful function was in bringing people together for formal conferences and informal, small gatherings, and in assembling investigators with either common or diverse interests for the exchange of ideas, exchanges which sometimes developed into confrontations and sometimes had the salutory effect of cross-fertilization. The proceedings of these gatherings, faithfully recorded by the NFIP, could not help but be of immense value.

Of inestimable value also were the international conferences, inaugurated in 1948 (see fig. 43). Subsequently they were held every three years until the demise of the National Foundation for Infantile Paralysis in 1962. They filled a sizable gap, particularly at first, although this function was also furthered by the European Association against Poliomyelitis and Allied Diseases (as it is now called), which was established in 1948 by Dr. Laruelle of Belgium. But the NFIP international poliomyelitis conferences set both the stage and the American standard for a global type of representation that had not existed before, and was especially welcomed in the immediate post–World War II period.

As far as pioneer research on poliomyelitis was concerned, European laboratories had been slow to recover from the effects of World War I, let alone World War II, except for the redoubtable Kling and his colleagues.

Thus in the years preceding and immediately following World War II, the United States had more or less preempted the field of poliovirus research. This was not solely because epidemic poliomyelitis had become

16. Letter from B. O'Connor to J. R. Paul, Feb. 17, 1944.

such a tremendous threat in North America and the demand that something be done had increased. Nor was it a matter of the United States being the only country that was in a position to support the expensive experiments required for such research. Rather, it was that the situation

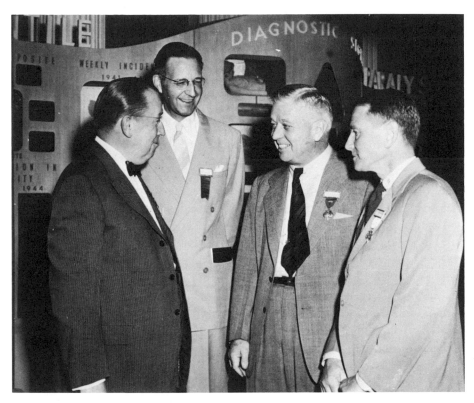

FIG. 43.   Group at the First International Poliomyelitis Conference, New York City, July 1948. Left to right: Mr. Basil O'Connor, Drs. Hart Van Riper, T. M. Rivers, and the author.

was critical, and interest in poliomyelitis was at an all-time high in this country. The NFIP international conferences, although heavily weighted with American representatives, were not put on "to show the world," but as a result of them the interest of many scientists in many countries had been aroused as never before. This was particularly true of countries outside of Europe. The astounding progress that was apparently being made in the fields of pathogenesis, virology, immunology, and therapy contributed heavily to this awakening.

These five international conferences were conducted in a lavish manner, and it was obvious that they could not have been put on without the unique financial backing of the NFIP. It was the so-called American way of doing things, which to some European scientists must have given the appearance of being "slightly, if not moderately, overdone," particularly in the years immediately following World War II. If the spectacle of medical science being closely allied to fund-raising and fund-spending techniques was to cause the raising of eyebrows in the United States, it is safe to say that it induced a far greater reaction in European medical scientists.

The conferences were nevertheless an immensely valuable undertaking on the foundation's part. It is to the credit of Morris Fishbein, ex-editor of the Journal of the American Medical Association and a long-time associate and committee member of the foundation, that they were so carefully planned and organized, and especially that the proceedings (Papers and Discussions)[17] were published in such distinguished and elegant fashion. Dr. Fishbein had a particular flair for publicizing information that was timely. He did it at the right moment and in the right way. Records of what transpired at these international conferences were important from an educational standpoint in that they constituted up-to-the-minute summaries of current information about most important aspects of poliomyelitis; moreover, they were promptly made available to practically all medical libraries in the world and institutions for medical research. Much of the data was scientifically newsworthy. Assuredly this information might not have been known so quickly had it not been for these NFIP conferences. Current incidence records, tissue-culture methods, diagnostic tests, new techniques in therapy, viremia, and discussions of the two types of vaccine, both inactivated and live attenuated varieties, reached a lively pitch during the last three conferences.

The NFIP was not the only agency that had a corner on the exchange of ideas between nations on poliomyelitis. As mentioned, the European Association against Poliomyelitis and Allied Diseases had been established in 1948, and it continues to this day (1970), having held eleven symposia in twenty years. This association has succeeded in maintaining its conferences almost annually, except in the years when the NFIP international conferences were held.

Another agency that promoted international aspects of poliomyelitis was the World Health Organization (WHO). This had come into being soon after the establishment of the United Nations in 1945 as one of its most important branch organizations. WHO was dedicated to providing medical care to populations of certain developing and needy nations and to the collection, dissemination, and standardization of medical information. The WHO Expert Committee on Poliomyelitis did not get under way until the 1940s, but beginning in 1952 it held a series of meetings

17. *Poliomyelitis; Papers and Discussion of the 1st–5th International Poliomyelitis Conferences.* 5 vols., Phila., Lippincott, 1949–61.

which in the eyes of the world had a truly authoritative ring. Reports of these meetings also received the widest kind of international circulation, and in the long run they proved to be formidable rivals to the reports of the NFIP's international conferences. The reason they carried such weight was that it was immediately recognized that WHO opinions were not personal ones but had been hammered out around a table by an international committee composed of scientists who represented different scientific backgrounds, politically and academically. It was an example of an international agency being able to settle its differences on the basis of a common aim that had worldwide appeal. No matter what different political views were entertained by individual committee members, when the subject of the control of infantile paralysis was brought up, this received universal endorsement. The means of achieving this control might differ, but the goal was the same.

CHAPTER 31

Therapeutic Methods
The Iron Lung

So far in this account methods of treating patients suffering from acute poliomyelitis and its aftereffects have received relatively short shrift. They have been mentioned only in chapter 7, where therapeutic ideas of the 1870s and 1880s are described, and in chapter 19, where serum therapy is discussed. Until now, most of the emphasis in this volume has been on the behavior of poliomyelitis as an infection, primarily with the idea of trying to understand its nature, and secondarily, of trying to decide what, if anything, might be done about controlling it.[1] With regard to a successful cure of the disease, from earliest times this had seemed futile and discouraging; no remedies had ever been found that were really effective in stopping the acute infection once it had started. There was also relatively little to be done about treating the residual paralysis, except by measures which could be called palliative. The best that could be said is that the physician of the nineteenth and early twentieth centuries generally had faith in his remedies—faith which he sometimes was able to instill into his patients. Even now, in the late twentieth century, no specific drug therapy is available, and no antimicrobials such as those which are so effective against bacterial infections are known. It would seem that until some virucidal agent is discovered or practical advantage can be taken of biologic approaches such as are presented by the interferon phenomenon, virus diseases like measles, chicken pox, and poliomyelitis still must run their course once the infection is established. Since the turn of the century wise medical opinion has held that powerful drugs or drastic therapeutic methods in the acute stages of poliomyelitis are apt to be harmful, and unless such measures are given for very specific purposes or are definitely life saving, they can be regarded as "risky or meddlesome therapy." The barbarous procedures proposed even as late as the 1870s, examples of which are given in chapter 7, are a case in point.

1. I am especially grateful to two individuals: Dr. Philip Drinker, Emeritus Professor of Industrial Hygiene, Harvard School of Public Health, for having provided the illustrations for this chapter and for his valued review and criticism of the text; and Dr. James L. Wilson, emeritus professor of pediatrics and communicable diseases at the University of Michigan, for providing me with his *Memoirs of the Respirator,* which constitutes a personal decription of the development of the use of respirators in poliomyelitis.

But with Dr. William Osler's teachings came a real reform. Although he was regarded by many contemporary physicians as a therapeutic nihilist, the treatment of acute infantile paralysis took a distinct turn for the better when, in 1892, in the first edition of his famous textbook he advocated the sensible policy that it was far better to use the least innocuous of remedies or to *do nothing* than to run the risk of aggravating the disease by drastic treatments. With his customary courage, he said: "No drugs have the slightest influence upon acute myelitis. The child should be put to bed and the affected limb or limbs wrapped in cotton"—a wise statement for that day.

Some twenty five years after this was written it looked for a time as if serum therapy was going to be the answer, but after two decades of trial, it too fell by the wayside. To this day, usually the advice during the acute febrile phase in an *uncomplicated* attack of nonparalytic or even mild paralytic poliomyelitis is to put the patient to bed and avoid doing anything that might prove harmful.

To continue in this vein would give the impression that there was nothing to be done about any variety of acute poliomyelitis. This is decidedly not the case. The patient with a complicated course requires an infinite amount of expert care and often round-the-clock attention by a whole battery of attendants. I am speaking here of patients who are severely paralyzed, including those who suffer from difficulties in urinating or in breathing. In caring for the latter, doctors were helpless until the 1920s. Then a discovery was made that hardly could be called curative but was one which revolutionized the treatment of this most serious form of the disease.

This was an invention which found clinical application by Dr. Philip Drinker of the Harvard School of Public Health,[2] the so-called Drinker respirator (see fig. 44). This life-saving apparatus was put to immediate use for patients who were unfortunate enough to be incapacitated because of difficulties resulting from paralysis of the muscles necessary for breathing, such as the intercostals and the diaphragm. Another and much more serious kind of respiratory difficulty often accompanies what is known as the bulbar form of the disease, in which there are lesions in that part of the brain (or bulb) that is adjacent to and leads into the spinal cord. Damage in this area is apt to involve the nervous centers that govern respiration, swallowing, and coughing. Patients with problems in these functions have a particularly poor prognosis.

Early pioneers in the design of an apparatus to aid respiration in polio-

2. Dr. Philip Drinker's immediate family has won distinction along various lines. To mention only two of its members, his father was president of Lehigh University, and his younger sister (Catherine Drinker Bowen), besides being an accomplished musician, is a distinguished writer and biographer.

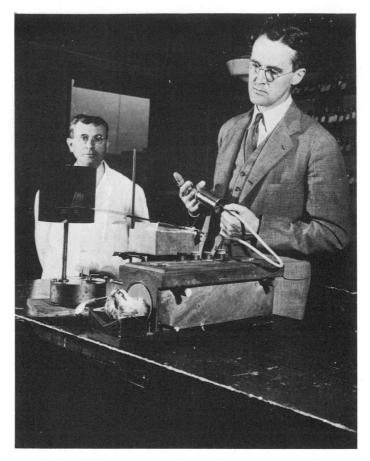

Fig. 44. Dr. Philip Drinker (with technical assistant at left) resuscitating a cat in the experimental laboratory of the Harvard School of Public Health as one of the necessary steps in preparing the respirator for human use. Reproduced by permission of *Life Magazine,* from a photograph taken by Hansel Mieth.

myelitis patients were Dr. Drinker's colleagues at the Harvard School of Public Health: L. A. Shaw, a physiologist;[3] and C. F. McKhann, a pediatrician.[4] It goes without saying that poliomyelitis was—and is—not the only disease in which mechanical assistance with breathing is necessary, but it quickly became the major disease in which the respirator was used.

The so-called Drinker respirator consisted of a rigid cylinder into which a patient could be placed, and at short regular intervals negative and positive pressure could be applied within the apparatus (see fig. 45).

3. P. Drinker and L. A. Shaw: Apparatus for prolonged administration of artificial respiration; design for adults and children. *J. clin. Invest., 7*: 229, 1929.

4. P. Drinker and C. F. McKhann: The use of a new apparatus for the prolonged administration of artificial respiration; a fatal case of poliomyelitis. *J. Amer. med. Ass., 92*: 1658, 1929.

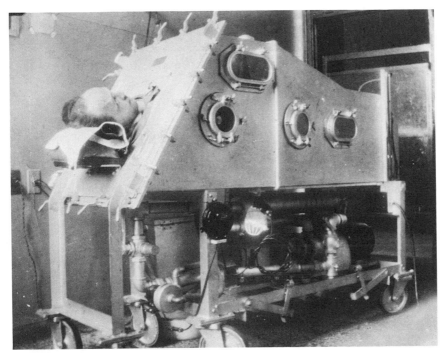

Fig. 45. An early model of the Drinker Respirator known as the "iron lung." Kindness of Professor Drinker.

It was promptly dubbed the "iron lung," a name which immediately caught on with all of its gruesome implications.

As to the early history of the respirator and the developments that attended its increasing use, Dr. James L. Wilson of the University of Michigan, who has been intimately connected with the story since the beginning, gives a far better account than any information that I would have been able to collect. In his "Memoirs of the Respirator," from which I have drawn freely and extensively, he says:

> I am not sure exactly who at the Harvard School of Public Health first got the concept of what was later developed into the so-called Drinker Respirator. It was certainly used by Louis Agissey Shaw there, for experimental work on small animals before it was used on a human being. Drinker certainly made the first one which could include a human. Drinker himself would, of course, remember the early developments. I was the first person to use the device for a small infant, I remember, and I put the baby in a "respirator," which was a little tank that Louis Shaw had for animal work. This was not for poliomyelitis. It was an attempt to get small infants and premature infants to breathe better. The results were dubious. This was some time after the first child with polio was treated. I do remember an early

discussion about the possible place of the device for poliomyelitis by a group of people on the lawn in the court of the Children's Hospital of Boston. Doctor Bronson Caruthers was one of the discussants. The question was one of the moral justification for using it, based on the question whether respiratory muscles could spontaneously recover so that once we saved a polio life with the machine the patient would not have to live in it for the rest of his life. There was no experience to guide us but there was a feeling that since some muscle power did come back in the arms and legs it might come back in the respiratory muscles and therefore the attempt was justified, and besides the concept of the value of rest to aid recovery of partially paralyzed muscles was considered.

The first patient was a little girl treated in a tank with household vacuum cleaners as pumps. One could hear it running for a quarter of a mile away because it was summer and the windows were all open. All of the residents, including myself, took turns sitting up with this child day and night until she died. The second patient was a man treated in a newer machine at the Peter Bent Brigham Hospital. We at the Children's Hospital had no responsibility for him though we went over to watch him. He seemed almost totally paralyzed and the use of the respirator demonstrated several things. One, the great difficulty of caring for a big man. The thing was closed with multiple clamps on a hard rubber gasket so there was no access to the man's body to clean him, or to do anything to him. To bathe him took an heroic effort with six men and nurses in an organized team. The important thing that this man, whose name I still remember, taught us, was that some months later, perhaps it was a year, he could walk with braces on his legs and with a cane. He came down to address an audience at the Massachusetts General Hospital; an experience which, of course, further justified the use of the respirator since this man was quite a useful person in spite of residual handicaps. Right away we could say, even then, that the moral justification of the use of this machine was that we could not give an exact enough prognosis at the initiation of respiratory paralysis to deny anyone the chance of using this life saving procedure.

Anyway at first the machine posed a lot of mechanical and physiological problems and those were the ones that I tackled, with enormous help, of course from Philip Drinker and also from Mr. Warren Collins who helped us in making these machines and who later was the first manufacturer of them. He spent a great deal of money and time on this before he ever sold one.

It took me some time, too, to realize that it was not an exact "physiological" machine; in fact, all patients, practically, had some ability to control their respirations. I remember very early, learning that by simple observation of the patient, that I could run the machine more wisely than by blood chemistry, as by seeing if he made attempts at little extra breaths when underventilated, or that he made a little grunt during inspiration to avoid deeper ventilation. We didn't have to run the machine with exactly determined pressure and rates for success.

To anticipate the story a little later we built a room respirator, the only one that was ever built except one many years earlier, in France I think, by a surgeon for different purposes. In my room respirator, I had space for four patients all sticking their heads out from this room with their bodies inside, and we could get inside with them and care for them without being influenced by the machine ourselves. The point that surprised many was that we could care for different sized children with the same pressures and rate and they all easily adjusted themselves from a 12 year old down to a one year old.

Very early in the development of the machines the inaccessibility of the patient bothered me and I remember, with Phil Drinker's advice, buying some portholes made for boats and having them welded on to the machine so that we could open them, fit them with rubber collars through which we could put our hands and so manipulate our patient without taking him out of the tank, nor interrupting his respirations. This really was a most important advance and was absolutely necessary for any kind of decent care.

A great deal of confusion occurred in the understanding of the different mechanisms of respiratory distress. In my first epidemic where I treated quite a few patients with many different kinds of respirators I soon learned to make the differentiation. With intercostal and diaphragmatic paralysis, the first always associated with shoulder paralysis and the last with neck weakness, the machine was ideal. But if there was a so-called "bulbar" paralysis associated with the pharyngeal paralysis with the less clearly established central respiratory disturbance, we had a more complex problem. I soon learned that respiratory distress due to pharyngeal paralysis was a counter-indication to the use of the respirator unless the pharyngeal paralysis, was combined with respiratory muscle paralysis as it often was. It prevented any effective use of the machine, in fact made it worse for the patient to get rid of his secretions. We soon began making tracheostomies, but with great conservatism.

Apparently a few others used the machine besides us in Boston, and after a while, it soon began to be used in a New York epidemic. As a result, a paper, very disappointing to me, was published, I don't remember by whom, indicating the futility of this procedure because practically every patient that they used it on there had died. We went to New York, Philip Drinker and I, to see what the trouble was, and we found it. Two things were happening. In the Willard Parker Hospital where they had only two or three machines during an epidemic, a new visiting man would come, see someone apparently in greater distress than the one in the machine, and so took one out and put the other one in—even sending some patients home too soon. Another problem that they didn't realize there was that not all people with respiratory distress should be in a respirator. So all bulbar polios were put in without any successful attempt to keep the airway clear and, of course, they died of aspiration or fatigue fighting the machine which didn't synchronize with their own respiratory efforts, and couldn't, of course, as long as there were pharyngeal secretions. That made me feel better but I think that the machine got a very bad reputation from that experience.[5]

To digress from Dr. Wilson's "Memoirs" for a moment, in the 1930s, the Willard Parker Hospital in New York City was not the only place that was having trouble with the respirator and difficulty with decisions as to whether to use it. There was little question that this apparatus, if expertly handled, could serve as a life-saving device in some cases and under some circumstances. Results were especially salutary when the respiratory difficulties began to improve of their own accord, due to the healing of a not-too-severe myelitic lesion, thus allowing the patient to emerge from the confines of the iron lung—miraculously saved. But in the 1930s there were few experts, and when a patient who had been subjected to this form of artificial respiration could not be weaned from it, the accusation was frequently made: Why had the doctor seen fit to use this contraption if he was aware of the possibility that the patient would have to be immured within it for the rest of his life? Far better to die, some thought, than be doomed to a fabulously expensive existence in a highly artificial environment with specially trained nurses in attendance around the clock. This was the reaction of a minority. On the other hand, a greater number of physicians and parents of patients alike recognized the justification of a decision to put the patient into the iron lung when inability to breathe threatened his life.

There were also innumerable difficulties of a logistic nature that beset the use of the respirator in its early days: the supply of machines was limited, trained physicians and assistants capable of running them properly were hard to come by, and emergencies were particularly apt to arise in small-town hospitals. In my own experience during the 1930s, several times when I had gone out to observe and study a given epidemic in a rural area of the United States, I ended up spending most of my time as a not-

5. J. L. Wilson: "Memoirs of the Development of the Respirator." Feb. 1968, unpublished. Extensive sections of these memoirs have been transcribed in this chapter with a minimum of editing. Most of the editorial changes represent deletions.

too-well-trained supervisor directing nurses in the use of the respirator. Also, in the event of an epidemic agonizing decisions had to be made; for instance, although three or four patients with respiratory difficulties might be on hand and waiting, there often was only *one* respirator available— what to do? whom to choose?[6] the patient with the severest disability, who possibly would die anyway; or the patient with lesser disability and a better prognosis? These and other troublesome questions had to be faced during the early days. Difficult also in the 1930s and 1940s were decisions as to when to call in the surgeon to perform an emergency tracheostomy, i.e. opening the windpipe, thus allowing free access of air to the lungs without its having to pass through the upper respiratory passages, which were obstructed by an excess of secretions and by paralysis of the pharyngeal and laryngeal muscles. And yet through it all, the life-saving capacities of the iron lung began to be appreciated more and more. The number of respirators available gradually increased. There were also refinements in design and especially improvements in the training of physicians as to what to do if they were called upon to handle respirator patients by themselves, perhaps only with the assistance of nurses who might or might not be experienced.

Dr. Wilson continues the story from this point:

Not much was done about the machines nationally, I believe, until I got to Detroit, in 1937. About that time the National Foundation began to get interested. I had nothing to do with the situation at first, but I do remember that the Foundation asked me to write a report at the request of the then Governor of Michigan as to what could be done with this problem of respiratory failure in an epidemic, should it occur. This is when I developed the concept of a respirator center so that we could bring patients to the center rather than machines to the patient; as I thought experience was worth a great deal in their care. Also, at the Foundation's request a year or so later, I made a survey, by letter, of all the tank respirators in the United States at that time, with some details about them, I believe, and of the number of patients who were treated.

I don't know whether this report was ever used or not but the concept of the respirator center was there, and later, Ken Landauer, one of the Medical Directors of the Foundation, came to me about this whole matter, and we developed a concept together of the respirator center, not just for emergency care, which was my earlier idea, but for complete rehabilitation and weaning from the tank. This was a very difficult task and many of the patients were so severely handicapped that often we felt guilty at saving their lives. About that time several

6. This was the main situation which prompted Drinker and Wilson to build a four-bed respirator.

respirator centers had been established and I got one going too, in Ann Arbor. Then we organized national meetings on "respiratory physiology." These meetings were held by all of us who were interested in this problem over the nation but financed by the National Foundation. Their purpose was not only to understand respiratory physiology, but to solve many of the problems of rehabilitation, as well as running the respirator. I know that at the time I felt like the old man on the subject, as there we were, studying anew some of the things that I thought I had already solved. My conceit runs through this report, I see.

There became a tendency, particularly with the urgency of Doctor Baker in Minnesota, to do tracheotomies on all patients with pharyngeal paralysis. I disagreed with this because I thought that with enough tilting of the machine, and careful aspiration of the throat, and cooperation of the patient, that we could often avoid this, particularly as the functional pharyngeal paralysis lasted sometimes only a few days. Nevertheless, as Baker said, his staff wasn't equipped to do all this all night with every patient and it became customary over the nation to do these tracheotomies.

I think, as a whole, from the national point of view it was probably a good thing to do tracheotomies early, since it is difficult to get enough people sophisticated and calm enough to choose the right patients and to get the right equipment to keep them from aspirating their oral secretions. One episode of aspiration could, indeed, be very serious, though I was conceited enough to think that with my hands and my experience we could avoid a lot of tracheotomies. I remember getting some children to suck out their own throats, those of course who had little arm paralysis.

I suppose in this record I should mention the patent that was obtained for the respirator. Philip Drinker didn't want it but since a lot of money had been contributed to develop the device by the Consolidated Gas Company of New York which thought that the machine would be useful to them in resuscitation of asphyxiated people, they agreed to hold the patent, and it was to them that the patent was finally assigned. However, they didn't really want the patent. They tried to give it to Harvard University who didn't want it, and it was finally assigned to Warren Collins, who was then the only manufacturer of the machine. He had showed enormous sincerity and energy and generosity in developing a practical machine, which never failed. When I was still at the Children's Hospital, in the early days I got Jack Emerson, who was Dr. Haven Emerson's son, the past Commissioner of Health of New York City, as you know, to help me build some oxygen tents. There were none available particularly for children, and this was another one of my gadgetering ideas. He did so, and showed a great deal of practical ingenuity. He could do things with a piece of tin and a pair of pliers that a regular manufacturer would need a blueprint for. But he saw my struggle with the Drinker respirator and immediately said he could make one better. I tried to advise him not to because I said Warren Collins was cooperative enough and he holds the patent. The patent, by the way, was taken out with the advice of some, through a fear which I think, in retrospect, was foolish, that the machine might be used in some quackery attempt at treatment, and that the use of it should be protected. It was not in any way taken out for any financial profit by anyone. Anyway, Jack Emerson went ahead and began making respirators and did make some improvements. This was typical of his ingenuity; however, the thing came to a lawsuit. At that time it was brought out that the concept of rhythmical negative pressure over the thorax and body of the patient with the head outside was certainly developed before we had made our own respirators. Both Jack Emerson and Warren Collins have always been most cooperative in developing new ideas and in selling the machines without exorbitant profits, in my opinion.

Later, in Detroit I helped develop the cuirass respirator. I think it was not my idea first. I think someone first fitted a box over a persons chest, I have forgotten who did it, and ventilated the box without having the legs or arms or head in it, with some rubber device fitted around the shoulders, but I got the idea of the cuirass and had it developed by a friend of the father, of a patient who was suffering from extreme respiratory distress and was brought half way round the world with this apparatus.[7]

Along here the Rocking Bed should be mentioned. This I had nothing to do with. It was, of course, a mechanical development of a very old concept for artificial respiration, a plank over a barrel on which a patient was placed and then rocked so that the abdominal contents pushed the diaphragm up and pulled it down to produce a tidal air. This rocking bed played a big part in the rehabilitation of patients with mild respiratory muscle paralysis and was a very useful device. I believe Jesse Wright of Philadelphia played a big part in this development and in its use before it was taken up by all the people in the respirator centers.

Dr. Wilson's memoirs provide a vivid and intimate account of the story of the respirator and other mechanical aids as they were developed and

---

7. Dr. Drinker has added to Dr. Wilson's "Memoirs": "The objection with the cuirass was that the patient suffered a certain amount of discomfort and had to be strapped up tight more or less like cinching up the saddle of a horse."

used in the United States. Other countries, faced with similar problems in handling patients with respiratory complications, developed similar approaches. In Denmark, during a severe epidemic, a relatively simple positive pressure apparatus was used in which air was pumped into the lungs through a tracheostomy tube. This was developed to take care of a special emergency when large numbers of patients suffering from respiratory distress were all admitted to the hospital around the same time, constituting an unprecedented load. The device served as a life-saving measure for many of the more than one thousand paralytic cases during the extensive epidemic in Denmark in 1952.[8] On this occasion many students volunteered for hospital work and took turns in the heroic effort of pedaling a bicycle day and night to supply the necessary leg power to keep the respirators going and the patients alive.

In England Professor W. Ritchie Russell of Oxford University became a leading expert on the use of various machines in the treatment of life-threatening types of poliomyelitis. While serving with the Middle East Forces in 1943–44, Brigadier Russell had treated numerous patients with poliomyelitis contracted in Egypt and North Africa, a wartime experience that was to stand him in good stead. He was peculiarly expert in assaying the particular needs of a given patient and deciding what machine was appropriate in his case.[9]

Here in the United States it is to the infinite credit of Dr. Wilson and the National Foundation for Infantile Paralysis that in the 1930s order was brought out of what promised to be a most difficult, chaotic, and distressing situation. The foundation was not only a pioneer in the establishment of respirator centers for the care of patients and for the special training of physicians, technicians, and nurses, but it also organized mobile expert teams which could be rushed to the scene when epidemic aid was needed.

The spectacle of havoc wrought by this form of the paralytic disease—the degree of disability and suffering undergone by patients with serious and chronic respiratory difficulties—was enough to leave a deep impression on the sympathetic visitor to one of these centers in the 1950s. It was indeed a godsend that within the next ten years the need to provide facilities for new cases with this kind of disability quickly lessened and then almost completely stopped. The iron lung with its gruesome connotations found its way into the basements of most hospitals instead of occupying a place on the wards as an important piece of apparatus that it once was.

8. H. C. Lassen: Discussion of papers by J. L. Whittenberger and H. L. Hodes at the session on acute medical care, in *Poliomyelitis; Papers and Discussions presented at the Third International Poliomyelitis Conference*. Philadelphia, Lippincott, 1955, pp. 97–98.

9. W. R. Russell: *Poliomyelitis,* 2nd ed. London, Edward Arnold, 1956.

CHAPTER 32

Therapeutic Methods
Sister Kenny's Orthopedic Ideas

Besides mechanical devices to aid respiration, many more orthopedic and other rehabilitative measures were also necessary in the aftercare of paralyzed patients. Medin and his pupil Wickman, during the period of 1900–10, were almost the last physicians who felt competent to deal with the entire course of the clinical disease from start to finish. But the idea that any one physician might be able to handle all therapeutic aspects, all orthopedic and other types of management required in chronic care, began to be outmoded at the turn of the century. This was not surprising, considering that a complicated case might need surgical treatment as well as the use of various skills in what is today called *physical medicine*.

Orthopedics had its beginnings in the dim past as far as the fitting of braces and other aids to standing and locomotion were concerned. But orthopedic surgery for the correction of disabilities due to poliomyelitis received a great boost starting with Strohmeyer in Germany in the 1830s. The procedures used were generally in the nature of salvage operations performed to aid patients in their endeavor to live with their disabilities. The orthopedic surgeon appreciated that the long-drawn-out care of the paralytic patient constituted an entirely different sort of problem than that posed by the acute or subacute disease. He had to think in terms of years instead of days.

Long before the time of Underwood it had begun to be recognized that the paralyzed child needed support in the form of splints and braces not only to aid him in standing and walking but also to avoid muscle contractures and a twisted or shrunken body. This called for the sort of talent that bracemakers had and that in due time orthopedists could best supply; so, early in the mid-nineteenth century orthopedic surgeons assumed a role of great prominence as major specialists in the overall care of paralytic poliomyelitis—a position maintained to this day. Because large numbers of disabled patients flocked to them in the early days, they were the first to collect sizable numbers of sporadic cases of the disease and to analyze them in a semistatistical fashion. The famous and capable Dr. Heine of Cannstadt, Germany had made his reputation in this way. He devised all sorts of splints, trusses, and mechanical aids to locomotion as well as exercise machines. His concept of the aftercare of the patient was modern in that it covered the broad field of rehabilitation, with recommendations for massage, hydrotherapy, and carefully controlled exercises. But it was not until advances due to the introduction of antisepsis and anesthesia and the consequent great developments in surgery in the latter part of the nineteenth century that real progress was made in the field of corrective operations for paralyzed limbs. Taking advantage of the vast improvement in techniques, surgeons began to test their skills and to explore possibilities in various procedures aimed at restoring function, e.g. cutting tendons (tenotomy) and suturing them and transplanting them as well. The general regimen of the patients who suffered from paralytic poliomyelitis consisted first of immobilizing the affected limb or limbs in splints, followed by massage and hydrotherapy, and later, surgery if needed.

The surgical efforts of the German doctor, Walter, who had emigrated to Pittsburgh in the mid-nineteenth century (see chap. 4) were pioneering examples in this direction. Much later, in the 1900s, the orthopedic surgeons DeForest Willard of Philadelphia[1] and J. W. Goldthwait of Boston became actively identified with what might be termed as the beginnings of the modern aftercare of patients who had suffered from paralytic poliomyelitis.

Since the days of Heine and before, besides the use of "irons attached to the legs" and all the other ancillary and supportive measures employed, there had been a sustained enthusiasm for electrical "treatments," an enthusiasm that was hardly justified considering their lack of real efficacy. In the beginning the approach was more or less exploratory but was urged both in the acute and chronic stages. French physicians were particularly partial to this method. Faradic current was advised as a measure superior to massage, and there seems little doubt that European and American physicians of the nineteenth century ascribed certain magical curative qualities to electricity. This form of therapy is still revered in some parts of the world, even considered necessary if a cure is to be achieved. It must be admitted, however, that electrotherapy has been, and still is, used much more to impress the patient from a psychological point of view, which has its place, than with any real conviction on the part of the physician of its effectiveness in actually restoring function to damaged nerves and wasted muscles. After 100 or more years of trial in the developed countries, almost the only use of electricity now is a diagnostic one in assaying the state of damage that muscles have undergone. Rarely is it resorted to therapeutically.

A completely different aspect of long-term treatment was the task of

---

1. DeForest Willard: Infantile spinal paralysis, chap. 26, in *The Surgery of Childhood including Orthopaedic Surgery*. Philadelphia, Lippincott, 1910, pp. 607–41.

morale building by judicious encouragement of the patient to use everything he had, including his muscles, regardless of how little there was left.
The results which early orthopedic surgeons obtained were in some measure due to their ability to encourage their patients and constantly, to im-
part confidence to them in reeducating themselves in the matter of locomotion, as well as helping them adjust to the changes in their lives neces-
sitated by physical limitations. Early in the twentieth century the British
orthopedic surgeon Sir Robert Jones had made the point that paralyzed
patients needed the utmost in the way of encouragement and surgeons
were not to expect that their operations would be necessarily successful
unless they too took an active, even a militant, part in forwarding the
patient's desire to get well. Sir Robert wisely said, "Pessimism as to prognosis causes lack of interest in treatment." It was a dictum often forgotten
when a young surgeon put entirely too much faith in his mechanistic procedures, overlooking the psychological impact of his therapy.

On the other hand, even before psychiatrists had come on the scene it
was clear that attempts to build up the morale of a paralyzed patient required a certain amount of judgment and finesse. Each case was a law
unto itself. At the First International Poliomyelitis Conference, held in
New York in 1948, Dr. Edward Strecker, a psychiatrist of Philadelphia,
noted pitfalls in store for the surgeon, or even a member of the patient's
family, who attempted to practice amateur psychiatry during the aftercare
of the paralyzed child or adult. He stressed that the situation is infinitely
more complicated than meets the eye. His remarks here were directed
not to morale building but to the ego of the patient. He said:

> Polio is of course, a major insult to developing personality, and nota-
> bly to the ego of the child. . . . It provides severe psychic temptations
> for the child, the mother and for the whole family. For the child, it
> offers the opportunity to thwart emotional maturing or to distort it
> very seriously. . . . its disabling effects provide a splendid opportunity
> for the retention of the so-called power stage of the child. . . . The
> problem psychiatrically is to set the stage for the child and for the
> family so that polio interferes as little as possible with the emotional
> growing process.[2]

It was Dr. Robert Lovett of Boston who probably had more to do in the
early years with placing the treatment of paralytic poliomyelitis in the
United States upon a good foundation. He had been writing on the orthopedic aspects of this subject since 1907 and finally came out with a
small but timely volume in 1916, which was devoted almost entirely to the

2. E. Strecker: Discussion of paper by W. T. Green: The Management of Poliomyelitis; The
Convalescent Stage, in *Poliomyelitis; Papers and Discussions Presented at the First International Poliomyelitis Conference*. Philadelphia, Lippincott, 1949, pp. 189–90.

care of the paralyzed patient.[3] He divided the disease into three stages—acute, convalescent, and chronic—pointing out that treatment varies tremendously with each stage.

He described the *acute* stage, otherwise known as the sensitive phase, as persisting until muscle tenderness disappears. In this period, Lovett maintained that rest in bed was to be strictly enforced in all cases, with adherence to whatever rules of isolation and quarantine that were advocated by the local health department. Physical therapy was not to be neglected, and for a patient with early paralysis, warm baths were advised with gentle massage to the affected limbs. But of greater importance were efforts to prevent contraction of muscles and deformity, which might occur early and were on the whole, Lovett said, evidences of neglect and lack of proper care.

In the *convalescent* stage, he maintained that one must carefully consider by what means the restoration of maximum function to affected muscles could be most rapidly brought about. He did not advocate immediate and prolonged rigid splinting of limbs, which became an accepted measure soon afterward. Lovett advised cautious encouragement in the use of residual muscle power, aided by massage, heat, and electricity. Eventually training with the help of braces was indicated.

In the late or *chronic* stages operative procedures to improve muscular function were advised, including tendon and nerve transplantation. Lastly, came admonitions on the use of exercise in improving gait and muscle power to combat a desultory, passive attitude into which some patients were so apt to sink.

This is a very cursory review of the principles set forth in Lovett's book, but it is enough at least to give some idea of the type of orthopedic treatment which was in vogue in 1916 at the time of the most extensive epidemic that the American nation had ever seen. Centers for the aftercare of paralytic poliomyelitis such as were set up at Warm Springs, Georgia, with elaborate equipment and a concentration of various specialists, had not yet come into being, but that there was a crying need for them was becoming increasingly evident.

It was inevitable that the general handling of patients who required special care was apt to change with the medical fashions of each passing decade. Twenty years later, Lovett's views had undergone a certain amount of distortion. The 1930s was decidedly an era when early and prolonged splinting of paralyzed limbs was carried to excess, in spite of efforts on the part of the U.S. Public Health Service to combat this tendency,[4] for the

3. R. W. Lovett: *The Treatment of Infantile Paralysis.* Philadelphia, P. Blakeston's Sons, 1916.

4. H. O. Kendall and F. P. Kendall: Care during the recovery period in paralytic poliomyelitis. *Publ. Hlth Bull. (Wash.),* No. 242, 1938, pp. 14–23.

view had been popularized that plaster casts should be applied at the slightest indication and should be kept in place for longer periods than Lovett had advised. It was during this period that the Los Angeles epidemic of 1934 occurred. There, I witnessed a prime example of how this form of treatment miscarried. During the epidemic a large number of nurses (totaling about 140) who were serving at the Los Angeles General Hospital were admitted to that hospital as patients. They were suffering from symptoms that might or might not have been due to poliomyelitis, although it turned out that very few of them had fever and none had any true paralysis (see chap. 21). The nurses were left to the earnest ministrations of a group of young interns who felt it their duty to give them especially good care since they were in a sense colleagues. Accordingly, when the nurses started streaming into the hospital as patients, the young doctors followed the current method of treatment for paralytic poliomyelitis with more enthusiasm than discretion. They immediately applied plaster casts and sometimes erected a frame over the bed, equipped with ropes and pulleys. The nurses may not have had "polio" at the time of admission, but by the time the interns got through with them they certainly were surrounded by all the earmarks associated with the paralytic form of that disease, along with the frightening thought that they might never be able to walk again.

How long these patients were kept encased in plaster I do not know, but in Gilliam's account of the events in Los Angeles in the summer months of 1934, he said that prompt immobilization sometimes for long periods of time made the evaluation of muscle weakness difficult, and he made this point clear in a footnote:

> One or more extremities were splinted, at some time during the illness, in 74 per cent of the patients; and 46 per cent of the patients were immobilized on a Bradford frame for varying periods of time.[5]

Yet the proportion of cases developing severe weakness at any time during the period covered by Gilliam's observations was only 26.5 percent. The word *paralysis* is not mentioned at all in this section of Gilliam's report! The handling of the Los Angeles nurses is an example of an approved method of treatment of a given disease going completely awry because of its excessive use. The interns were not to blame; they did the best they knew how, but owing to the exigencies of the epidemic and the confusion among staff members of a relatively new hospital they did not have the proper guidance.

By 1940 it had become obvious that the fashion of treating weak limbs by early and prolonged immobilization had gone too far. Incredibly, *im-*

5. A. G. Gilliam: Epidemiological study of an epidemic, diagnosed as poliomyelitis, occurring among personnel of the Los Angeles County General Hospital during the summer of 1934. *Publ. Hlth Bull. (Wash.)*, No. 240, 1938, footnote p. 26.

mobility had become such a fetish that it was proposed even as a preventive measure for "keeping the paralysis away." This absurdity did more harm than good. Obviously it could not last, and an inevitable reaction set in. But it was not inevitable from whence this reaction would come: When it did arrive, it came from an unusual source.

One thing *was* evident. It was going to take a vigorous personality to show that the prevailing system of rigid and prolonged fixation of paralyzed limbs was not having the desired effect, and could be harmful. Physicians and surgeons do not like to have their methods suddenly impugned, particularly by a nurse from Australia, which is exactly what happened when Sister Kenny (see fig. 46) emerged on the scene in 1940. This redoubtable figure, who found a campaigning ground in the United States, wasted no time in expressing her disapproval of the treatments then in vogue.[6] In her first book, published in this country in 1941, she said:

> My reasons for the condemnation of the principles of immobilization as generally accepted are as follows:
> 1. Immobilization prevents the treatment of the disease, that is, the symptoms of the disease, in the acute stage.
> 2. It prolongs the condition of muscle spasm and prevents its treatment.
> 3. It prevents the treatment for the restoration of coördination of muscle action, a serious error.
> 4. It promotes the condition of stiffness which according to all reports prevents satisfactory treatment for the symptoms that brought about the condition (muscle spasm) or the development of muscle power by reëducation, or re-awakening of impulse.[7]

Sister Kenny mentioned eight more items which she felt were worthy of condemnation, including the last (no. 12), which was to the effect that "It gives the patient an adverse psychological outlook."

The year (1940) was optimal when Sister Kenny wrote these harsh words condemning prevailing therapeutic methods. She knew very little about the concept of poliomyelitis as an acute viral disease which must inevitably run its course. But she certainly knew about the business of handling the paralyzed child. In this she was well ahead of current orthopedic fash-

6. A part of Sister Kenny's antagonism for this rigid immobilization of a limb may have stemmed from the therapeutic admonitions of a local rival in the form of Dr. (later Dame) Jean Macnamara who preached the doctrine of rigid immobilization in her native Australia. The latter's visit to the United States in the mid-1930s in which she was given considerable publicity, included an exhibit of Dr. Macnamara's methods at a meeting of the American Medical Association. R. K. Ghormley: *History of Treatment of Poliomyelitis. Lectures on Regional Orthopaedic Surgery and Fundamental Orthopaedic Problems.* Ann Arbor, J. W. Edwards, No. 3, 1947.

7. Elizabeth Kenny: *The Treatment of Infantile Paralysis in the Acute Stage.* Minneapolis, Bruce, 1941, pp. 21–22.

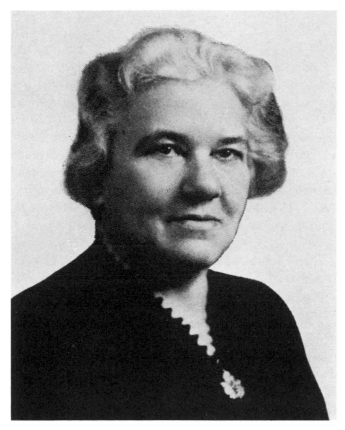

FIG. 46. Sister Elizabeth Kenny (circa 1890–1952).

ions in the United States. In Australia, orthopedic surgeons had already lined up in two groups pro and con, and by 1940 she was well accustomed to preaching her doctrine before a skeptical audience and using her vigorous powers of persuasion. Her watchword was "Let my record speak," and she usually demonstrated a patient in testimony of the effectiveness of her methods.

What was the history of this remarkable woman? In 1910 she had already finished nursing training and gone out to the Australian bush country far from the nearest physician. There she is supposed to have encountered her first cases of poliomyelitis. Left entirely to her own devices she is said to have brought these cases back "to normalcy." Upon returning to her headquarters hospital she was told that her concepts and methods had violated all accepted rules of the medical profession for the treatment of the disease. Nevertheless, convinced that she had made an important medical discovery, she started a crusade that was to carry her to far places and was to end in a bitter struggle.

At first Sister Kenny won immediate support in the United States, particularly in Minneapolis. In a second book, by Pohl and Kenny, published in 1943,[8] which included aspects not only of the treatment of the acute case but also of the aftercare, the authors went further into intricate descriptions of the ways to relax muscle spasm by the use of warm moist packs. And especially they went to great lengths to emphasize that intimate and constant attention must be given to a paralyzed child in reeducating what muscles he had left.

At the time of Sister Kenny's first visit and during the three years which elapsed until she became established as director of the Elizabeth Kenny Institute in Minneapolis, Minnesota, her ideas and methods, some cautious and some otherwise, were received with enthusiasm by certain orthopedists in this country. Prominent among these supporters were Dr. Philip Lewin of Chicago, Dr. F. H. Krusen of the Mayo Clinic, and Dr. Frank R. Ober, clinical professor of orthopedic surgery at Harvard and at the time, president of the American Orthopedic Association.

At the Medical School of the University of Minnesota Sister Kenny was cordially received, and Dr. Miland E. Knapp, who became director of the training course in Kenny techniques, contributed the following commentary:

> Just what the true physiologic explanation for these phenomena will be, I do not know. However, Sister Kenny's observations of symptomatology are absolutely correct and regardless of future developments this much I do know: she has knocked us so completely out of our complacent groove of thought about infantile paralysis that some worthwhile advance is bound to result from both the revolutionary ideas and the frantic efforts of her opponents to refute them.[9]

Mr. O'Connor, the president of the National Foundation for Infantile Paralysis, called a meeting of his advisers early in 1943, at which some of the group of consultants acknowledged that Miss Kenny's ideas had some basis in fact and were beginning to pay off. Following this meeting O'Connor wrote: "The National Foundation for Infantile Paralysis has sponsored and directed a broad program of research in connection with Miss Kenny's work. Not only has it supported Sister Kenny and her staff at the University of Minnesota, but it has financed other investigative and instructional programs in many laboratories, medical schools and hospitals throughout all of the United States."[10]

It was inevitable that the indomitable spirit possessed by Sister Kenny would soar too far and that ultimately a counterreaction would set in. The first episode was touched off when the government of Argentina requested

---

8. J. F. Pohl and Elizabeth Kenny: *The Kenny Concept of Infantile Paralysis and Its Treatment.* Minneapolis, Bruce, 1943.

9. Ibid., p. 355.

10. The National Foundation was to issue a pamphlet at about this time (1942–43): *Principles of the Kenny Method of Treatment of Infantile Paralysis.* Publication No. 41, undated.

President Roosevelt to send Sister Kenny to aid in its efforts to combat an epidemic of poliomyelitis. The National Foundation for Infantile Paralysis requested that its own clinical experts should accompany Sister Kenny's team on her trip. It is easy to see that differences in attitudes and policies between the two groups would arise. This was the beginning of a breach that soon widened into a true schism.

Although the National Foundation had been ready and willing to take Sister Kenny under its wing so to speak, this was not the way that this powerful lady viewed the situation at all. Her hopes were that she might succeed in taking the NFIP under her own wing. The story is a familiar one, with proponents lined up on both sides in maneuvers to explain and defend their respective points of view. The blame can even be partially put on some prominent American orthopedic surgeons who attempted to discredit Miss Kenny's reputation—almost, it would seem, out of professional jealousy. Sister Kenny became the persecuted martyr. A sizable group rallied to her support, and this it was that brought the rival Sister Kenny Foundation into being. And so the fight continued for some years. By this time the principles and practice of the *treatment* of poliomyelitis had become lost in the shuffle.

When I had occasion to visit Sister Kenny at her Minneapolis institute a few years after World War II, I found her in a shaken mood, embittered at the treatment she had received from an illiberal group of American orthopedists who had sent her an insulting telegram and were not going to let a nurse from the Australian bush show them the error of their ways.

And yet to give some idea of the degree of fanaticism that had been reached in support of the Kenny treatment, an incident in the 1940s is worth recording. It involved a boy of fifteen or sixteen who had been taken ill with poliomyelitis at a New England boarding school. Although the patient was in the early acute febrile stage of the disease and there were plenty of good physicians on the spot and good regional hospitals where the Kenny concepts of treatment could have been carried out, the parents of the boy, who lived in Minneapolis, acting on the advice of local medical authorities, dispatched instructions that local doctors in New England were to keep hands off, and he was to be sent immediately by air to the Kenny Institute in Minneapolis. A private plane was hired, and the ill boy was sped on his way. Unfortunately the plane had to make a forced landing before it reached the halfway mark, and although adequate care was available at a local hospital near where the plane had landed, the parents urged that he continue his journey by whatever means available. He was still alive on arrival some days later, but more severely paralyzed than when he had started the journey. Perhaps this harrowing trip had nothing to do with the extent of the eventual paralysis, but considering that it is universally agreed that the treatment of acute poliomyelitis consists of complete rest in bed and freedom as far as possible from physical and mental trauma, the extent to which this incident violated those therapeutic principles is a measure of the extent to which both lay and professional people had been led to worship Sister Kenny. It would seem that they acted in the fixed belief that there was something magical in her personality as well as in her treatment of the acute disease; it is equally easy to see that the opposition was far from convinced.

In retrospect there is no denying that Sister Kenny's ideas and techniques marked a turning point, even an about-face, in the aftercare of paralytic poliomyelitis. By determination and sheer willpower she helped to raise the treatment of paralyzed patients out of the slough into which it had sunk in the 1930s. The system which prevailed before her advent, i.e. prolonged immobilization of affected limbs which in some instances led to a certain amount of calculated neglect, militated against involving the patient in early efforts to aid return of muscle function. It also eliminated the element of continued encouragement, which Sir Robert Jones had felt was so important as a psychological asset to rehabilitation. There was little use in exhorting a patient to exert himself physically if he was in a plaster cast.

Sister Kenny herself was not without blame, for instead of sticking to her daily work in the hospital wards, caring for and rehabilitating her patients, work for which she was eminently qualified, she became busy with all of the paraphernalia of publicity campaigns and press agents, who, needless to say, loved a fight. It is said that Sister Kenny played directly into the hands of the press by the aggressive manner in which her ideas were presented, a way that was calculated to antagonize physicians. If the spectacle of a physician, supposedly dedicated to the healing art, is apt to become tarnished when he shows himself publicity and power minded and engages too heavily in medical polemics, how much more tarnished is the image of a nurse who, forsaking her natural duties, becomes similarly embroiled.

Sister Kenny died in 1952 but her followers carried on. The Sister Kenny Institute (later known as the Kenny Rehabilitation Institute) had been established in Minneapolis in 1942, and the Sister Kenny Foundation, supported by contributions given by advocates of her cause, was launched three years later, after an unsuccessful effort on the part of the institute to obtain a grant of some $840,000 from the National Foundation. Once launched the Kenny Foundation took on some of the features of the NFIP and made project grants in the broad field of poliomyelitis not only for therapy but also in virology, epidemiology, and prophylaxis.[11]

The Kenny Foundation was even drawn into the field of oral poliovirus

11. For an account of the Sister Kenny Institute, the Foundation, and the Rehabilitation Institute, as well as the methods and personality of its original central figure, I am greatly indebted to Dr. E. J. Huenekens of Minneapolis, and to Dr. Paul M. Ellwood, who has written

vaccines by one of its own staff members. This was during the period when the Salk-type vaccine was being tried with great success; but to some investigators the idea of a live virus vaccine seemed more appealing, and accordingly many oral vaccine trials were carried out in the years 1957–59. Among them was one planned and conducted under the auspices of the University of Minnesota by Dr. Martins da Silva, a pediatrician from Brazil. The Lederle oral vaccine was used, in a trial which involved more than 100,000 persons. The Kenny Foundation supported the study, and in addition a similar program, which enjoyed the participation of the Health Department of the State of Minnesota, was launched. By this time Martins da Silva had joined the Pan American Health Organization (PAHO), and there he discussed the need for an international conference to obtain an overall picture of worldwide experiences with live poliovirus vaccines. Washington offered excellent opportunities for such a gathering, and in due time PAHO assumed the official role of the sponsoring organization. The Kenny Foundation contributed approximately $60,000 to each of the two PAHO conferences, held in 1959 and 1960. These week-long meetings[12] were singularly significant, as it turned out, in the cause of the prevention of poliomyelitis. They provided an arena for protracted and intimate discussions on a truly international basis, dealing with pros and cons of the oral poliovirus vaccines. To say that they were helpful in paving the way for the eventual licensing of this vaccine by the U.S. Public Health Service would be an understatement.

The National Foundation for Infantile Paralysis on the other hand, although it continued to support several projects in the live poliovirus field, was by this time to all intents and purposes concentrating its energies on promoting the inactivated Salk-type vaccine as the standard one in the United States, to the exclusion of oral vaccines, and on launching the Salk Institute. Its attitude has been interpreted as reflecting the belief that to all intents and purposes poliomyelitis had been conquered in the United States, and the American people were not going to support a prophylactic measure that happened to be more effective in controlling polio in Ethiopia, let us say. But here we are anticipating our story, which will be recounted in due time.

---

at some length about the history of these institutes following Sister Kenny's death. See letter from Paul M. Ellwood to Dr. J. R. Paul (unpublished), March 23, 1968.

12. First and Second *International Conferences on Live Poliovirus Vaccines*, Washington, D.C., Pan American Health Organization, 1959 and 1960.

CHAPTER 33

Military Significance of Poliomyelitis in World War II

Prior to the outbreak of World War II there had been no intimation that poliomyelitis was a disease of military significance. Its incidence had been very low among the U.S. armed forces personnel during and immediately following World War I; in fact, before 1920 in the United States infantile paralysis was still predominantly a disease of early childhood. But between 1920 and 1940 a marked shift was to take place. This is illustrated in table 7, which lists the age distribution of cases in New York City beginning with the great epidemic of 1916 and including the years thereafter as far as 1947. The name infantile paralysis was strictly suitable for the 1916 era, but by 1947 in the United States the term poliomyelitis had become more appropriate. The disease was no longer strictly infantile, and few of those infected became paralyzed.

During the years between the two world wars the age distribution of cases had shifted. Both British and American troops had become more susceptible to clinical poliomyelitis than their fathers had been during World War I. This was totally unexpected, and even as late as 1941 military medical authorities had not only been almost completely unaware of the change but when informed, they refused to believe it. The first indication of the military importance of poliomyelitis was the recovery of strains of the virus from central nervous system tissue obtained from fatal cases of a "strange" disease that had been attacking soldiers in United Kingdom forces serving in the Middle East. The virus isolations were made in Cairo in 1941 by Maj. C. E. Van Rooyen, RAMC (Royal Army Medical Corps), who published his findings two years later.[1] CNS material from these Middle East cases had also been sent to Dr. Rivers at the Rockefeller Institute (in 1942) for confirmation of the diagnosis, largely so that other neurotropic viruses could be eliminated. At the institute, Schlesinger and his colleagues also recovered poliovirus from these specimens.[2]

Later, aided by the copious use of hindsight, another fact came to light in the early 1940s when it was found that military cases of poliomyelitis

1. C. E. Van Rooyen and A. D. Morgan: Poliomyelitis; experimental work in Egypt. *Edinb. med. J.,* 50: 705–20, 1943.

2. R. W. Schlesinger, I. M. Morgan, and P. K. Olitsky: Transmission to rodents of Lansing type poliomyelitis virus originating in the Middle East. *Science, 98*: 452, 1943. From one of these isolations came the MEF[1] strain of poliovirus.

TABLE 7. The shift in age incidence of poliomyelitis cases occurring in
New York City between 1916 and 1947

	Percent of Total Cases in Three Age Groups (Years)		
Year	0–9	10–19	20+
1916 (epidemic year)*	95	3	2
1931 (epidemic year)	84	13	3
1938	74	14	12
1940	65	24	11
1944	63	32	5
1947 (epidemic year)	52	38	10

Data from the New York City Dept. of Health, as recorded in the
New York Herald Tribune, July 27, 1949.
* Estimates during epidemic years are presumably more accurate
from the standpoint of statistical significance than in nonepidemic
years.

could indeed occur in the tropics. This state of affairs might have been
predicted on the basis of an unexpected occurrence of the disease in soldiers and their dependents in the Philippines in 1936.[3] There Lt. Col.
(later Brig. Gen.) C. C. Hillman, MC, described 17 patients with poliomyelitis who had been admitted to the Sternberg General Hospital in Manila. Of these, 3 were in U.S. military personnel, and the remaining 14
were in their families. All 17 cases occurred in American visitors (i.e. "immigrants") to this tropical area. Coincidentally, the number of cases
among the local Filipinos had been extremely small, presumably only 9
in a population that numbered several millions. Not only had a discovery
been made that the disease existed in tropical areas, but immigrant military personnel might be particularly subject to it. This was a new idea
but considered as just a curiosity in 1936. Colonel Hillman commented
that in view of the vastly greater number of natives compared to Americans in the community, there was a striking discrepancy between the incidence rates in the two groups.[4] That age-specific immunity differed in Filipinos and Americans had not been considered at the time. Moreover, even
in the early 1940s experts on military medicine could not believe that
poliomyelitis had become, overnight so to speak, a threat to military personnel, especially in the tropics.

When in January 1941 the United States Army sensed the imminent
threat of war, its medical department laid plans by establishing a board

3. C. C. Hillman: Poliomyelitis in the Philippine Islands. *Milit. Surg., 79*: 48–58, 1936.
4. These observations have been confirmed time and again. For instance, in epidemic times
the Caucasians in the Hawaiian Islands' population have suffered far higher rates of poliomyelitis than have the native Hawaiians.

to deal with epidemics and problems of infectious disease generally.[5] But, although the Army Epidemiological Board created a separate unit known as the Neurotropic Virus Disease Commission to cope with virus infections of the central nervous system, this commission was charged primarily with the duty of investigating viral encephalitis. The possibility that it might also be concerned with poliomyelitis had been lightly dismissed.

Current events in the Middle East provided a rude awakening. There the first cases of poliomyelitis among soldiers occurred in British troops, and not only were sporadic cases noted but there was an epidemic! This was in 1940–41. The outbreak was in all probability the first sizable military epidemic of the disease ever to be reported. It occurred among United Kingdom troops at their base camps in Egypt. Unfortunately, due to reasons of military censorship this historic event was not reported until some six years later[6] and thus did not receive the attention it deserved. The epidemic consisted of 40 cases, 4 of them fatal, among a contingent of New Zealanders which altogether numbered about 18,000 men. It was unusual in that it lasted over a period of nine months, with two distinct waves. Of the 40 cases, 38 occurred in the base camps located just outside of Cairo and 2 on the north coast of Egypt—one at Alexandria, and another in the Western Desert. The remarkable thing was that the outbreak occurred within an entirely adult population.[7] All of the recorded cases were between 20 and 40 years old!

Caughey and Porteous in reporting this military outbreak were understandably puzzled. They concluded that "poliomyelitis may arise and be widely propagated among an adult male population." They added further that although the disease was endemic in Egypt, there had been no significant increase in cases in the local native Cairo population during the 1940–41 outbreak among the troops (see n. 6).

Actually, Van Rooyen and Morgan, who were colleagues of Caughey and Porteous in the same military hospital, were the first to publish on the remarkably high incidence of poliomyelitis in United Kingdom troops in the Middle East. They almost hit on the explanation for this unexpected state of affairs, but as their report (see n. 1) indicated they too were distinctly puzzled:

In the M.E.F. [Middle East Forces] during the years 1941 and 1942,

5. First known as the Board for the Prevention of Influenza and other Diseases in the Army, it eventually became the Armed Forces Epidemiological Board, which continues to this day.

6. J. E. Caughey and W. M. Porteous: An epidemic of poliomyelitis occurring among troops in the Middle East. *Med. J. Aust.*, 1: 5–10, 1946.

7. This high age-specific susceptibility to poliovirus infection in adults was also reflected in an earlier epidemic due to an unknown type of poliovirus that occurred in New Zealand in 1937. In that outbreak the number of reported cases was 806; 20.4 percent of the patients were over the age of 15.

106 cases were diagnosed as poliomyelitis, and of these 33 died. As mentioned, such a high mortality excites curiosity as to whether mild cases passed unrecognized. The high death rate may be due to increased susceptibility of the twenty to thirty-five age group to poliomyelitis, or alternatively, to the infection of British troops with Egyptian strains of virus against which our men possess no immunity. Neither of these explanations is adequate, . . . space forbids further discussion of this interesting subject, but one is left with the most unsatisfactory impression that poliomyelitis in Egypt among both children and adults may assume a non-paralytic abortive illness, whereas British troops between the third and fourth decade of life who become infected, develop the typical disease.

It is a tribute to Major Van Rooyen and other medical officers of the Fifteenth Scottish Hospital in Cairo at the time that they were able to discern what was happening and to perform careful work on the isolation of the virus under the most trying conditions, while the desert warfare swept back and forth over North Africa until the culmination of the struggle took place in the battle of El Alamein in October 1942, a scant sixty miles west of Alexandria and a little over one hundred miles from Cairo.[8] It was a close thing.

Actually, during the years of 1941–42 Van Rooyen and Morgan were able to isolate 6 strains of poliovirus from 7 fatal military cases; and furthermore, by enlisting the services of the Rockefeller Institute in New York, they were able to determine that various other encephalitic viruses known at that time were not involved. Indeed Van Rooyen and Morgan were the first to suspect that as far as the prevalence of polioviruses was concerned, something was amiss about "polio" in Egypt—and indeed perhaps in the whole of the Middle East.

In the meantime American medical officers in Washington, particularly those attached to the Army Epidemiological Board, had begun to sense what might be going on, and in view of the sizable numbers of U.S. troops which had been dispatched to North Africa and the Middle East in late 1942 and early 1943, they were anxious to find out more about the situation. The U.S. troops consisted of combat units that had participated in the landings in North Africa in early November 1942 as well as military supply units that had been dispatched later and were distributed over a wide area including Egypt, Palestine, Iran, the Persian Gulf area, and as far south as Eritrea. The decision was therefore quickly made to send an epidemiological team to continue the work started by Van Rooyen in the Middle East. Objectives were to investigate the neurotropic (and other)

8. A. Moorhead: *The March to Tunis; The North African War 1940–43.* New York, Harper and Row, 1965.

viruses pathogenic for man, which were prevalent in this semiarid and tropical area, and the diseases they might cause. Not only did the situation deserve study; it called for recommendations as to what, if any, were the possibilities of preventing such infections as sand-fly fever (to which American soldiers had never been exposed before), viral hepatitis, and last but not least—the board having seen the light by this time—poliomyelitis. Accordingly, three members (including myself) of the Army Epidemiological Board's Commission on Neurotropic Virus Diseases, to be known later as the "Virus Commission" (see fig. 47), were dispatched to Cairo in 1943.[9] This ten-month-long activity came about as a result of the discernment of those who guided the board's early activities.

Dr. Rivers' interest in poliomyelitis in the Middle East also continued unabated. He had much to do with the sending of this team, and it was he who persuaded Mr. Basil O'Connor that the commission's project deserved a financial contribution from the National Foundation for Infantile Paralysis. This amounted to $10,000 and enormously facilitated the experimental work of the Virus Commission in the Middle East.

Almost immediately upon our arrival in Cairo in April 1943, we began to see cases of poliomyelitis among American troops. Indeed from the time that the men started to arrive in the latter part of 1942, and for many months subsequently, it was noted that the rate for this disease rose to more than ten times that recorded for soldiers of the same age in the United States. By pooling American and British observations the problem of poliomyelitis was again (in 1944) brought to the attention of military authorities of both nations.[10] Most of the cases were sporadic, but in the meantime at least two further small outbreaks had been noted among United Kingdom forces in Libya.

Several of the U.S. Medical Reserve officers in Cairo who had had wide experience as neurologists in civilian practice were quite emphatic in maintaining that these adult military cases were *not* examples of poliomyelitis, certainly nothing like the cases they had encountered at home. This attitude was understandable since before 1940 the clinical picture in adults had received scant notice in American textbooks of medicine. Only reluctantly did these neurologists accept the diagnosis when poliovirus was demonstrated at the Virus Commission's laboratory, using pathological material obtained from fatal cases in American soldiers. The official

9. Members of this so-called Virus Commission, Army Epidemiological Board (AFEB) who were attached to U.S.A. forces in the Middle East (USAFIME) consisted of: Major A. B. Sabin, MC, Maj. C. B. Philip, Sn.C., and Dr. J. R. Paul, director. Later, Capt. W. P. Havens, MC joined this group which had established its base laboratory and its experimental ward for patients at the 38th General Hospital, 17 kilometers outside of Cairo.

10. J. R. Paul, W. P. Havens, and C. E. Van Rooyen: Poliomyelitis in British and American Troops in the Middle East; the isolation of virus from human faeces. *Brit. med. J., 1*: 841, 1944.

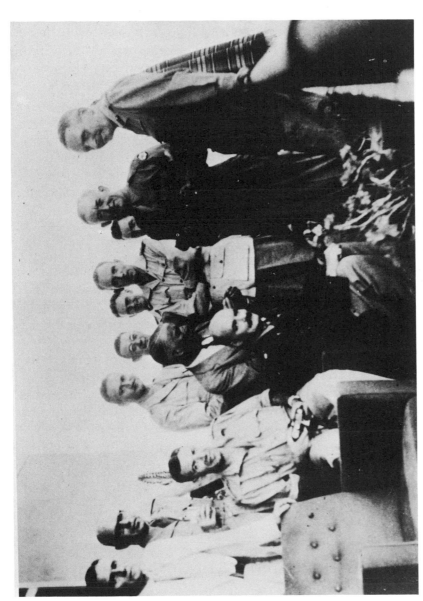

FIG. 47. Group at the Middle East billet of the "Virus Commission," Cairo, Egypt, Sept. 1943. Seated, left to right: Maj. C. E. Van Rooyen, RAMC, John Marquand (author and war correspondent), Maj. C. E. Philip, Sn.C. Standing: the author, Major Theodore, RAMC, Maj. A. B. Sabin, MC, Col. D. W. Billick, MC, Maj. J. Caughey, New Zealand, MC, Lt. Col. Eliott, South Africa, MC, Lt. Col. F. K. Sewell, MC (partially hidden), Brig. Gen. J. S. Simmons, MC, and Col. J. S. K. Boyd, RAMC.

Picture taken by Brigadier Sydney Smith, RAMC.

account of this episode, published almost twenty years later, is given in the history of the Medical Department, United States Army, World War II.

At the 38th General Hospital near Cairo, Egypt, this author, in consultation, saw at least a dozen cases of poliomyelitis, several of which were fatal. In the majority of patients, the disease was characterized by insidious onset with 2 or 3 days of malaise, relatively little fever, but severe pain in the back. This is in some contrast to the textbook picture seen in children with an acute onset with fever and usually a biphasic course. Fortunately, at the 38th General Hospital, a virus laboratory had been established in the summer of 1943. Monkeys were obtained locally and from Eritrea, where they had been trapped by members of the Army Veterinary Service, and the isolation of poliomyelitis virus by monkey inoculation with material from a number of these cases during the summer of 1943 supported the diagnosis.[11]

The findings of Van Rooyen and Morgan (see n. 1) together with those of the U.S. commission (see n. 10) proved unquestionably that sporadic (or even epidemic) cases of poliomyelitis could occur in the Middle East in immigrant military populations and established the fact that they were not rare in certain areas where poliomyelitis had been supposed not to exist or at least not be prevalent in native inhabitants.[12] Although the complete explanation of this state of affairs was not worked out until some years later, suspicions were aroused in 1943 that cases of true infantile paralysis had been grossly underreported in the civilian population of Egypt. For instance, I had occasion to discuss the question in the summer of 1943 with two prominent Cairo pediatricians and found that in their experience paralytic poliomyelitis was *not at all uncommon* in Egypt. As a matter of fact, the number of cases diagnosed annually in the outpatient department of a single hospital in Cairo, the Children's Hospital, during 1938 and 1939 had been 96 and 41 respectively. However, almost none of these had been officially reported. Such an incidence decidedly contradicted the statistics put out by the Egyptian Ministry of Health (see n. 12). Something was wrong somewhere. Information about the ages of the patients was scanty except it was said that most of them were children under five years old. Poliomyelitis in native Egyptian adults was decidedly rare;

11. J. R. Paul: "Poliomyelitis," in *Internal Medicine in World War II,* vol. 2, *Infectious Diseases.* Office of the Surgeon General, Dept. of the Army, Washington, D.C., 1963, pp. 91–99.

12. According to a report from the Ministry of Finance, Kingdom of Egypt, 1941, there were only 3 cases of poliomyelitis and 2 deaths in 1938; and in 1939, 8 cases and 8 deaths. Thus over a period of two years only 11 cases had been reported among a total population of 16,000,000 people. This was an infinitesimal rate.

no cases had been seen at the local Egyptian Military General Hospital for the past several years.

From a diary I kept in Egypt in that summer of 1943, I find the following excerpt under the date of August 20:

> In the morning came Dr. Ibrahim Shawki Bey, Director of Medical Services at the Children's Hospital and Dispensary in Cairo, to take me to his hospital. He was accompanied by a small dog (rare for an Egyptian) full of affection, wet mouthings and—fleas.
>
> "Poliomyelitis," he said, "is not rare in Egypt. It is never epidemic —always sporadic. It is a disease of poorer classes. Never have I seen a case in my private praxis (sic). The cases are as a rule mild, involving only one limb—rarely a fatality. The patients are seldom seen during the acute phase of the illness. Instead the child is brought to the Hospital weeks after the onset with the complaint that its leg is weak and doesn't seem to be getting better. The acute illness has been long forgotten by this time."
>
> In the course of our hospital visit we passed a huge hall full of murmuring women and children—the Out-Patient Department (OPD). There must have been from 500–1000 persons all waiting to be seen. Dr. Shawki Bey said: "We have 160,000 admissions in this clinic a year." With this large daily admission rate and in view of the apparent dearth of dispensary physicians, it is small wonder that sometimes both diagnoses and therapy suffered.

Shawki Bey's account explains why the discrepancy was so great between the official number of cases and the children with paralysed limbs seen at the Children's Hospital. In the majority of instances when persistent weakness or paralysis followed an initial short fever, the tendency was for the earlier, transient acute phase to be forgotten. It seems probable that the cases officially listed as poliomyelitis by the Egyptian Ministry of Health included only those few that were successfully diagnosed in the acute phase or those that were fatal early in their course. The patients who survived and came to the hospital late in convalescence for treatment of their paralysis were *not* reported as poliomyelitis.

Some of the officers of the RAMC in the Middle East and more than a few U.S. Army medical officers were not to be won over by any demonstration such as a diagnostic laboratory test, which might after all be subject to all kinds of errors. They stoutly opposed the diagnosis of poliomyelitis in military personnel, especially as some of the cases were atypical. They also had the idea that if poliomyelitis did indeed exist in the troops, the men had not contracted it from the local population, where the disease was extremely rare; but rather, these officers supported the official Egyptian view that our troops, acting as carriers, "had brought their own disease with them."

Despite such protests, a growing tide of opinion in the opposite direction soon gained ascendancy. Similar cases of poliomyelitis began to be recorded elsewhere in British forces, notably in India, by McAlpine[13] and by Illingworth.[14] The latter commented that the disease was particularly severe in foreign troops whereas coincidentally it was uncommon and mild in Indian natives.

An equally important observation was made during an epidemic on the island of Malta in 1942–43, while it was occupied by British forces.[15] Here again the case rate in adult Maltese was almost nil, and there were no cases in native-born soldiers. In contrast, British military personnel suffered an astronomical rate for poliomyelitis in an adult age group, of 2.5 per 1,000!

Later, in 1944–45, this same experience was encountered by the U.S. military forces over and over again on the other side of the world, both in tropical and temperate zones. For example, when American soldiers first invaded the Philippines there was an outbreak on the island of Leyte. This occurred in November 1944, when 47, 37 paralytic and 10 nonparalytic, cases occurred within 16 days of the landings.[16] Apparently word had not yet gotten around of the comparable experiences among British and United States forces in the Middle East. So, in keeping with older points of view, it was assumed that the virus had been brought in by the troops from the United States. Sabin, in his history of preventive medicine in World War II, quotes Col. Henry M. Thomas, Jr., MC, the medical consultant who had responsibility for the military patients on Leyte, as stating that "certain facts seem fairly sure, however, and these point to the introduction of the reservoir into Leyte with the troops."[17] According to Colonal Thomas' information, no recent cases had been uncovered among Filipinos, and furthermore a case had developed as early as 5 days after an American soldier had arrived in Leyte. Fifteen years later Sabin (see n. 16) gave five reasons why Colonel Thomas' interpretation was incorrect and presented evidence that favored the *local native population* of Leyte as the actual reservoir of the virus.

13. D. McAlpine: Epidemiology of acute poliomyelitis in the India Command. *Lancet, 2*: 130–33, 1945.

14. R. S. Illingworth: Poliomyelitis and meningismus; a hundred cases. *J. roy. Army med. Cps, 84*: 210–17, 1945.

15. H. J. Seddon, T. Agius, H. G. G. Bernstein, and R. E. Turnbridge: The poliomyelitis epidemic in Malta, 1942–43. *Quart. J. Med., 38*: 1–26, 1945.

16. A. B. Sabin: *Poliomyelitis; Preventive Medicine in World War II,* vol. 5, *Communicable Disease through Contact or by Unknown Means.* Office of the Surgeon General, Dept. of the Army, Washington, D.C., 1960, pp. 367–400.

17. Letter from Col. Henry M. Thomas, MC to Chief Surgeon U.S. Army, Services of Supply, Dec. 29, 1944. Quoted in n. 16.

The same higher incidence of poliomyelitis in our troops abroad than in the United States prevailed in China, Burma, and India; later when American soldiers occupied the territory of Japan and Korea, army rates in these areas underwent an immediate upsurge. A chart illustrating this is shown in figure 48. It compares the rates in soldiers within the confines

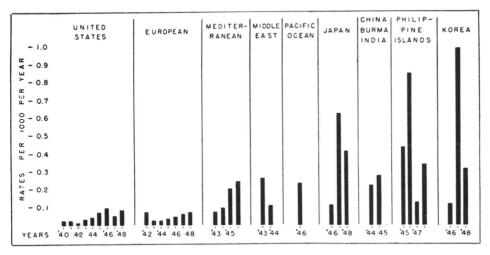

Fig. 48. Annual rates (per 1,000) at which poliomyelitis was acquired by U.S. troops stationed in nine different geographical areas during various periods between 1940 and 1948 (from Paul, n. 18).

of the United States and European countries during 1940–48 with the rates at which American troops contracted the disease in the places where they were stationed in seven foreign areas throughout the world.[18]

Previously it had been observed by military medical men that when troops from a developed country occupy an area inhabited by a population with unsanitary habits where the environmental sanitation is primitive, military personnel are likely to suffer from a variety of infections common to the natives of that area, particularly within the first few months after their arrival. These include all kinds of dysenteries, hepatitis, and other acute viral and parasitic infections, even typhoid fever. During World War II poliomyelitis was added to this group. It had suddenly become a disease with which the armed forces had to reckon. After 1945, U.S. military hospitals were equipped to handle acute cases, and, of course later, preventive measures (vaccination) were adopted by the armed services.

It had taken a cruel war to bring these new facts about poliomyelitis to the surface—but one more stepping-stone had been placed in position

18. J. R. Paul: Poliomyelitis attack rates in American Troops (1940–1948). *Amer. J. Hyg.*, *50*: 57–62, 1949.

to explain the behavior of the disease in different parts of the world.[19] The stage was set to find out why certain adolescents and young adults living in one environment were susceptible while those from another were immune. The discovery that poliomyelitis had now attained the status of a military disease was interesting enough and not without practical consequences, but of far greater importance was the emergence of an understanding of the behavior of the infection in civilian populations in different environments. Such knowledge contained the roots of the explanation as to why in the late nineteenth century the disease suddenly began to appear in epidemic form. But this is for a chapter in which another visit to Cairo is described. On this occasion investigators came armed with more sophisticated and accurate methods to search out and measure the circumstances that accounted for the differences in immunity between one population and another.

19. In 1947, Sabin, who had been one of the original members of the Neurotropic Virus Disease Commission, expressed his views somewhat as follows: Prior to World War II, we were in possession of totally inadequate statistics on poliomyelitis and its actual prevalence in most parts of the world including both tropical or semitropical areas. A. B. Sabin: The epidemiology of poliomyelitis; problems at home and among the Armed Forces abroad. *J. Amer. med. Ass., 134*: 749–56, 1947.

CHAPTER 34

Serological Surveys and Antibody Patterns
Endemicity versus Epidemicity

With the Lansing strain established in mice, a way was open at last to perform practical serologic tests; the neutralizing antibody content of sera
could be readily determined now that it was no longer necessary to use
the cumbersome and often prohibitively expensive method of monkey
inoculation. Not only did this mean that the test could be used for clinical
diagnosis and that the immune status of an individual could be tested,
but large scale serologic surveys of many individuals and the immunity
of different population groups could be compared. Although at first antibodies to only one type (II) could be measured, this was an immense step
forward. It may be recalled that serologic tests employing monkeys had
been performed since the time of Flexner's first efforts. One to three (later
five) monkeys per serum had been required. Expense was not the only
drawback, for in due time the "monkey neutralization test" had been
strongly challenged as unreliable.

An antecedent of the new mouse test had been devised by Dr. L. T. Webster of the Rockefeller Institute in the early 1930s for work with infections caused by St. Louis encephalitis virus. So it was not difficult to adapt
the same neutralization test method for use with the Lansing strain of
poliovirus in mice. The test provided a means of mapping out the age-
specific pattern of a given population's immunity to poliomyelitis. In order
to do this one had to collect sera from scores of healthy children, adolescents, and adults and to determine the percent with and without antibodies in each age group, i.e. the proportion of immunes and susceptibles. An early effort in this direction, using the monkey neutralization
test, had been made by Aycock and Kramer in 1930; their results have
been shown previously in table 4. Five years later the Yale Unit constructed a similar chart, which illustrated an age-specific global pattern
of poliovirus antibodies, using its own data together with results reported
in the literature.[1] Admittedly it was a hodgepodge which is valid reason
for its not being shown here. Several strains of poliovirus had been employed in these tests in monkeys, using sera collected in many cities and

1. J. R. Paul and J. D. Trask: The neutralization test in poliomyelitis; Comparative results
with four strains of the virus. *J. exp. Med., 61*: 447–64, 1935.

rural areas and even in many lands. But it was perhaps the first chart ever published that illustrated age-specific immunity to poliomyelitis on a worldwide basis—and also the last. Data from the Yale laboratory had been obtained with blood specimens from recent convalescents affected during the epidemic of 1931 and from normal persons sampled at the same time. Moreover the use of multiple polyglot populations obscured the issues at stake. But despite these inadequacies—immunological, statistical, and demographic—the pattern was sufficient to determine certain basic features that subsequent, more sophisticated studies confirmed. These included the firm demonstration that most infants are born with short-lived, passive antibodies, derived from their mothers. Having lost these by about six or seven months of age, a certain number begin to acquire active antibodies and immunity through inapparent infection. These percentages increased either slowly or rapidly until generally by the age of fifteen between 80 and 100 percent of children are antibody positive and presumably immune.

A crucial point was that the speed at which this acquisition of active poliovirus antibodies went on proved to be an indication of the kind of environment in which the children had lived. Also uncovered was the unexpected finding that the highest percent positive was recorded universally in normal adolescents and adults from tropical areas, where, according to some "authorities" in the 1920s and 1930s, poliomyelitis was not supposed to exist! This observation started a trend of thinking which led to the idea that the natural home of poliomyelitis might after all be in the tropics and other warm weather areas, and only occasionally might this disease stray into northern and southern temperate zones during summertime.

The advent of the mouse neutralization test employing the Lansing strain contributed mightily to the whole field of poliovirus research. Hammon and Izumi[2] were among the first to attempt to use it as a specific diagnostic measure in human poliomyelitis. It was their practice to obtain two or more serial samples of blood from the patient, i.e. one taken very early in the disease and another one or two weeks later. The test's clinical usefulness, however, proved limited, primarily because it was applicable only to infection with Type II poliovirus, the one least often associated with paralysis; but also because patients often have maximum antibody levels at the time their disease is recognized, and it is thus impossible to demonstrate significant rises in titer.

Three years later, Dr. Thomas B. Turner and his colleagues at the Johns Hopkins School of Hygiene took advantage of the mouse test to survey

---

2. W. McD. Hammon and E. M. Izumi: Poliomyelitis mouse neutralization test, applied to acute and convalescent sera. *Proc. Soc. exp. Biol. Med. (N.Y.)*, *49*: 242, 1942.

the immune status of different age groups in an urban population, namely residents of the east side of the city of Baltimore, which is one of the poorer and less favored sections of that area.[3] The curves that they constructed indicated a rising incidence of Lansing antibodies during childhood. This was an infinitely more exact measure of immunity, and more adequate statistically, than previous surveys. In due time, during the decade that preceded the vaccination era, this graph became a standard pattern for urban underprivileged populations in many parts of the world. Only later did it turn out that there was a correlation between the rate of antibody acquisition and the type of sanitary environment; in populations with poor standards of hygiene, the steepest rise in antibody prevalence occurred in the youngest age group, while in more favored areas, with higher socioeconomic levels, the steepest part of the curve tended to be in older children (of school age) or even adolescents.

Anyway by the use of the serologic survey technique it gradually dawned on those interested in the way resistance to poliomyelitis was acquired that in some, indeed most, urban populations immunization was going on at a surprising rate in infancy and early childhood without accompanying disease. Such observations confirmed another first for the Swedes, for, just as Wernstedt had predicted thirty years before, populations inevitably became immune when exposed to poliovirus under conditions which favored its dissemination.

It was natural to try to determine whether antibody patterns elsewhere conformed to those of lower socioeconomic groups in Baltimore To this end Sabin used the mouse neutralization test to survey populations in the Far East,[4] to which he had access in the early post–World War II period. Similar surveys were made by Hammon in the Pacific Islands and in the United States;[5] Melnick, in various places in the United States;[6] and Gear in southern Africa.[7] From these determinations it was found that in certain parts of the world, including the Far East and particularly in tropical areas, most children had acquired antibodies to the Lansing strain before they had reached the age of five years; whereas in contrast, most children in the United States did not acquire this antibody until between the ages of five and ten years.

3. T. B. Turner, L. E. Young, and E. S. Maxwell: Mouse-adapted Lansing strain of poliomyelitis virus: neutralizing antibodies in serum of healthy children. *Amer. J. Hyg., 42*: 119–27, 1945.

4. A. B. Sabin: "Epidemiologic patterns of poliomyelitis in different parts of the world," in *Poliomyelitis; Papers and Discussions presented at the First Internat. Poliomyelitis Conference,* Philadelphia, Lippincott, 1948, p. 24.

5. W. McD. Hammon: Immunity in poliomyelitis. *Bact. Rev., 13*: 135, 1948.

6. J. L. Melnick: Unpublished data, collected in 1947–49 by the Yale Poliomyelitis Study Unit.

7. J. H. S. Gear: Poliomyelitis in Southern Africa. *Proc. 4th Internat. Congress Trop. Med. & Malaria, 1*: 555, 1948.

A golden opportunity existed for exploring still another type of population, namely the peoples living in the Arctic. This idea was touched off by events described by Canadian observers in the winter of 1948–49, involving an isolated district of the Hudson Bay region where it was believed that the natives had not previously been exposed to poliovirus.[8] In this area a sharp epidemic of the paralytic disease had erupted; it was particularly severe, with an especially high attack rate in one community, Chesterfield Inlet, where in a population of 275 Eskimos, 51 came down with paralytic poliomyelitis and of these, 14 died—an unprecedented death rate! But the high mortality was not the only or even the main significant feature of this disastrous epidemic. Of greater concern was the number of Eskimos left with residual paralysis. A paralyzed patient in the United States has some chance of making his way in our industrial environment, where attempts are made to rehabilitate him by teaching him a trade for which he is suited. But in the Arctic, a paralyzed Eskimo has virtually no chance of coping with his environment. And if brought south to an urban setting, he has even less chance of survival because, being so accustomed to Arctic ways of living, he is apt to succumb to diseases of civilization, of which tuberculosis leads the list.

Another indication of heightened susceptibility to poliomyelitis of the Chesterfield Inlet Eskimo population was that the disease was not confined to children or even to adolescents, but appeared in all ages. Indeed it was most frequent and most severe in the age groups above forty years, suggesting a complete absence of immunity in the whole population. One would have to conclude that it must have been a long time since polioviruses had penetrated this remote region. The pattern of the outbreak suggested that if anyone had measured the age-specific prevalence of Lansing poliovirus antibodies in 1946 or 1947, before the epidemic broke, the findings might well have revealed a complete absence of these antibodies in all ages. So the task of the investigator was to locate an Eskimo population similar to the Chesterfield Inlet one, but one in which there had been no evidence of a recent poliomyelitis epidemic. A serum survey of such a population might answer a number of pertinent questions.

Accordingly, an Eskimo population was selected, and a serum survey was carried out by the Yale Poliomyelitis Study Unit in villages on the north coast of Alaska during the summer of 1949.[9] Two such adjacent vil-

8. A. F. W. Peart: An outbreak of poliomyelitis in Canadian Eskimos in wintertime. *Canad. J. Publ. Hlth, 40*: 405, 1949.

9. J. R. Paul and J. T. Riordan: Observations on serological epidemiology. *Amer. J. Hyg., 52*: 202–12, 1950; and J. R. Paul, J. T. Riordan, and J. L. Melnick: Antibodies to three different antigenic types of poliomyelitis viruses in sera from North Alaskan Eskimos. *Amer. J. Hyg., 54*: 275–85, 1951. This project was conducted under the auspices of the Armed Forces Epidemiological Board at the Arctic Research Laboratory, Point Barrow, Alaska and with the cooperation of the Office of Naval Research. It was partially supported by funds granted by the NFIP.

lages (Barrow and Wainwright) were chosen; together they boasted a population of about 1,000 Eskimos at the time. The medical history of these villages was understandably scanty, but that gleaned from a physician and from other tenuous sources indicated that although they had experienced disastrous epidemics of whooping cough, measles, and influenza, there had been little evidence of poliomyelitis.[10] Actually the greater part of the medical story was found in a review of death certificates. The diagnoses of fatalities had been listed regularly since 1915 by local representatives of the Alaska Native Service; also, brief clinical records were found in a "Morbidity Book" kept by Dr. H. W. Greist. Two deaths from infantile paralysis, and only two, were found in the entire list covering a period of thirty-four years; both were in young children (aged 4 and 3) and both occurred in Barrow in October 1930. There were also two other deaths in the same village in that summer and fall of 1930, which attracted my attention. One was that of a boy of fifteen years diagnosed as having "sleeping sickness"; another was a boy of nine whose death was ascribed to "spinal meningitis due to an injury of the spine." It is possible, but not in any way definite, that these could have been cases of encephalitic or paralytic poliomyelitis that were misdiagnosed. Apart from the two definite cases, no record either verbal or written could be obtained from natives, schoolteachers, missionaries, or nurses, with whom I had contact, which indicated that acute cases of poliomyelitis had occurred on the north coast of Alaska within the last nineteen years. Admittedly, however, one could not claim that poliomyelitis had not been present in this remote Arctic area, either prior or subsequent to 1930. All that one can say is that there is no record of it.

Samples of blood were collected from 243 inhabitants of Barrow and Wainwright villagers, representing a range of ages from 5 to 60 years. The sera were examined for antibody by means of neutralization tests performed with the mouse-adapted strain of Lansing poliovirus. As might have been expected, the age-specific antibody pattern in this population was decidedly different from that obtained in Baltimore by Turner and colleagues (see n. 3) and, in fact, did not conform to any pattern that had yet been described. It is illustrated in figure 49 as the Alaskan curve. Its unique quality is shown by the fact that of the 129 Eskimos under 20 years of age whose sera were tested and who had not been outside the community, there was a universal absence of poliovirus (Lansing) antibod-

For the original suggestion that an investigation be carried out in the Arctic Research Laboratory I am indebted to Dr. M. C. Schlesnyak of Columbia University, N.Y.

10. I am indebted for much valued information about medical conditions in the area to the late Dr. Henry W. Greist of Monticello, Ind., who had been the medical missionary at the Presbyterian Hospital at Barrow Village since 1921; with his wife, a registered nurse, he had remained there until World War II.

ies; whereas 80 percent of individuals over that age possessed such antibodies. The shift from negative to positive coincided with the year 1930, when poliomyelitis was known to have visited Barrow Village. But what was not expected was the persistence of substantial levels of neutralizing

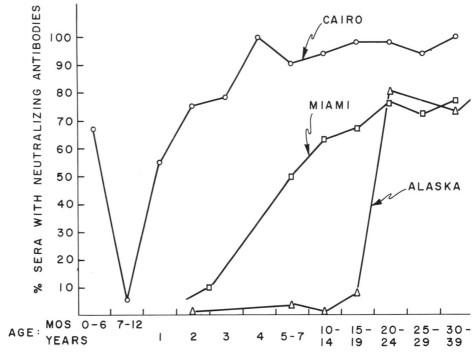

Fig. 49. Age-specific percentages of antibodies to Type II poliovirus as determined in collections of sera obtained in 1949–51. Three population groups are shown. Not only are they geographically separated but also they represent very different ways of living (unpublished and published data from the Yale Poliomyelitis Study Unit).

antibody in adults over the age of 20—especially in the 20–40 group. Presumably no exposure to polioviruses had occurred since 1930, and yet the antibody content of 80 percent of the entire adult population had been maintained over the twenty-year period, 1930–49. This meant that once these Eskimos had been exposed and infected, the resulting immunity *was* lasting! Prior to 1950 there had been many an argument as to how long human immunity after a single infection persisted, and whether it was necessary to have reinforcement by multiple infections with the same type of poliovirus or different types. Indeed, the reinforcement theory had been suspected as an explanation of the usual way in which the vast majority of adults gained their immunity to poliomyelitis—namely, bit by bit. But now it was apparent that a single subclinical or inapparent infection could produce lasting immunity, perhaps for life. It was fortunate indeed that the 1930 epidemic in both villages happened to have been caused by a Lansing-like (Type II) strain of poliovirus.[11]

The implication of this unexpected finding of long persistence of antibodies to poliovirus was not wholly academic. It contained indications of the way in which artificial immunization with a live virus might be expected to work, if and when such immunization became a reality. For, if an inapparent infection with an attenuated strain of poliovirus could be induced, it *could* result in *permanent* immunity. If, on the other hand, immunization was to be achieved by methods other than by the production of an actual infection, the question was open as to how long such immunity would last, and whether one would have to look forward to its constant reinforcement.

The Eskimo serum survey was the harbinger of a series of such investigations that was conducted in populations and areas which differed widely from the Arctic. In 1950, the year after the Alaska project, the Yale Unit decided to try its luck in a population as far removed from Eskimo land as possible, not only from a geographical but also from a sociological point of view. This time the choice fell on a group of villages on the outskirts of the city of Cairo, Egypt, an area which had become familiar to me during the war years.[12]

The results of tests on sera from this Egyptian population revealed, as had long been suspected, that the age-specific antibody pattern was very different from that of the Eskimo population. Not only among adults, but among children and adolescents as well, there was a very high percent with antibodies to poliovirus. This finding explained why the bulk of the population enjoyed immunity to the disease, and why paralytic cases had been confined to the infantile age group.

The comparative findings for the Eskimos and the Egyptians are illus-

---

11. A year later (1951) the same collection of sera was tested for antibodies to Types I and III polioviruses, using monkey neutralization tests (see n. 9). The results indicated that Type I had been present in the area about the year 1915, and only persons 35 years or older possessed Type I antibodies. Similarly only those 45 or more had evidence of previous infection with Type III virus. There was no evidence that infection with any poliovirus type had occurred since 1930.

Twelve years later, in 1963, the Yale group repeated some of these determinations. The tests were performed with all three types of poliovirus in a much more sophisticated manner using tissue-culture techniques. In spite of the sera having been frozen for 14 years at –20° C, and in spite of their having been dipped into several times, the results came out exactly as had been determined back in 1949–50 (see n. 9). See also Third Annual Report of WHO Reference Serum Bank, Yale University, 1963, unpublished.

12. J. R. Paul, J. L. Melnick, V. H. Barnett, and N. Goldblum: A survey of neutralizing antibodies to poliomyelitis virus in Cairo, Egypt. *Amer. J. Hyg.,* 55: 402–13, 1952.

This project was also carried out by the Yale Unit under multiple auspices, i.e. the Armed Forces Epidemiological Board; the National Foundation for Infantile Paralysis; the Rockefeller Foundation (notably through the agency of John M. Weir); and the Naval Medical Research Unit No. 3 (NAMRU-3), where some of the laboratory work was done.

trated in figure 49. The curve for the Egyptian population indicates that almost all individuals over five years of age had already been infected and acquired antibodies to the Lansing strain and thus were solidly immune to paralytic poliomyelitis due to Type II for the rest of their lives. A certain small percentage of infants did develop paralysis, but even if recognized, the chances were that a different name had been applied to their disease. Hence the dearth of officially reported acute poliomyelitis cases. Just as Shawki Bey had described to me six years earlier, young children with paralysis were usually brought for treatment long after the acute symptoms had subsided—and been forgotten.

By 1950 the numbers of infants and young children diagnosed as having paralytic poliomyelitis and admitted for treatment at the Children's Hospital in Cairo had risen in the brief period of six years to the relatively high level of 235 per year for 1948–49.

Comparing these statistics with serologic surveys, it was thus possible to confirm what had previously been only an impression and theory. One did not have to search far to determine that exposure to polioviruses was very frequent in the Egyptian environment. Infection (inapparent or otherwise) was extremely prevalent among native infants living in the vicinity of Cairo, and not, as had been once thought in 1938, exceedingly uncommon. Moreover, the extensive dissemination of virus provided an explanation for the military cases of the years 1941–43.

But what was of more importance to the natural history of poliomyelitis was that it immediately became apparent that as long as crude sanitation prevailed in most parts of the world, as it did in the nineteenth century and long before that, poliomyelitis had existed as a worldwide *endemic* infection of infancy and such a situation resulted in an absence of epidemics. What the serum surveys revealed was that where primitive environmental sanitation still persisted, as in many semiarid or semitropical climates, there *endemic* poliomyelitis continued to prevail.

In contrast to Egypt, and many other comparable regions, the circulation of polioviruses in the Scandinavian countries, the United States, and elsewhere underwent a change, coincidentally with the era which followed Pasteur. When sanitary methods began to be introduced and practiced, the habits of the population were profoundly altered in the direction of higher standards of public environmental and personal hygiene. In the United States, by 1900 the recently introduced improvements were enthusiastically hailed, almost as a new religion. Comparatively pure food and water became the order of the day in many of the developed countries. Yet the result was paradoxical with respect to poliomyelitis. Although the incidence of endemic, enteric bacterial diseases was markedly reduced, the effect on enteric viral infections such as poliomyelitis was less favorable. In fact it was the reverse and had the effect of transforming a situation which favored endemic infection into one that encouraged epidemics. What happened was that the circulation of polioviruses became more spotty and intermittent as the twentieth century progressed; children arrived at school age and even adolescence without having been exposed or infected, i.e. they remained as susceptibles. Accordingly, they became increasingly vulnerable, and when, inevitably, the virus was introduced after an interval of some years, it spread rapidly through an awaiting susceptible population much as happens with measles. The result was periodic *epidemics* of the disease.

In the 1930s it had been categorically stated that "No circumstance in the history of poliomyelitis is so baffling as its change during the last two decades of the nineteenth century from a sporadic to an epidemic disease."[13] It may be remembered that earlier in this volume the idea had been entertained that poliomyelitis was a *new* disease which had come into being at about the turn of the twentieth century. To solve the mystery, a number of other unsatisfactory explanations had been invoked. It had even been suggested that polioviruses prevalent in North America and Europe in the twentieth century had taken on a new and special type of increased virulence, perhaps with a greater tendency to involve the central nervous system; or, possibly totally new strains of the agent had made their appearance and had spread throughout the civilized world. At first the unfair accusation was made that these strains had arisen and emanated from Scandinavian countries where epidemics had suddenly made their sinister appearance in the 1870s and 1880s. It was not until serologic surveys were carried out in different types of populations that a satisfactory explanation of the shift from *endemic* to *epidemic* poliomyelitis became apparent. This shift continues today in the developing countries of the world where profound changes in the environment are occurring, much as they did at the turn of the century in the Scandinavian countries, the United States, and elsewhere.

Another feature associated with the changing age patterns of susceptibility was equally important in bringing paralytic poliomyelitis more out into the open, so to speak. This has to do with the effect of age on the manifestations of the infection. The older a susceptible individual is when infection is acquired, the more likely is the illness to be serious. When poliovirus infection is restricted to the youngest age group (0–4 years) more than 95 percent of such infections are inapparent. On the other hand, when school children and adolescents represent the most susceptible groups, the percentage of inapparent infection falls off progressively with age and far more individuals experience a paralytic attack. Thus as older

13. E. F. Hutchins: "Historical summary," in *Poliomyelitis.* International Committee for the Study of Infantile Paralysis, Baltimore, Williams & Wilkins, 1932, p. 18.

and older susceptibles begin to get infected, it follows inevitably that more and more clinical evidence of the infection comes to the surface. The disease becomes easier to diagnose, more cases are reported, and the incidence of paralytic poliomyelitis increases. This serves to reemphasize the point that endemic poliomyelitis remains under cover as long as primitive sanitation prevails amid crowded areas, and the great bulk of poliovirus infection thus remains undetected.

The way in which the problem of the shift from endemic to epidemic poliomyelitis was elucidated through comparative serologic studies is illustrated by the results of three surveys conducted between 1950 and 1952 (see fig. 49).[14] When immunity patterns in the three populations were examined it was clear that the differences observed were not based on geography alone; primitive hygiene and crowded socioeconomic conditions shared in producing the high incidence of infection and immunity in the young children in Egypt. In northern Alaska, notwithstanding the primitiveness of the sanitation, the remoteness of the geographical location, and the small size of the population groups (which could not support endemic circulation of the virus) accounted for the infrequency of the infection and the lack of immunity in children and teen-agers. During periods of freedom from virus dissemination in this sparsely settled area, children were born and grew up as susceptibles until the inevitable reintroduction of the virus occurred, and exposure to polioviruses finally caught up with them. Profiting from the ever-expanding number of nonimmune hosts, the virus spread readily and an epidemic resulted. Not so in Cairo, Egypt, where infection remained endemic, as it had for centuries. An endless supply of new susceptibles born into the population and living in crowded cities and villages where sanitation was primitive kept the agent in continuous circulation. Young children were exposed, infected, and acquired their immunity early in life, and under these circumstances the clinical disease remained sporadic and concentrated in the youngest age groups. In Miami, Florida, which is on the same latitude as Cairo and yet has markedly different ways of life, circulation of virus was more variable, and periodic epidemics in preschool and school-aged children occurred every 7 to 10 years in the prevaccination era.

The importance of environmental as opposed to geographic features was confirmed by Melnick and Ledinko, who compared immunity patterns in the population of a single city, Winston-Salem, North Carolina, by examining the antibody status of upper and lower socioeconomic groups.[15] They found that children from the lower socioeconomic segment

14. Partially from unpublished data from the YPSU.
15. J. L. Melnick and N. Ledinko: Social serology; antibody levels in a normal young population during an epidemic of poliomyelitis. *Amer. J. Hyg., 54*: 354, 1951.

acquired infection and antibodies at an earlier age than did those in the upper stratum; but by age fifteen, close to 100 percent of both groups were immune.

A rough measure of the hygienic factors operative in the shift from en-

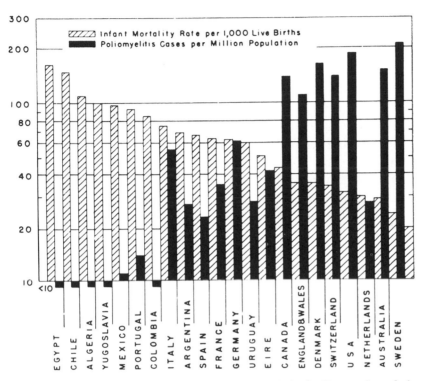

FIG. 50. A comparison of infant mortality rates and the incidence of paralytic poliomyelitis in different countries. Both rates in individual countries have been calculated simultaneously as five-year medians (from A. M.-M. Payne, n. 17).

demic to epidemic poliomyelitis is *infant mortality*.[16] The rate must have been appallingly high in the early nineteenth century, as it still is in some places today, where 75 percent of children die before reaching the age of 5. An inverse relationship between infant mortality and the incidence of poliomyelitis has been established for many countries of the world. This relationship reflects a number of features other than improved sanitation, as for instance the increased reporting of cases when the public health facilities of a given country improve. But as a generalization, when infant mortality rates fall below about 75 per 1,000, experience has shown that not only are first epidemics likely to occur within a few years, but also a

16. Infant mortality rate represents the number of deaths in the first year of life per 1,000 live births per year.

general increase in the number of cases can be expected (see fig. 50) as well as an increase in the ages of the patients.[17]

The World Health Organization was quick to adopt serum surveys as part of its program. In the field of poliomyelitis and a number of other, particularly viral, diseases such an approach proved to be a far more accurate indicator of how widespread a given infection might be in a population than was revealed by reports of clinically diagnosed cases, especially in developing countries where such reports are likely to be inadequate.

From these small beginnings in 1945, when the mouse neutralization test was first employed as a means of determining the poliovirus antibody status of the children of Baltimore, the techniques and the science of *serological epidemiology* have been developed to an impressive degree in a remarkably short period. The approach has contributed greatly not only to an understanding of neurotropic virus infections such as poliomyelitis but to many other infectious diseases as well.

17. A. M.-M. Payne: "Poliomyelitis as a world problem," in *Poliomyelitis; Papers and Discussions presented at the Third Internat. Poliomyelitis Conference.* Philadelphia, Lippincott, 1955, pp. 391–400.

CHAPTER 35

Enders and His Colleagues
The Growth of Poliovirus in Tissue Culture

Ever since viruses were first known, vigorous—almost frantic—attempts had been made to culture them in the manner that had been so successful with bacteria. The difficulty, which virtually amounted to a complete roadblock, was that viruses are dependent upon living and multiplying cells for their growth. No inanimate cell-free media such as supported the growth of various bacteria, regardless of how it was enriched, could suffice. Historically, this was one of the major characteristics that placed viruses in an entirely separate category from bacteria. Other distinctive features were that viruses were filterable and invisible (prior to the development of the electron microscope); also, infections they caused could only be identified by special types of lesions that differentiated some of them from those of bacterial origin. This was sufficient to render them mysterious agents of infection.

Today viruses are hardly considered as microorganisms in the strict sense of the word at all, but are regarded as well-defined molecular assemblages whose multiplication processes are known in considerable detail, thanks to the dramatic discovery in 1953 of the double-helical structure of desoxyribonucleic acid (DNA).[1] The complex physicochemical differences which place viruses in a special category as infectious agents may not sound so basic to some, but to the biologist, biochemist, and cell geneticist they are fundamental.

It was not until biologists had actually begun to cultivate living cells in vitro early in the twentieth century that an opportunity came of culturing viruses in the laboratory. Cell cultures were first achieved by Ross G. Harrison of the Biology Department at Yale University, who in 1907 used nervous tissue to perform this tremendous feat.[2] Shortly thereafter the

1. Such a characterization has been made because, in their physicochemical makeup, viruses contain either only RNA (ribonucleic acid) or DNA (desoxyribonucleic); whereas all microorganisms contain both types of nucleic acids. Microorganisms multiply by binary fission (division) whereas viruses do not; they are completely dependent for their replication on the ribosomes of the host cell, that is, the protein-synthesizing machinery of the cell which is subverted to the synthesis of viral nucleic acid and protein. In contrast all microorganisms contain their own ribosomes.

2. R. G. Harrison: Observations on the living developing nerve fiber. *Proc. Soc. exp. Biol. Med. (N.Y.), 4*: 140, 1906–7; Ibid., Embryonic transplantation and development of the nervous system. *Anat. Record, 2*: 385, 1908.

principle and the method were taken up by Alexis Carrel of the Rockefeller Institute. Carrel, a commanding figure in the world of science at the time, was so successful in the cultivation of embryonic chicken heart cells that he created the startling concept, that provided the cultured tissues received the proper nourishment, they could be made to survive indefinitely. As they continually multiplied, whole sheets of cells could be produced, enough to cover a few square miles, if one were so inclined.

This astounding new idea, namely that one could capture living cells, put them into a test tube, and make them live and multiply forever, was enough to signalize the use of tissue culture as a method suitable for the examination and analysis of vitalistic forces. Carrel's chicken heart cultures became famous overnight—a symbol of immortality. Together with his new discoveries in the field of the suturing of blood vessels, it won for him a Nobel Prize in 1912. As a postscript, Carrel's original tissue culture of embryonic chicken heart cells was kept going at the Rockefeller Institute for many years, possibly to see if it really could go on forever. When the cultures were finally discontinued, "on October 2, 1946 the New York Herald Tribune reported in stricken tones the death of Carrel's culture as if some great man had passed away."[3]

With the outbreak of World War I Carrel returned to his native France and there began work on eminently practical and timely wartime problems. He and Dakin, an Englishman, developed the Carrel-Dakin method of irrigating infected war wounds with weakly antiseptic solutions. In this manner they succeeded in reducing the putrefying and gangrenous effects produced by the wound infections which were so prevalent and so fatal in World War I. Carrel had reached the high point in his career.

Immediately after the United States had declared war on Germany, in April 1917, a French delegation which included Carrel and General (Papa) Joffre came to this country, ostensibly, among other reasons, to add fuel to our newly found enthusiasms. When the delegation reached Baltimore, Carrel was asked to address the students of the Johns Hopkins Medical School. I can well remember him on this occasion when he mounted the podium clad in a bright blue suit, and the inevitable yellow shoes with pointed toes, and began speaking in perfect English. Here was a Nobel laureate in medicine who had gone on to further scientific and technical achievements leading to a wartime triumph which was said to have saved the lives of countless wounded soldiers. The student audience gave him a delirious ovation.

After Carrel's postwar return to the Rockefeller Institute, he carried on, as a collaborator of Dr. Rivers, some unsuccessful attempts to grow

---

3. G. W. Corner: *The History of Rockefeller Institute for Medical Research.* New York, The Rockefeller Institute Press, 1964, p. 533.

viruses in tissue culture. However, he accomplished more spectacular things during this period.[4] During the late 1930s his reputation became more that of a philosopher and mystic than a productive scientist. Eventually he "returned to France to end his days there amid the confusion of World War II and Vichy, France and its aftermath."[5]

Once the technique of culturing cells in artificial media had been established it might seem that it would have been easy to grow viruses in vitro. But it did not turn out that way at all. In Rivers' *Filterable Viruses,* a textbook published in 1928,[6] he expressed grave doubts that viruses had ever been actually cultivated, although there were many established claims to the contrary. In the book, there is a special section written by Carrel, who goes into great detail in describing techniques then in use.[7] While he admits that Levaditi was successful as early as 1913 in maintaining the virus of poliomyelitis in nervous tissue placed in drops of human plasma, Carrel was doubtful whether the virus had actually multiplied, i.e. *la fabrication,* as he put it. Carrel was also skeptical about the very existence of viruses as biological entities, preferring to regard them not as infectious but rather as toxic agents of a chemical nature. Nevertheless he admitted that the 1923–25 work of Parker and Nye in Boston, who succeeded in carrying vaccinia virus (cowpox) through 11 generations of tissue culture, was of "great interest."

The first solid advance came in 1928, when the husband and wife team of the Maitlands at the University of Manchester in England succeeded in growing vaccinia virus in a medium containing minced hen's kidney tissue and serum. Their method speedily underwent various changes. Many other techniques and modifications were soon proposed, so that by 1936 no less than a dozen or more animal viruses had been cultured in vitro. By this time Rivers had come around to the belief that viruses could actually be grown in cultures of embryonic tissue; and with his clever assistant Dr. Li he went so far in 1930 as to recommend a technique for their cultivation which, although it was to undergo modifications, proved to be the basis of procedures used during the next few years.[8]

One modification later thought to be vital was the addition of serum ultrafiltrate by several investigators, including Dochez, at the College of Physicians and Surgeons in New York. By using serum ultrafiltrate in

---

4. It was during this period that Carrel collaborated with Charles Lindbergh, the hero of transatlantic flights, on an apparatus designed to keep certain organs of the body alive. This apparatus simulated the action of the heart in inducing circulation of the blood.

5. See n. 3, pp. 340–41.

6. *Filterable Viruses,* ed. by T. M. Rivers. Baltimore, Williams & Wilkins, 1928.

7. Ibid., pp. 97–109.

8. C. P. Li and T. M. Rivers: Cultivation of vaccine virus. *J. exp. Med.,* 52: 465–70, 1930. For an appreciation of the somewhat complicated tissue-culture techniques known as the Rivers' method, the reader is referred to this article.

the media, Simms and Sanders[9] claimed that they had grown not only the neurotropic viruses of St. Louis, western, and eastern encephalomyelitis but also the Columbia Sk strain of which was subsequently identified as the EMC virus. These experiments were interrupted by World War II.

So quickly did further modifications of various tissue-culture methods take place during the decade of 1934–44 that no attempt will be made to trace this evolution. Mostly embryonic tissue was employed, but adult animal cells came into use more and more. A signal advance during this period was the addition of a bacteriostatic agent, such as one of the sulfonamides. This was of immense value in keeping bacterial contamination down to a minimum.

Meanwhile in a parallel development the practice of growing viruses in the developing chick embryo, i.e. using the whole hen's egg (in vivo), was introduced by Goodpasture and quickly taken up by Burnet in Australia.[10] The method was at once put to extensive use. Prior to 1936 the number of viruses that could be cultured in this truly biological medium was to prove quite large, although poliovirus was not among them. Inoculation on the chorioallantoic membrane of the fertile egg was the route most generally employed. An added advantage was that the method could be used for quantitative determinations; with vaccinia virus, for instance, after 2–3 days of incubation, discrete lesions (plaques) could be readily observed on the chorioallantoic membrane and even counted. Success in the use of hens' eggs for the growth of a special strain of poliovirus did not come until after the cultivation of polioviruses in tissue culture had become common practice, and so this aspect of the story will not be considered further at this time.

It is important historically to know, however, when poliovirus was *first* grown artificially. The original attempts were Levaditi's in 1913. Next it might even be considered that Flexner's interpretations of his globoid bodies could have meant that poliovirus had been propagated in contaminated cultures by this means. At least these experiments were to prove an uneasy and, eventually, unsatisfactory effort in this direction. In the next two decades repeated attempts were made to grow polioviruses.[11] By far the most sophisticated one, which succeeded, was made in 1936 by Sabin and Olitsky at the Rockefeller Institute. These investigators started with the premise that prior to their attempt there had been no "unequivo-

9. H. S. Simms and M. Sanders: Use of serum ultrafiltrate in tissue cultures for studying deposition of fat and for propagation of viruses. *Arch. Pathol., 33*: 619–35, 1942.

10. F. M. Burnet: *The use of the developing egg in virus research.* Med. Research Council (Brit.), Special Rep. Series, No. 220, pp. 3–58, 1936. For a later and full description see W. I. B. Beveridge and F. M. Burnet: *The Cultivation of Viruses and Rickettsia in the Chick Embryo.* Spec. Res. Ser. Med. Res. Council, No. 256, 1946, London.

11. C. E. Van Rooyen and A. J. Rhodes: "The virus of poliomyelitis," in *Virus Diseases of Man.* London, Oxford Univ. Press, 1940, p. 798.

cal evidence that the virus of poliomyelitis has as yet been successfully cultivated outside of the body."[12]

Their approach was to obtain tissues from two human embryos, 3–4 months old, which had been made available through surgical operations and to carefully separate the tissue or organs—brain and spinal cord, kidney, liver, spleen, etc. Once divided, each type of tissue was placed in a flask containing the appropriate culture media. Success was achieved with the MV strain of poliovirus, which by the way represented the standard and most eminently respectable strain of that period. This strain, which had been subjected for more than 20 years to intracerebral passages from monkey to monkey, was shown by Sabin and Olitsky's experiments to have the capacity of multiplying in human embryonic nervous tissue, but not in any of the visceral tissues. The choice of the MV strain was unfortunate. The results served to strengthen the idea that polioviruses were more neurotropic than they actually were. Also, as MV was probably the most highly neurotropic strain of poliovirus in existence, its use jeopardized the chances of growth in nonnervous tissue. In other words the selection of another strain might have made the whole task of cultivation easier. Obviously Sabin and Olitsky's findings were of academic interest, but hardly of practical usefulness because not only was human embryonic nervous tissue difficult to come by, but the monkey was quite essential in proving whether the virus had grown or not.

The next milestone in the story of the cultivation of polioviruses scored such a triumph (and is so well known) that it hardly bears repeating. However, the *manner* in which the new discoveries of Enders, Weller, and Robbins came about may not be so familiar.

The first intimation that I had of their success came on a weekend visit, in November 1948, to John Enders' summer home in Waterford, Connecticut. During the course of this visit, casual but confidential mention was made by Enders that he and his colleagues had succeeded in growing Lansing poliovirus in human embryonic nonnervous tissue. The results were to be published in a few weeks.[13]

For the moment, I was stupidly unaware of the implications that this finding held. At least it did not appear to me as an electrifying piece of news. Instead, I visualized it as just another, but obviously more exciting, repetition of the results which Sabin and Olitsky and Simms and Sanders had reported twelve and seven years earlier. After all, I assumed that monkeys would be necessary to prove that poliovirus was actually present in the cultures. However remarkable the technical triumph was, it hardly

12. A. B. Sabin and P. K. Olitsky: Cultivation of poliovirus *in vitro* in human embryonic nervous tissue. *Proc. Soc. exp. Biol. Med.* (N.Y.), *34*: 357–59, 1936.

13. J. F. Enders, T. H. Weller, and F. C. Robbins: Cultivation of the Lansing strain of poliomyelitis virus in cultures of various human embryonic tissue. *Science, 109*: 85, 1949.

seemed to me to be a trick which could be put to any special or practical diagnostic use. How utterly mistaken was my preliminary judgment of this discovery to prove!

In the subsequent unfolding of this remarkable story during the period of 1948–50, the team of Enders, Weller, and Robbins and their associates produced a series of observations which came thick and fast. Strains of polioviruses representing each of the three serotypes were cultivated in a variety of extraneural human tissues, both embryonic and otherwise. Most significant of all—and this was a feature which crowned the whole tissue-culture story—was the highly practical discovery that multiplication of polioviruses was accompanied by a characteristic kind of change within the infected cells. It represented a specific injury that could be readily recognized under the high power of the light microscope, and thus only simple observation of the cultures was required to detect whether viable and growing poliovirus was there or not! This was the characteristic which made all the difference. It opened the door to quantitative determinations as to how much poliovirus existed in a given culture; to a way in which neutralization tests could be performed in vitro, and to countless other advances. In brief, it led to an enormous increase in the facility with which polioviruses and other viruses could be handled for a variety of purposes.

And, wonderful to say, came the realization that at long last monkeys, which had been so essential in the poliomyelitis laboratory, could be replaced by tissue cultures, for certain purposes at least. This marked an end, at least partially, of the monkey era.

For a running account of this story I have followed a firsthand report that was prepared for me by Dr. Thomas H. Weller and in fact by both of the other members of the Enders team.[14] As a description of events which revolutionized the direction of poliovirus research, it deserves a more detailed account, but in the cause of brevity, its high points only will be reviewed.

It would seem that long before 1948 the idea of maintaining a tissue-culture laboratory for viruses for diagnostic purposes had been entertained by all three of the participants of this team, two of them (Weller and Robbins) when they were still members of the class of 1940 at the Harvard Medical School. Another member of that class, Lawrence C. Kingsland, had also become interested in one of the newer improvements in tissue-culture techniques that had been recently introduced by Dr. George Gey at the Johns Hopkins Medical School. This was the practice of gently rolling over and over again the flasks or tubes containing viable

14. I am greatly indebted to Dr. Weller of the Harvard School of Public Health, and to his two fellow members of this research team, Drs. Enders and Robbins, for this account of events leading up to and through the period of their discovery that poliovirus could be cultivated and identified in vitro.

cells and fluid media. In the meantime (1939–40) in Dr. Enders' laboratory, he with his two colleagues Feller and Weller had started work with cultures of embryonic chick tissue in an effort to grow vaccinia virus. Later Kingsland and Weller, while they were interns on the services of pathology and bacteriology at the Children's Hospital in Boston (in 1940–41) set up a small tissue-culture laboratory. Their objective was to grow a variety of viruses and to handle them in a manner similar to bacteria, which meant that these viruses might be isolated from patients and put to use in numerous diagnostic tests. A children's hospital which furnished many patients suffering from a variety of infections was an optimum source of common viruses. But the program was to suffer a rude interruption due to World War II, which caused a lapse of some six years. Remarkably, however, this lapse was not enough to divert the members of the original team from their primary objective.

Shortly after the war had drawn to a close, Dr. Enders, on the death of Dr. Zinsser, resigned his position in the bacteriological department of the Harvard Medical School to become director of the Research Division of Infectious Diseases at the Children's Hospital of Boston. With this new-found release from the exigencies of teaching and administration which a senior university post required, he immediately set up facilities suitable for a tissue-culture laboratory. He was soon joined by his former student and colleague, Major Weller, MC, and subsequently, within a year (January 1948), by Major Robbins, MC. By this time the task of growing viruses in tissue culture had become somewhat easier due to the use of the new antibiotics (penicillin and streptomycin) for controlling bacterial contamination. It was a considerable advance over the sulfonamide technique that had been previously used for reducing bacterial contamination to a minimum.

Early in March 1948 Weller had inoculated mumps virus into cultures containing fragments of chick amniotic membrane and, using the method of rolling the tubes and changing the nutrient fluid at intervals of 3–4 days, had succeeded in producing evidence that this virus could indeed be cultivated in vitro. The success encountered in this model led Weller to use human embryonic skin-muscle tissue in his next trial. On March 30, 1948, 12 tissue culture flasks were set up: 4 were inoculated with oral washings from a case of chicken pox, 4 with the Lansing strain of poliovirus, and 4 were kept as controls. Varicella virus proved recalcitrant, but it was with the historic cultures inoculated with the Lansing strain that proof was obtained that poliovirus could be grown in nonnervous, human embryonic tissue. Mice were used as the test animal to indicate whether the agent had actually multiplied. The evidence was so convincing that an early report, which appeared in *Science* in January 1949 (see n. 13), could be made. Others soon followed.

In May 1948 Robbins set up his first poliovirus tissue-culture experiments and shortly thereafter obtained evidence that Lansing virus would also grow in human embryonic intestinal tissue. Events from that time forward came crowding in. One was the demonstration that the Brunhilde strain of poliovirus (a Type I) could be grown in similar cultures. The other was that the infected cells underwent pathologic changes—exhibited "cytopathogenic effect," or CPE, a term coined by Enders. By the summer of 1951, 13 strains of poliovirus had been isolated and typed in cultures of living cells. As an improved technique for the practical study of polioviruses, tissue culture had been quickly established and was well on its way to becoming a standard method.

In view of all of the important observations which came out of the tissue-culture experiments in the three subsequent years one might have thought that Enders would predict rhapsodically about all of the vistas to which he and his team had opened the door. Yet, in 1954 at the International Poliomyelitis Conference held in Rome, he chose to be unexpansive and said with all modesty:

> The application of the tissue culture method as modified in these various ways has facilitated the accumulation of data within various areas of poliomyelitis research, many of which had been defined previously but explored incompletely. In addition, opportunities for new lines of investigation have been revealed such as the analysis of biochemical factors involved in the multiplication of the virus, the study of its mode of attachment to the cell or of changes in pathogenicity that may occur during cultivation *in vitro,* as well as other variations in biological properties.[15]

Considering all the advances which stemmed directly or indirectly from Enders, Weller, and Robbins' discovery, and considering the resulting expansion of the field which enabled a great variety of viruses to be cultivated in a similar manner, indeed the above was a conservative prediction for polioviruses, or for that matter for virology in general. Enders was possibly aware even at this time that he was describing crucial events which had changed the course of poliomyelitis research from that time forward. Channels had been opened up which led directly down the road that made both the inactivated and attenuated poliovirus vaccines possible.

15. This almost amounted to a brief progress report; for Enders had described this development three years before at a previous international poliomyelitis conference in 1951. This second, 1954 report contains an important bibliography of key articles covering the period of 1949–1954. See J. F. Enders: "Developments in tissue culture," in *Poliomyelitis; Papers and Discussions presented at the Third Internat. Poliomyelitis Conf.,* Philadelphia, Lippincott, 1955, pp. 221–23.

John Franklin Enders (see fig. 51) was born in Hartford, Connecticut in 1897 into a family with banking interests, a career that his father and brother both followed. He entered Yale College in 1914, to have his course interrupted by World War I during which he served from 1917 to 1919

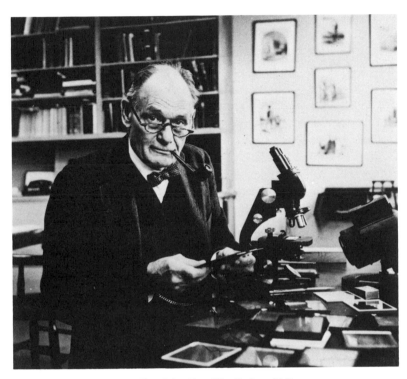

FIG. 51. John Franklin Enders, M.D.

as an officer in the U.S. Naval Reserve Flying Corps. The war over, he was able to return to Yale and graduate with an A.B. degree in 1920. Originally his ambition was to pursue studies in English literature at the Harvard Graduate School. He started on this course, but after a year switched to medicine. And so it was that Enders began to study the medical sciences. Early in his Harvard medical school course he had fallen under the spell of the dynamic personality of Prof. Hans Zinsser, a man with great charm and many talents, who besides being one of the leading microbiologists of the day was an articulate medical statesman, philosopher, author, and musician. So persuasive was Zinsser's influence, and so attractive was he as a man and as a symbol of the science which he professed, that the first year medical student decided to give up the study of medicine, choosing instead to try for a Ph.D. degree in microbiology, a decision that some members of his family viewed with considerable dismay. During his postgraduate years when he was studying and working for his degree, which he obtained in 1930, he was able to join Zinsser's department, at first as an assistant. Later, he ascended the academic ladder to reach the rank of associate professor. Also, it was during this stage in his career that Enders and others in the department collaborated with Dr. Zinsser in the writing of *Principles of Immunity.*

In the decade that followed, Enders devoted much time to the study of viruses—their behavior, their growth in hens' eggs, and other methods for their cultivation. So when World War II came he was well equipped to serve as a member of the Commission on Measles and Mumps of the Army Epidemiological Board. The tasks of this commission during wartime were dedicated to practical ends—devising diagnostic tests and methods of immunization—and here it was that Enders worked with a group of pediatricians, including Joseph Stokes, Jr., of Philadelphia, and others. Possibly at this time the plan of setting up a pediatric virus laboratory gained strength, and the idea evolved that various problems relating to quite a number of common human viruses such as measles, mumps, and poliovirus could be solved more readily by investigating their behavior in children rather than in adults. So once again Enders made a break with tradition in turning away from a course which presumably would have led him to the top of the academic hierarchy and accepted instead a post at the Children's Hospital of Boston as director of the Laboratory of Infectious Disease.

It is possible that his path was smoothed by the fact that he was not dependent entirely upon his salary from the university; but here again a far greater influence was that of the instinct of the true scientist with vision, who will always go for those subjects in his chosen field of interest that have the best chance of succeeding. So in 1947, Enders stepped off the academic ladder. Most ambitious scientists would have considered this step as a comedown or at least as a step in the wrong direction, but not so with Enders. He was aware of his own talents and was anxious to get on with his *own* work.

The work that he and his two young colleagues accomplished was to gain for them a well-merited Nobel Prize (see fig. 52). In 1953, a year before Enders became a Nobel laureate, Yale University recognized its distinguished son with an honorary Sc.D. degree.

A graduate of Yale College in the Class of 1919, microbiologist and investigator who has discovered new possibilities for the prevention of virus diseases, you have revolutionized the study of infantile paralysis. The lives saved from this dread disease will be the measure of your researches. In recognition of your inestimable service to humanity, your Alma Mater confers upon you the degree of Doctor of Science.

Later, not content to rest on his laurels, Enders set himself once more to explore the problems of another virus disease, measles. Here he embarked anew not only at the laboratory bench but also took part in the agonizing clinical decisions necessary to put into practical use a live measles

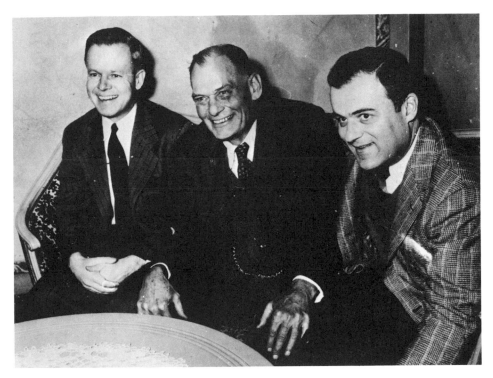

FIG. 52.   Trio of Nobel laureates. Left to right: Thomas H. Weller, John F. Enders, and Frederick C. Robbins.

vaccine. Would the attenuated strain produce measles encephalitis, for instance? The virus had been tamed through serial passage in tissue culture, the same method which had proved so successful in producing a live poliovirus vaccine. The successful measles vaccine, which is used in many countries throughout the world today, will stand as another of Enders' achievements in preventive medicine, worthy of a second Nobel Prize, or so it might seem. John Enders may have forsaken the field of medicine early in his career for a career in the basic medical sciences, but he was eventually to come back to it through the side door of preventive medicine.

Not the least of John Enders' qualities has been his ability to attract young men of high caliber to work with him. From his laboratory a host of disciples have gone out to occupy responsible posts in various universities. In 1966 at a celebration in his honor, a reunion of colleagues, foreign professors, and former research fellows who had worked under Dr. Enders was organized in Boston. The men who were invited were designated as the "Enders Alumni." Some ninety received invitations to attend, eighty of whom came from far and wide for the occasion.

As regards other members of the team, Dr. Thomas H. Weller was born at Ann Arbor, Michigan in 1915, the son of the professor of pathology at the University of Michigan Medical School. After attending the University of Michigan, Tom went on to the Harvard Medical School. Soon afterward his postgraduate activities at the Children's Hospital of Boston were interrupted by World War II. During the war years of 1942–46 he saw service in the medical corps, ending up with the rank of major. Either by good luck or for other reasons he obtained a military assignment that must have suited him eminently, as he was appointed to head the military Laboratory of Parasitology, Bacteriology and Virus Diseases of the Antilles Department, located at San Juan, Puerto Rico. This apparently served to get Weller's interest aroused permanently in the direction of tropical medicine.

During his entire wartime service, however, Major Weller never could rid himself of the urge to have another go at viruses and tissue culture in the clinical laboratory; so when released from military service he sought a return to Dr. Enders' laboratory and participation in the activities of which we have just heard. In 1947 his academic title was that of a research fellow in tropical medicine and pediatrics at the Harvard Medical School. Within a few short years he became the Richard Pearson Strong Professor of Tropical Health at the Harvard School of Public Health. It was partially due to Dr. Weller that the well-established concept of tropical medicine was transformed into the new and timely concept of tropical public health of which he has been an ardent champion ever since.

But Weller with all of his far-flung interests in the tropics and elsewhere had by no means deserted explorations in the field of viruses. His work did not end with poliovirus for he has the distinction of having been among the first to establish the pathogenic potential of cytomegaloviruses in man, and to devise new methods of studying these agents.

The third member of the team, Dr. Frederick C. Robbins, was born in Auburn, Alabama in 1916, the son of Dr. William J. Robbins, a distinguished man with a wide diversity of talents; besides being a botanist of considerable note and onetime head of the New York Botanical Gardens, the elder Robbins was a member (and treasurer for a time) of the National Academy of Sciences.

Frederick Robbins obtained his college degree at the University of Missouri in 1936 and graduated in medicine from the Harvard Medical School in 1940. Shortly thereafter he entered the Medical Corps of the U.S. Army and spent some time serving as chief of the Laboratory of Virus and Rickettsial Diseases at the Sixteenth Medical General Hospital in Italy. This was a time in 1943–44 when hepatitis epidemics were rampant in British and American troops in Sicily and Italy, and Robbins no doubt had ambitions to try his hand at the growth of hepatitis viruses.

Four years later Major Robbins was also to be reunited with his colleagues in Boston to form the team of Enders, Weller, and Robbins at the Children's Hospital. Of their activities we have already heard.

After several years in research activities Robbins, following in the steps of many students of poliomyelitis, chose the field of pediatrics as a career. It was a fortunate decision. After working for several years more on the staff of Children's Hospital in Boston with an appointment on the Harvard faculty in pediatrics, he became the director of the Department of Pediatrics and Contagious Diseases of the Metropolitan General Hospital of Cleveland, a position that John Toomey had formerly held. This post carried with it the appointment of professor of pediatrics at Western Reserve Medical School; eventually he became chairman of the department. In 1967 Robbins' talents not only as a clinician and investigator, but as an administrator as well, had come sufficiently to the fore that he was appointed dean of Case-Western Reserve Medical School.

So in concluding this brief review of the lives of these three men who made history in poliovirus research, one can recognize that John Enders, besides being a genius in his own field, was a keen judge of young men. He chose two of extraordinarily high caliber.

CHAPTER 36

The Bloodstream as a Pathway in the Human Body

For a generation, starting with Flexner's early experiments in monkeys, scientists had been wedded to the idea that strict neurotropism was an outstanding property of poliovirus. This interpretation was understandable in light of practices then current at the Rockefeller Institute and elsewhere, of using so-called standard strains to induce the experimental disease. A familiar strain was MV, which, like several others, had been passed from one monkey to another, year after year, always by the intracerebral route. In the process, the virus had become highly neurotropic and had lost some of the properties which it possessed when first isolated. As recounted earlier this exclusive use of laboratory-manipulated strains was the basis for an untold number of misconceptions which quickly translated themselves into hypotheses and even laws about the pathogenesis of poliovirus infection in man. Observations on the behavior of the MV strain in monkeys gave rise to considerable literature supporting the view that in the human disease once the virus gained a foothold in the body, it immediately made its way via nervous pathways, i.e. by peripheral nerves, to the central nervous system. Needless to say this included the olfactory nerves along which the virus was supposed to go straight into the brain. This concept held sway for a generation and even provided the rationale for a preventive approach—the spraying of various chemicals into the nose, which was supposed to block the virus and thus prevent its becoming established (see chap. 23).

In 1942, Howe and Bodian set for themselves the task of reexamining the problem of how poliovirus reaches the central nervous system.[1] In their treatise on the subject, which was rightly regarded as a contemporary classic description of the pathology and pathogenesis of poliomyelitis, they started out by strongly emphasizing the neurotropic character of the virus, but in the end they qualified this view, as follows:

> Despite the fact that there has been demonstrated an almost unbelievable dependence of poliomyelitis virus upon the nervous system,

---

1. H. A. Howe and D. Bodian: *Neural Mechanisms in Poliomyelitis.* New York, Commonwealth Fund, 1942.

it must be recognized that this situation has so far been shown to apply only to the rhesus monkey.[2]

This statement represented the authors' growing awareness of differences in the way the monkey, the chimpanzee, and man respond to poliovirus infection. They acknowledged that the more they studied the pathways which the virus traveled from the nasopharynx and the intestinal tract to the central nervous system, the more mysterious these became.

A militant proponent of the strict neurotropism of poliovirus was Dr. Harold K. Faber, professor of pediatrics at Stanford University Medical School in San Francisco.[3] He conducted a long series of elaborate experiments in monkeys between 1931 and 1947, in an attempt to prove that after entering the nasopharynx the virus moved along nerve fibers to peripheral ganglia and thence to the central nervous system. In 1937 at a meeting of the American Pediatric Society he was to challenge Dr. Trask, who gave some convincing evidence that he and his colleague Dr. German had demonstrated experimentally that poliovirus did indeed travel via blood and lymph channels in the monkey to the central nervous system.[4] But Faber maintained that Trask's technical maneuvers cast little doubt on the "absolute neurotropism" of the virus.[5]

In 1960, long after the controversial question of the pathogenesis of the human infection had been temporarily settled,[6] Burnet wrote:

> It is quite impossible to review the literature without accepting the existence of such movement [along nerves] and almost equally impossible to believe in its physical reality.[7]

In line with broader issues involved, one of the crucial dicta accepted in the 1930s was that once the virus had entered the human host it rapidly was absorbed into the cells of the nervous system and was accordingly no

---

2. Ibid., p. 207.

3. H. K. Faber: Acute poliomyelitis as a primary disease of the central nervous system; a reconsideration of the pathology, symptomatology and treatment, based on the hypothesis of axonal propagation of the infective agent. *Medicine, 12*: 83, 1933; see also H. K. Faber: *The Pathogenesis of Poliomyelitis*. Springfield, Ill., Thomas, 1955.

4. W. J. German and J. D. Trask: Cutaneous infectivity in experimental poliomyelitis; increased susceptibility after neurosurgical procedures. *J. exp. Med., 68*: 125–45, 1938.

5. H. K. Faber and R. McIntosh: *History of the American Pediatric Society, 1887–1965*. McGraw-Hill, 1966, p. 188.

6. A measure of how protracted the discussion on this point has been is the publication as late as 1968 by Johnson and Mims describing the manner in which they believe that viruses traverse or gain access to the central nervous system. See R. T. Johnson and C. A. Mims: Pathogenesis of viral infections of the nervous system. *New Engl. J. Med., 278*: 23–30 and 84–92, 1968.

7. F. M. Burnet: *Principles of Animal Virology*, 2nd ed. New York, Academic Press, 1960, p. 242.

longer accessible to the action of the body's natural defenses, including circulating antibody. Strict neurotropism seemed also to fit the facts because the virus had never been demonstrated in the bloodstream of patients with the disease, although admittedly, prior to 1946, it had not been looked for on a large scale. In addition there was the concept of the blood-brain barrier; a vast amount of experimental data indicated that many neurotropic viruses, poliovirus included, when inoculated intravenously did not penetrate or at least did not harm the central nervous system unless huge amounts were given.

Despite the firm hold that the concept of strict neurotropism exerted for thirty years, if one goes back to some of the earliest work, to the papers of Medin and Wickman, and certainly to the 1912 monograph of Peabody, Draper, and Dochez (see chap. 12), it is apparent that these clinical investigators were aware of a preliminary systemic or prodromal phase that preceded central nervous system involvement. This might have suggested to them a period of generalized infection including viremia, but such was not mentioned. On the other hand it might have been that early febrile symptoms were considered as part of an initial involvement of the central nervous system. Anyway, Peabody and his colleagues were not willing to abandon the view of Flexner and his associates that the virus entered through the nose and proceeded directly to the central nervous system via the olfactory pathway.

One of the authors, Draper, went a little further afield and expressed the idea that the prodromal illness had all of the earmarks of a generalized infection that *preceded* penetration of the nervous system. In the first edition of his book, published in 1917, this interpretation is illustrated in his diagram (see fig. 26) in which the prodromal, supposedly systemic, febrile illness represents the first "hump" in the dromedary course. What was the virus doing in the body at this stage? Was it in the lymphatic system? Could it possibly be circulating in the blood and thus widely distributed throughout the body? Draper almost grasped the significance of this important clinical observation, but not quite; the main theme eluded him, and in his second edition he had long ago repudiated the idea, claiming instead that the most important portal of entry of the virus was the nose (see fig. 35).

What makes these speculations of Draper all the more extraordinary were his conclusions in terms of treatment. During the period 1917–35, when convalescent serum therapy was very much in vogue, his eminently practical advice was that in order to be effective, the serum should be given in the early, preparalytic stage, *before* the virus had become established in the central nervous system or even in the network of nerves leading to the brain or spinal cord. Here he was suggesting that the "naked" virus, not as yet safely entrenched in the cells of the nervous system, might be more vulnerable to attack by specific antibody than was the case later, particularly after paralysis had developed. Although this therapeutic advice was followed, the principles upon which it originally had been based seem to have dropped from sight. Draper had gone over completely to Flexner's views on the nasal portal of entry. The clock had been set back about twenty-five years in poliovirus research.

Nevertheless in the late 1930s bits of evidence began to accumulate which indicated that strains of poliovirus recently isolated from patients were not so highly neurotropic after all, and could even induce paralytic poliomyelitis in monkeys by injection into the skin.[8] This was in contrast to the action of established strains, which had lost this property as a result of continuous intracerebral passage in monkeys. These observations encouraged Trask and other workers from the Yale Unit in their belief that by concentrating on "standard" monkey-adapted strains in experimental work, investigators had been led further and further away from the human disease, a circumstance which virtually destroyed the hope of discovering the manner in which the infection might spread within the human body. Some years were to pass before there were answers to such questions as where the nonneural sites of viral multiplication might be, and whether or not a viremic phase occurred before central nervous system invasion. Yet the discovery in 1938 of the "skin-taking" property of freshly isolated strains reawakened thinking along these lines.

During this period investigators were somewhat in a quandary as to how they might approach immunization against poliomyelitis. This was due in large measure to two features: first, there was no true evidence that the virus appeared early in the blood either in the experimental or the human infection; and second, it was clear that a high level of immunity, a level that was difficult to attain, was necessary to protect monkeys against intracerebral challenge. During the period 1945–50, however, Isabel Morgan of the Johns Hopkins poliomyelitis group conducted a series of excellent experiments in which she was able to achieve such high-level immunization in rhesus monkeys by 10 *intramuscular* injections of virus over a period of 4 months. Large amounts of antigen were used, in the form of a 20 percent suspension of infected monkey spinal cord, to produce large amounts of antibody. The nicety and exactitude of Morgan's experiments became apparent when she was able to define, as no one else had, the level of circulating antibody necessary to protect animals against intracerebral challenge.[9] And yet, partially because of the artificial nature of the challenge, some regarded Dr. Morgan's experiments in the light

8. J. D. Trask and J. R. Paul: The skin infectivity of poliomyelitis virus. *Science, 87:* 44–45, 1938.

9. I. M. Morgan: Level of serum antibody associated with intracerebral immunity in monkeys vaccinated with Lansing poliomyelitis virus. *J. Immunol., 62:* 301–10, 1949.

of academic interest, and remote from practical application in terms of immunization of man.

Also observations in the late 1930s and early 1940s had provided new insights which had shaken the old concept of the pathogenesis of human poliomyelitis in terms of strict neurotropism of the virus. These included the discovery of the skin-taking properties of newly isolated strains of virus and the rediscovery of the role of the alimentary tract—and the prolonged presence of the virus in the wall and contents of the intestinal tract (see chap. 27). More than ever, it seemed that there must be a systemic phase to the acute infection; quite probably the lymphatic system was involved, and possibly there was a period of viremia.

When at last an adequate search was made to detect virus in the blood at various stages of the human disease, a group of clinical investigators from the Yale Poliomyelitis Study Unit came up with somewhat discouraging results.[10] Of 111 blood specimens collected from patients during various stages of the acute disease in 1943 and 1944, only one yielded the virus! The positive blood sample was obtained early, within 6 hours of onset of a somewhat nonspecific febrile illness in a girl of 9 years, who never developed either central nervous system signs or abnormalities of the spinal fluid, but from whose stool, collected 2 days after the blood, poliovirus was also isolated. This finding, unfortunately but naturally enough, was regarded at the time as exceptional; no one suspected its true significance. Viremia had been found in less than one percent of the cases tested —enough to brand it as a fluke. Yet it should have alerted this group to search further for virus in the blood, concentrating on the incubation period or at least on the beginning of the symptoms of Draper's first phase (the minor illness).

In the year following this report, Koprowski and his colleagues at the Lederle Laboratories also reported the recovery of virus from the blood of a patient with presumed nonparalytic poliomyelitis.[11] However, the conditions of the isolation—blind passage in mice—were sufficiently unusual as to make some scientists critical.

Needless to say members of the Yale Poliomyelitis Study Unit and others, although discouraged by their meager positive results, still believed that a generalized infection, possibly accompanied by viremia, preceded involvement of the central nervous system. Nearly all of the members of the unit were clinical investigators who had seen too much of the acute disease in man to be willing to accept the experimental infection,

10. R. Ward, D. M. Horstmann, and J. L. Melnick: The isolation of poliovirus from human extra-neural sources; search for virus in the blood of patients. *J. clin. Invest., 25*: 284–86, 1946.

11. H. Koprowski, T. W. Norton, and W. McDermott: Isolation of poliovirus from human serum by direct inoculation into a laboratory mouse. *Publ. Hlth Rep. (Wash.), 62*: 1497–76, 1947.

particularly in the rhesus monkey, as an exact replica of the human disease.[12] By the late 1940s it was clear, however, that the behavior of the infection in cynomolgus monkeys and chimpanzees resembled human poliomyelitis more closely, since in these two species the disease could be induced by a natural route—by feeding the virus. The use of these animals in investigations of the pathogenesis of poliomyelitis therefore offered a more suitable model of the human infection than did the rhesus monkey.

Others had been thinking along similar lines even prior to 1946. In his Bela Schick lecture, delivered in New York in 1944, Sabin reported that in experiments performed before World War II, he had detected viremia in pooled blood from three cynomolgus monkeys.[13] But the exact time or phase in the infection when the virus had been found in the bloodstream was not recorded, so these results were of little help in telling when viremia had occurred in relation to the onset of central nervous system lesions.

A fresh attack of the problem was undertaken in the Yale laboratory early in 1951. By then it was clear from Hammon and Roberts' serologic investigations that by the time a patient enters the hospital with signs of central nervous system involvement, he already has a significant level of circulating antibody against the infecting strain of poliovirus.[14] Obviously in earlier efforts (see n. 8) the search for viremia had been made too late in the course of the infection, after the appearance of antibodies that would have neutralized any virus present.

Based on this line of thinking, cynomolgus monkeys infected by the oral route were examined daily for viremia, during the incubation period well before the onset of paralysis. The results were positive; and at the Second International Conference on Poliomyelitis in Copenhagen (held early in September 1951) it was clearly stated by Horstmann[15] (see fig. 53) that poliovirus did indeed enter the bloodstream during the incubation period of the experimental infection. On this occasion she said that in view of the "isolation of virus from the blood of a cynomolgus monkey

12. D. M. Horstmann and J. R. Paul: The incubation period in human poliomyelitis and its implications. *J. Amer. med. Ass., 135*: 11–14, 1947.

13. A. B. Sabin: Studies on the natural history of poliomyelitis. *J. Mt. Sinai Hosp., 11*: 185–206, 1944.

14. W. McD. Hammon and E. C. Roberts: Serum neutralizing antibodies to the infecting strain of virus in poliomyelitis patients. *Proc. Soc. exp. Biol. Med. (N.Y.), 69*: 256–58, 1948.

15. Dorothy M. Horstmann, born in Spokane, Washington of German parentage, had received her medical degree at the University of California in 1939. After three years of internship and residency, one of which was spent at the Vanderbilt University Hospital, she accepted a fellowship at Yale in the newly established section of Preventive Medicine, a branch of the Department of Internal Medicine. Her talents soon came to the fore and within a few years she became a trusted member of the Yale Poliomyelitis Study Unit. In due time she transferred to pediatrics and at present holds a full professorship with a joint appointment in the fields of epidemiology and pediatrics at the Yale University School of Medicine.

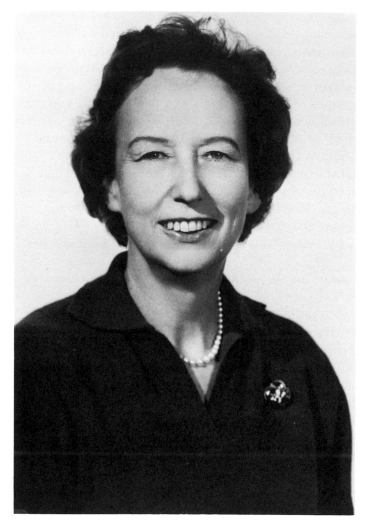

Fig. 53. Dorothy Millicent Horstmann, M.D.

5 days after virus feeding and 6 days before the appearance of symptoms, the possibility of viremia in human poliomyelitis, it seems, must be reconsidered."[16] These results were quickly confirmed by Horstmann herself in experiments in orally infected chimpanzees.[17] Similar findings were reported almost simultaneously by Bodian in 1952.[18] The next step, to show

16. D. M. Horstmann: "Discussion of Symposium 4," in *Poliomyelitis; Papers and Discussions presented at the Second Internatl. Poliomyelitis Conference* (held in Copenhagen, Sept. 1951). Phila., Lippincott, 1952, p. 336.

17. D. M. Horstmann: Poliomyelitis in the blood of orally infected monkeys and chimpanzees. *Proc. Soc. exp. Biol. Med. (N.Y.)*, *79*: 417, 1952.

18. D. Bodian: Pathogenesis of poliomyelitis in normal and passively immunized primates after virus feeding. *Fed. Proc., 11*: 462, 1952.

that the same pattern of viremia occurred in man, was accomplished promptly. In the summer of 1952, by testing blood collected from familial contacts of paralytic cases, who might still be in the incubation period or the minor illness phase of the disease, it was possible to isolate virus from the blood during the incubation period with some regularity in the human infection.[19] Furthermore, this demonstration of viremia was amply and convincingly confirmed after the use of attenuated strains of poliovirus as an oral vaccine had become a common practice, and it was possible to investigate the problem experimentally in man.[20]

Why was the discovery of viremia in the incubation period of the paralytic form—or indeed any form—of poliovirus infection so important? Because, theoretically, it meant that small amounts of virus which invaded the blood could probably be overcome by relatively small amounts of circulating antibody, and by this means could be blocked from gaining access to the central nervous system. With this reappraisal of the pathogenesis of human poliomyelitis and recognition of the role of viremia at the onset of infection, at one fell swoop the problem of immunizing man had been rendered easier than was expected.

That viremia plays an important part in the course of human infection is undisputed today. But it is still debatable whether more is involved than simple progression of the virus from its original sites of multiplication straight into the bloodstream and thence directly to the central nervous system.[21] Current views, however, are indeed a far cry from the earlier idea that the virus slipped directly up the nose and into the brain.

Coincident with this new evidence that poliovirus is present in the blood prior to invasion of the central nervous system, there was a revival of interest in the use of serum as a preventive, rather than as a therapeu-

19. D. M. Horstmann, R. W. McCollum, and A. D. Mascola: Viremia in human poliomyelitis. *J. exp. Med., 99*: 355–69, 1954; D. Bodian and R. Paffenbarger: Poliomyelitis infection in households. Frequency of viremia and specific antibody response. *Amer. J. Hyg., 60*: 83, 1954.

20. The use of live attenuated poliovirus vaccines has made the task of tracing the course of the virus much easier. In recent years the detection of Type II virus in the blood stream has been noted within a very few days of the administration of this type of oral poliovirus vaccine. It lasts sometimes 2–5 days. See D. M. Horstmann, E. M. Opton, R. Klemperer, B. Llado, and A. J. Vignec: Viremia in infants vaccinated with oral poliovirus vaccine (Sabin). *Amer. J. Hyg., 79*: 47–63, 1963.

21. This question has received extensive discussion in an authoritative article by Dr. Bodian and D. M. Horstmann: "Poliomyelitis," in *Viral and Rickettsial Diseases of Man,* 4th ed., ed. by F. Horsfall and I. Tamm. Philadelphia, Lippincott, 1965, pp. 430–72.

Still more recently, Miller and Horstmann used sensitive methods in cynomolgus monkeys to reaffirm that viremia, like bacteremia, results indirectly, via lymph channels. They and others have also presented evidence of a primary, transient viremia that results in distribution of the virus "to viscera and other sites where further multiplication occurs, followed by discharge of larger amounts of virus into the circulation during the visceral-viremic phase of infection," which precedes invasion of the CNS. D. G. Miller and D. M. Horstmann: The use of proflavine-tagged virus to study the pathogenesis of poliomyelitis in monkeys. *Virology, 30*: 319–27, 1966.

tic, measure. By this time, it was not convalescent serum that was used, but the gamma globulin fraction, which represented an approximately 30-fold concentration of serum antibody. This product had been demonstrated to be useful in preventing such diseases as measles and viral hepatitis. To be effective, however, it was necessary that it be administered during the incubation period, at least a week before symptoms appeared.

Davide in Sweden had originally proposed the use of convalescent (or parent's) blood for the prevention of paralytic poliomyelitis and had given it to 157 persons in the north of Sweden during an epidemic there in 1928. In the same year Flexner and Stewart had similarly suggested the prophylactic use of convalescent serum, based on the view that if given at the time of exposure, it might protect the child from a paralytic attack, or at least might render the infection less serious.

Acting on this principle Brebner, from W. H. Park's laboratory in New York City, had launched a small trial in the town of Bradford, Pennsylvania in 1932; Stokes and his associates put on a similar but larger experiment in Philadelphia during the same epidemic. In these two attempts not nearly enough of the juvenile population was inoculated to obtain statistically adequate results, and of course, homeopathic doses of the serum were given. Findings were reported as "encouraging though not conclusive."[22] Following these efforts, interest in this preventive method lapsed for some ten or twelve years. It was not revived again until the mid-1940s when a far more potent weapon had become available in the form of gamma globulin.

Gamma globulin was introduced as a result of the wartime experiments on the fractionation of blood under the direction of E. J. Cohn, professor of biochemistry at Harvard.[23] The concentration of serum globulins meant that a great increase in the amount of antibody could be administered in a small volume. Furthermore, the practice in fractionating blood was to pool hundreds of samples of human sera, and by this means a vast but unknown quantity of various antibodies was also concentrated.

It was inevitable that there should be a revival of interest in the use of gamma globulin as a preventive measure in poliomyelitis. One of the first to consider this possibility was Kramer, Aycock's former colleague,

22. J. Stokes, Jr., I. J. Wolman, H. C. Carpenter, and J. Margolis: Prophylactic use of parents' whole blood in anterior poliomyelitis; Philadelphia epidemic of 1932. *Amer. J. Dis. Child.*, *50*: 581, 1935.

23. This project, carried out under the auspices of the Committee on Medical Research of the U.S. Office of Research and Development (USORD), produced many remarkable results. The Harvard team succeeded in separating out, among other fractions, serum albumin and serum globulins. The former could be used as a blood substitute in the treatment of shock; the latter, which contained the majority of antibodies, could be used to great advantage in the prevention of certain virus diseases. See E. J. Cohn: "The history of plasma fractionation," in *Advances in Military Medicine* by E. C. Andrus et al., vol. 1 (chap. 28). Boston, Little, Brown, 1948, pp. 364–443.

who was then working in the laboratories of the Michigan State Department of Health. Kramer had proposed a small trial in 1944, using gamma globulin instead of parent's blood. He actually applied for support to the National Foundation, but it was felt that with the war on, it was not the time to be conducting such trials. Dr. Joseph Stokes, Jr. of Philadelphia also had his interest revived in passive immunization as a promising preventive measure and had even conducted a few preliminary trials. Years afterward he had occasion to write of this missed opportunity:

> Had the urgency of the theme of control affected authorities in the National Foundation for Infantile Paralysis as forcefully as it did Dr. Sidney Kramer and myself in the early 1940s again nature might well have been brought into balance at a considerably earlier date than actually obtained.[24]

In the meantime Dr. William McD. Hammon (see fig. 54), who was on the verge of emigrating from California to be professor of epidemiology at the School of Public Health of the University of Pittsburgh, began to show an interest in gamma globulin as a method of preventing paralytic poliomyelitis. Hammon was perfectly aware of what had gone before, and there were few keener contemporary students of the immunology and virology of neurotropic virus infections—including poliomyelitis. But Hammon did not arrive at his decision to try gamma globulin on purely theoretical considerations.

From his own account, as related to me on numerous occasions, his interest was aroused in the late 1940s, not in the laboratory but on one of his many visits to an area that was in the throes of a poliomyelitis epidemic.[25] As usual, as a visiting specialist, he was asked to speak at a meeting attended by the local medical profession. These doctors were in a difficult position because there was ever so little that they could do in the way of preventing or curing paralytic poliomyelitis. Yet even if the out-of-town specialist was a man who did not know the answers to all of the perplexing questions that were raised, at least this was an opportunity to get *some* advice. In the course of the meeting one doctor asked: "Why isn't gamma globulin used to treat the disease in its preparalytic stage? Why isn't it used in the prevention of poliomyelitis?" Dr. Hammon's answer was that this method had not been shown to be effective, and its use was therefore not recommended at present, or words to that effect.

That night Bill Hammon's conscience would not let him sleep. He was

24. J. Stokes, Jr.: Immunization in infants and children with particular reference to viral hepatitis. *Johns Hopk. med. J.*, *121*: 305–28, 1966.

25. I am greatly indebted to Dr. W. McD. Hammon of the School of Public Health, University of Pittsburgh, for reviewing the text of this chapter; and in particular, the section dealing with gamma globulin trials in the prophylaxis of poliomyelitis.

distinctly worried—so worried, in fact, that he soon applied to the National Foundation for Infantile Paralysis to support a field trial to test the effectiveness of gamma globulin as a control measure in an epidemic. In the end, Dr. Stokes collaborated on this project, and in his words the

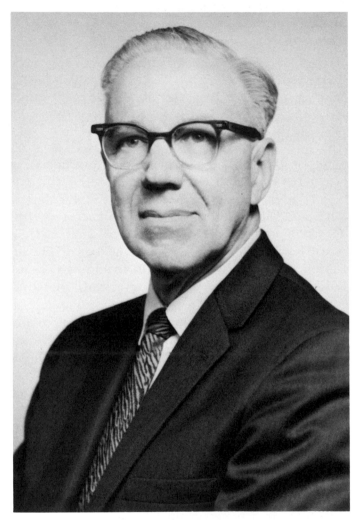

FIG. 54.   William McDowell Hammon, M.D.

two investigators agreed that an application should be submitted to the National Foundation by Hammon after he had moved to his new home in Pittsburgh. At first the foundation's advisory committees were unenthusiastic. The logistics of carrying out such a trial presented obstacles; and if it were successful, there never would be sufficient amounts of gamma globulin to go around. The ticklish business of control groups would also have to be provided for, if the results of the experiment were to be at all meaningful. The matter of trauma inflicted by injections was also brought up. This was indeed a theoretical menace. As far back as 1935 there had been speculations about a possible relationship between the local irritation caused by the Kolmer vaccine and the vaccine-induced paralysis that followed it. Later the situation came into sharp review when a disturbing observation was made in England during the summer of 1949. In that epidemic year, cases of paralytic poliomyelitis were reported to have occurred with increased frequency in children who had received routine inoculations for the prevention of diphtheria, whooping cough, and tetanus within the previous 28 days. The incidence of poliomyelitis in such children was greater than in those who had not received such inoculations; furthermore, the site of paralysis correlated with the site of antigen injection. Similar findings had been promptly reported from Australia. So with this background the conclusion was reached that inoculation with gamma globulin might have an effect similar to the irritant reaction of some immunizing antigens and might therefore bring an added hazard to the asymptomatic child who had already been infected with poliovirus. Would such injections have the effect of precipitating paralysis in a child who might otherwise have escaped? It was argued that until it was known how irritating gamma globulin was, how much trauma was involved, this was *not* the thing to do.

These problems were hotly argued back and forth, but in the end this expensive project was approved by the National Foundation for Infantile Paralysis. The initial trial was staged in Provo, Utah, during an epidemic in September 1951.[26] Two other field trials were conducted subsequently— one in Houston, Texas, and the other in Sioux City, Iowa. When the combined results were submitted to statistical evaluation it was evident that gamma globulin in the dose used had greatly reduced the incidence of the disease when administered within a suitable period preceding exposure.[27] It also turned out that gamma globulin injections were not irritating and could be safely given without fear of a provocative action. But the method was expensive and cumbersome, particularly since it had to be applied on an emergency basis. An immense amount of effort by a quickly assembled staff was necessary, and the large amounts of gamma globulin required might exceed the supply. In fact, attempts by the Public Health Service's Communicable Disease Center during a series of out-

26. W. McD. Hammon, L. I. Coriell, and J. Stokes, Jr.: Evaluation of Red Cross gamma globulin as a prophylactic agent for poliomyelitis. I. Plan of controlled field tests and results of 1951 pilot study in Utah. *J. Amer. med. Ass., 150*: 139, 1952.

27. National Advisory Committee for the Evaluation of Gamma Globulin in the Prophylaxis of Poliomyelitis; an evaluation on the efficiency of gamma globulin in the prophylaxis of paralytic poliomyelitis as used in the United States, 1953. *Publ. Hlth Monogr*, No. 20, 1954.

breaks in 1953 demonstrated that unless one was able to predict epidemics, an effective use of gamma globulin prophylaxis on a mass scale could not be made. So difficult were the problems that the proposed programs frequently led to wasteful errors. Furthermore by this time a new method was in the wind—active immunization by means of vaccination. This carried the prospect that the vaccinated child could produce his own antibodies. The method of passive protection with injected antibodies contained in gamma globulin was therefore used only occasionally during the next few years and then abandoned altogether. The trials had, however, served a useful purpose. Years afterward, in 1965, Dr. Stokes, in his Gudakunst lecture at the University of Michigan, quoted Dr. Thomas Francis as saying that experiences with the mass use of gamma globulin had placed the situation in its true perspective (see n. 24). Francis is reported to have said that these studies by Hammon and his associates:

> "showed in a well designed and well conducted field study that antibody, in the form of gamma globulin, was capable of providing protection against paralytic poliomyelitis of man during two to five weeks after administration. This demonstration that antibody alone, given presumably before infection, could prevent paralytic poliomyelitis was a clear invitation to active immunization."

The most important point here was that the amount of passive antibody required *need not be large;* indeed the presence of only a trace was still protective.

Thus, the discovery of viremia elucidated at least two significant features of the disease that paved the way to vaccination. One was a clearer understanding of the pathogenesis of the infection—how it behaves in man; another was the implication arising from the demonstration of virus in the blood early in the incubation period and during the minor illness phase—namely, if serum antibody were present, it could serve to block the viremia and therefore protect against subsequent invasion of the central nervous system.

CHAPTER 37

Polio's Cousins from Coxsackie

A noteworthy thing about developments in the late 1940s described in this chapter is that they produced not one new virus that in some ways resembled poliovirus, but a whole new family of such viruses.

In this story Dr. Gilbert Dalldorf was the central figure from the start, and he has maintained a dominant role ever since.[1] Prior to his remarkable discovery, Dalldorf had been working on polioviruses and related problems for about ten years. Only recently had he acceded to the directorship of the Division of Laboratories and Research in the New York State Department of Health at Albany. He had assumed this highly important position only with his own provision that he "wouldn't stop fiddling with viruses," and he firmly believed:

> that the most important function of the director was to be, by precept, in deadly earnest about research. No use talking about it. One should *do* it. It would color all the attitude of the staff. I still believe it. The director must express his conviction that administration is a minor issue, the work is what counts.[2]

Gilbert Dalldorf (see fig. 55) was born in Iowa in 1900. He received his college education at the University of Iowa and was graduated in medicine from New York University and Bellevue Hospital Medical College in 1924. After medical school his early training both in this country and abroad had been in pathology. He had worked in Freiburg, Germany under the contemporary dean of pathologists, Ludwig Aschoff.[3] So Dalldorf was well qualified to join Prof. James Ewing's pathology department at Cornell University Medical College in New York in the late 1920s. In 1930 he became the pathologist at the Grasslands Hospital in Westchester

The title of this chapter has been borrowed from a similar title of an editorial that appeared in the *Lancet, 1*: 123, 1950.

1. I am particularly indebted to Dr. Gilbert Dalldorf for his personal correspondence and conversations dealing with this chapter.

Also, I have drawn heavily on a *Chronicle of the Division of Laboratories & Research; New York State Department of Health. The First Fifty Years, 1914–1964,* by Anna M. Sexton. Lunenburg, Vt., The Stinehour Press, 1967.

2. Letter from G. Dalldorf to J. R. Paul, April 19, 1968.

3. Subsequently the University of Freiburg was to recognize Dalldorf's work by awarding him an honorary degree.

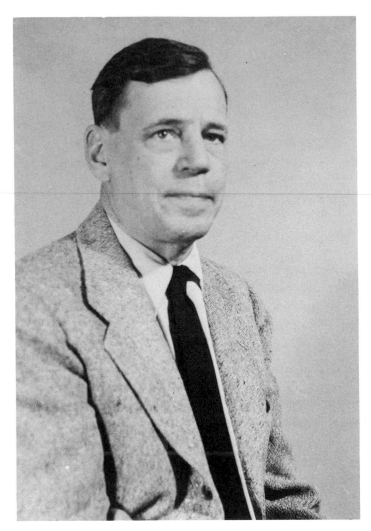

Fig. 55.   Gilbert Dalldorf, M.D.

County, New York but at the same time managed to retain his faculty position at Cornell, a position that enabled him to continue with teaching and
research.

It was during the Grasslands period that his research activities on poliovirus were begun, and it was here, during a 1942 poliomyelitis outbreak in
White Plains, New York, that he saw what he called "the footprints of
other viruses." It was also here that he received encouragement to explore
the whole broad subject of neurotropic viruses, from Dr. L. T. Webster
of the Rockefeller Institute, of whom we have heard previously. In addition, while at Grasslands Dalldorf discovered the sparing effect (later
called the interference phenomenon) that some other neurotropic viruses
had upon polioviruses.

Dalldorf gave the impression of a man keenly interested in multiple activities, with a degree of outward composure that seemed to belie his restless mind. Throughout his professional career he made a practice of shifting his field of activities every now and again: at first he concentrated on pathology; after that he became director, successively, of a laboratory devoted to general microbiology, to a state laboratory of public health, and then to one which had the special function of dealing with viruses as they relate to tumor growth. Yet during periods of heavy administrative responsibilities he never allowed his investigative work to be suppressed. His extracurricular explorations also took a number of forms. He was an expert yachtsman, and when his children had grown up and gone their own ways, the Dalldorfs spent many months living on their boat. In the 1960s he piloted his own plane in East Africa when he and his wife set out to explore Kenya from the air, examining the types of terrain, vegetation, and waterways, where the children suffering from Burkitt's tumor were coming from—patients whom he had occasion to examine at the hospital in Nairobi. This indeed was the jet-age variety of "shoe-leather" epidemiology.

It was in 1945 that Dalldorf went to Albany as the director of the New York State laboratory. This large institution had been built up through the efforts and talents of Dr. Augustus M. Wadsworth and was recognized as a model among similar state laboratories in the United States and abroad. In defining what services might be expected of such facilities and how to go about providing them, Wadsworth had compiled a book, *Standard Methods,* which appeared in 1927.[4] It was a landmark that described most of the up-to-the-minute procedures used in public health laboratories. With its appearance, the Albany laboratory had emerged into a position of undisputed leadership. Needless to say, *Standard Methods* went through several editions, the third (in 1947) under the editorship of Gilbert Dalldorf; this was another arduous duty he had undertaken at the start of his directorship.

With all these new responsibilities, administrative and literary, it was remarkable that the director should have found time to continue a search for polioviruses or polio-like viruses. Nevertheless, during the late summer of 1947, Dalldorf and his associate, Grace M. Sickles, investigated a number of small epidemics in upstate New York from which they hoped to find evidence of mouse-adaptable polioviruses or any other viruses which they could turn up from cases of poliomyelitis. It might well have been a wild goose chase. Indeed such efforts made little sense according to the views expressed in 1940, by Kessel and Stimpert. These authors maintained that the adaptation of poliovirus strains to mice was "so rare that such animals cannot be used for routine experimental work in isolation"

---

4. A. M. Wadsworth: *Standard Methods of the Division of Laboratories and Research of the New York State Department of Health.* Baltimore, Williams & Wilkins, 1927.

(see chap. 26). But despite the approach being unorthodox, it made sense, if only from the economic point of view, as mice were infinitely cheaper to work with than monkeys.

During the early part of the summer of 1947, Dalldorf had attended the Fourth International Congress for Microbiology in Copenhagen, where he had the opportunity of hearing Dr. Ørskov's paper with Miss Andersen, which dealt with an ingenious method of infecting very young mice with Theiler's (TO) virus.[5] In these investigations the nipples of the dams had been painted with TO virus, and in this way the infant mice that they nursed were successfully infected. Dalldorf maintains that it was this demonstration that put the idea into his head of using suckling mice.

And so it was that Dalldorf and Sickles began their experiments which turned out to contain the secret of a new technique—a new laboratory animal. It was a discovery that changed the course of research in the entire virus field as well as revolutionizing investigations in poliomyelitis and related human infections. Here was another proof of the oft repeated dictum: "Die Methode ist alles."

As early as 1929 Theiler had found that suckling mice could be infected with yellow fever virus by intraperitoneal and subcutaneous routes, whereas older mice were susceptible only on intracerebral inoculation. But nothing more had been made of this observation, and it had been largely forgotten. Almost twenty years later, by turning to the suckling mouse, the team of Dalldorf and Sickles made not only one major discovery; they made several. To begin with, from fecal suspensions obtained from two patients suspected of having paralytic poliomyelitis, they isolated what seemed to be a completely new virus, having certain unique features.[6] This agent, though it caused paralysis of the limbs of these tiny animals, could be differentiated from the Lansing strain of poliovirus and from Theiler's virus and several other neurotropic viruses, not only by its serological reactions but also by the pathological picture it produced. Indeed one of the most extraordinary things about the new agent was that the damage responsible for paralysis of the limbs turned out to consist of widespread lesions in the skeletal muscles rather than in the central nervous system. The abnormality was primarily a myositis instead of an encephalomyelitis. Another striking feature was that only suckling mice one to seven days old were susceptible, whereas animals more than one week of age were resistant to the infection.

Dalldorf and Sickles were unaware at first that they had opened a verita-

5. J. Ørskov and E. K. Andersen: Poliomyelitis in mice. *Acta path. microbiol. scand., 25*: 746–54, 1948.

Dr. Ørskov was at that time the director of Denmark's State Serum Institute.

6. G. Dalldorf and G. M. Sickles: An unidentified, filtrable agent isolated from the feces of children with paralysis. *Science, 108*: 61–62, 1948.

ble Pandora's box containing a huge family of new viruses. At one fell swoop they had introduced (and popularized) a new and inexpensive animal into the virologist's laboratory—the suckling mouse. Other workers, some of them in the Yale Unit, were not slow to exploit this novel approach; they took it up avidly, and even suggested a name for the new virus. This led Dalldorf in 1949 to state wisely that the time was not yet ripe for nomenclature and that certain issues should first be clarified. He said on this occasion:

> I have felt that the disease should not be named until something is known of the anatomic lesions in man and a good deal more is learned of the range of symptoms and the relationship, if any, to classical polio-myelitis. On the other hand, a provisional designation is needed and it is suggested that the agent be called "Coxsackie virus," since the first recognized human cases were residents of that New York village. Since a number of viruses may be involved, the term "Coxsackie group of viruses" seems especially suitable.[7]

This unique name, which was soon to attract worldwide attention, was of North American Indian origin and is pronounced Cock-sock-ee by residents of the Hudson River town which at that time boasted a population of about 2,500.

A dozen years later Dr. Max Finland of the Thorndike Laboratory of the Boston City Hospital and his associate Lerner were to state:

> The isolation by Dalldorf and Sickles of viruses which produced paralysis with destructive lesions of muscle in suckling mice and hamsters, from the stools of two children with signs of paralytic poliomyelitis was an achievement that may rank in importance with Landsteiner and Popper's production of human poliomyelitis in monkeys.[8]

As intimated earlier, things moved promptly after 1949, and within a year a number of other investigators had isolated related viruses from a number of different clinical syndromes, some of which bore a resemblance to mild forms of poliomyelitis and some of which did not. This course of events represented a reversal of the usual pattern in clinical investigation of infectious diseases. Usually, a disease is recognized first; then, if one is lucky, the discovery of its etiological agent or agents follows. But not so with the Coxsackie viruses: the discovery of an array of viruses came first, to be followed by the bewildering task of sorting out the types of illness from which they could be isolated.

Also, unlike the discovery of the virus of poliomyelitis, which could be

7. G. Dalldorf: The Coxsackie group of viruses. *Science, 110*: 594, 1949.

8. A. M. Lerner and M. Finland: Coxsackie Virus Infection. Editorial in *Arch. Intern. Med., 108*: 329–34, 1961.

identified promptly because it produced in the monkey an exact replica of the human paralytic disease, with Coxsackie viruses the experimental disease in the mouse proved to be puzzling and diffuse, sometimes producing a wide variety of seemingly unrelated lesions. This was confusing. But at least the pathological picture in suckling mice became the basis of criteria for an early division of the agents into Groups A and B. With Group A strains the major lesions were those of muscle inflammation and destruction with absence of abnormal findings elsewhere; Group B strains produced, besides myositis, lesions not only in the central nervous system but also in the brown fat (the hibernation gland) and, less frequently, in the liver, heart, and other viscera.

Yet, although Coxsackie viruses were antigenically and pathologically distinct from the poliovirus family, the more they were studied the more they came to resemble polioviruses in their other characteristics, such as physical properties—resistance to chemicals and small size; their biological behavior, particularly the manner in which they invaded and persisted in the human intestinal tract; and in their epidemiological aspects. Indeed, these viruses cropped up again and again in places where polioviruses abounded. The illnesses they caused turned out to be summer diseases, at least within the temperate zones. From individual patients they could be isolated not only from the same anatomical sites as poliovirus, but also from feces, sewage, and flies—again in keeping with the behavior of polioviruses.

By 1951 it had become apparent that the large and still growing family of Coxsackie viruses could be recovered from patients suffering from a wide variety of different diseases or clinical syndromes. Few of the illnesses were severe; some had heretofore been considered to be "specific" infections notwithstanding the fact that such clinical "entities" had been created by man as diagnostic concepts to satisfy an understandable desire to identify and pigeonhole diseases by characteristic symptoms and lesions. A major group in which there were central nervous system signs was typical of nonparalytic poliomyelitis or "aseptic meningitis," a term coined by Wallgren some twenty-five years earlier for what eventually was recognized as a syndrome with a variety of viral and other causes. There was one clinical syndrome of a unique kind which in Europe had gone under the name of Bornholm disease, and in the United States as "devil's grippe" or pleurodynia—a kind of epidemic myalgia. It was a shock to European physicians to learn from the work of Curnen and Melnick that their Bornholm disease, which had seemed so specific, was just another of the large number of illnesses caused by the American family of Coxsackie viruses.[9]

9. G. Finger: Epidemic myalgia or Bornholm Disease caused by Coxsackie Virus in Europe from 1931–1952. *Welt-Seuchen Atlas*, E. Rodenwaldt, ed. Hamburg, Falk. 1954, vol. 2, pp. 95–100.

Many another syndrome or minor illness soon came into the picture, some characterized by short fevers and some by skin rashes, particularly in younger children. Also identified was a type of febrile illness with lesions in the pharynx known as "herpangina," which Huebner and his colleagues at the National Institutes of Health found was due to Coxsackie A viruses.

Almost immediately it became apparent that the family of Coxsackie viruses and the clinical syndromes they caused were practically worldwide in distribution. Thus strains soon began to be isolated in Canada, Cuba, Scandinavia, and Israel. So quickly did the word spread around that during the decade following the original discovery by Dalldorf and Sickles more than two thousand articles dealing with the newly discovered agents appeared in the medical literature. Within a few short years the family of Coxsackie viruses had come to occupy a major place in the sun.

The expanding use of tissue-culture methods also led to the recovery of large numbers of hitherto unknown cytopathogenic agents from the human intestinal tract. In the process of sorting them out still another new group of viruses was discovered. These agents did not infect suckling mice, or other experimental animals, yet they grew well in cell cultures of human and simian tissues. The isolation of numerous different strains and serotypes came so rapidly that an improbable descriptive nomenclature arose which quickly caught on: "viruses in search of disease." Naturally, or unnaturally, this led to the name of *orphan viruses*,[10] however farfetched the linking of a man-created concept of a disease to a biological virus may sound. Eventually the term *Enteric Cytopathogenic Human Orphan (ECHO)* was concocted.[11] This unlikely etymological masterpiece was derived from the fact that these viruses which could be readily isolated from human feces and caused cytopathic effects in tissue culture were not polioviruses, nor Coxsackie viruses, and their potentialities to cause human disease were only partially known. The name ECHO virus, which has recently been downgraded to echovirus, farfetched though it may sound, was at least one that could be easily remembered, and accordingly it caught on. As of 1969, the family had grown to number 34! Many of its members have since graduated from the orphan estate to being associated with relatively respectable disease syndromes.

The similarities of polio, Coxsackie, and echoviruses in terms of their

A graphic description and a history of this syndrome going back to 1856 can be found in W. H. Pickles: *Epidemiology in Country Practice*. Baltimore, Williams & Wilkins, 1939. Chap. 8, "Epidemic Myalgia."

10. In May 1955, The National Foundation for Infantile Paralysis held a major "Conference on Orphan Viruses" in New York City, which led to this new classification.

11. Committee on the ECHO Viruses. Enteric cytopathogenic human orphan (ECHO) viruses. *Science, 122*: 1187, 1955.

predilection for the human intestinal tract, their shared physicochemical properties, and clinical and epidemiologic behavior eventually led taxonomists to unite them under a new banner—the *enteroviruses,* which constitute a broad category of agents. And so, to the amazement of certain diehards in the neurotropic virus field, the ultimate fate of polioviruses was that they were embraced by the new and huge family of enteroviruses. By 1969, the 24 Coxsackie A viruses and 6 Bs together with the 34-odd echoviruses made a total of 62, a somewhat unmanageable number. Considering that most of the agents can be distinguished from one another only by laboratory tests, no one would expect the average physician or pediatrician to keep them straight.

It presently became evident that a veritable host of viruses had preempted polioviruses from its former unique position of being the only viral inhabitant of the human intestinal tract. Soon surveys revealed that in temperate climates in the summer season as high as 20 percent of normal children might be harboring various enteroviruses. In tropical and subtropical areas the figure reached as high as 70 percent! The evidence indicated that the new agents, like polioviruses, caused acute infections —whether apparent or inapparent—and then generally disappeared when immunity had been established.

Questions as to the possible interaction between the various enteroviruses in human infections also arose. Simultaneous inapparent infection with several virus types had been demonstrated, and epidemics caused by a combination of polioviruses and Coxsackie viruses had been found to be not uncommon. There was some evidence that in a single patient concurrent infection with both agents seemed to give rise to unusually severe illness, which led to the inevitable question: Does one virus sometimes fortify the other instead of interfering with it?

As to interference, the question was raised as to whether Coxsackie and echoviruses play a role in the human intestinal tract, or elsewhere in the body, as interfering agents that could act as barriers to infection with either wild or attenuated polioviruses. The practicality of this point was realized when attenuated poliovirus vaccines came into increasing use, and interference, caused by other enterovirus infections, became a significant factor in preventing satisfactory immunization. Thus on occasion the oral (Sabin-type) vaccine simply would not take when given in the presence of an *established* infection caused by some other enterovirus. This led in temperate climates to the practice of administering the vaccine in winter or at least not in the summer, when enteroviruses might be rampant. But the task of successfully immunizing young children by means of attenuated poliovirus vaccine has not been easy in either semitropical or tropical areas, where enteroviruses are prevalent the year round.

On a more academic basis, the elimination of poliomyelitis and poliovirus infections by vaccination in developed countries during the early 1960s soon gave rise to many speculations in theoretical epidemiology. What was going to happen next? Would other enteroviruses take over partially or completely? Would these quickly burgeon into prominence in an alarming manner as polioviruses had apparently done in the first half of the twentieth century? Or would the flooding of a population with attenuated vaccine strains of poliovirus have a dampening effect on the other enteroviruses?

Dalldorf considered these questions in 1961 from the ecological aspect, pointing out that the massive introduction and dissemination of strains of attenuated poliovirus, as is currently the case with the Sabin-type oral vaccine (to be discussed later on), "may be presumed to be a huge experiment, unique in size and boldness and rich in opportunity for the study and understanding of the ecologic relationships of human viruses."[12]

While these speculations were still rife, Dr. Sven Gard of Stockholm wrote an article with the provocative title of: "Exit poliomyelitis—What next?"[13] In it he posed the question, With the demise of poliomyelitis will the world be so flooded with different kinds of enteroviruses that these agents will soon take the ominous place of polioviruses? He chose to answer this question in the negative. In the years which have elapsed since Gard's prediction, his thesis has certainly stood the test.

12. G. Dalldorf: A great experiment. *Yale J. Biol. Med., 34*: 234–38, 1961–2.
13. S. Gard: Exit poliomyelitis—What next? *Yale J. Biol. Med., 34*: 277–88, 1961–2.

CHAPTER 38

Decks Cleared for Action on a Vaccine

To describe the stage that research on immunization had reached by 1950, I will quote from an article, written by myself, with the high-sounding title of "Controlling Poliomyelitis." It appeared in the *Yale Review* and focused on most of the well-worn issues that had been reiterated time and again. The article ended on this familiar note:

> In the present state of our ignorance, it is questionable whether we know how to handle the situation at all. Apparently what is needed most in this disease is some means, not of partially eliminating the virus from a community, nor of quarantine, but of bolstering up the immunity of children. That is, we would combat poliomyelitis as we now combat smallpox, diphtheria, and whooping cough, by vaccination.
>
> Since no vaccine of this kind is now known, it is, of course, impossible to foretell exactly what the nature of such a preventive might be, . . .
>
> Without attempting to comment on the chances for or against the development of such a vaccine, I believe it is valid to say that this is the great quest to which the energy of many laboratories is being turned. The path is dangerous and difficult.[1]

One excuse for the pompous note on which this article ends is that if premature and glowing predictions had been made at this point, indicating that a vaccine was imminent, they might just have been taken seriously. This in turn would have kindled false hopes and evoked a rash of inquiries about the new vaccine, which was still hypothetical or at least had not left the drawing board. What some of the gentlemen of the press could not understand was that letting the public in on every new development would not help the cause and might even hinder it: a safe and effective vaccine could not be produced hastily, pressure from the public not withstanding. As it turned out, the story was one of the worst kept secrets of the early 1950s.

For by 1950 the hour was already late; several investigators had been hard at work and actually a vaccine was just around the corner. By this

1. J. R. Paul: Controlling Poliomyelitis. *Yale Review, 39*: 647–53, 1950.

time success in dealing with the Typing Program had given the National Foundation the confidence to go after bigger game. It had prompted that organization to assume, in addition to its function as a granting agency, the role of chief strategist, almost an active implementer, in a campaign to develop and promote methods of immunization. Indeed, progress toward a poliovirus vaccine had been barreling along for some time, although not nearly as swiftly as the National Foundation desired. This was natural, particularly in view of the NFIP's avowed aim to "conquer polio," even though a deadline for this had not been set.

Meantime the prevailing attitude among most investigators, who would eventually do the actual work, was that things were not to be unduly hurried. One prominent grantee of the foundation wrote to me at this time: "Are we now employees who are ordered about?" The Foundation, however, was following its own course: it was making the most of its own talents, and I may add, its leverage, in promoting the good cause.

In any event the time was ripe. Sufficient years had elapsed since the fiasco of 1935, and much progress had been made since then. Recent accomplishments with inactivated influenza vaccines among American troops during World War II and in the postwar years had blazed the trail as far as logistics, statistical criteria, and effectiveness in this kind of clinical research were concerned. Key developments which had brought the poliovirus vaccine closer were several. The discoveries by the team of Enders, Weller, and Robbins led the way; and the polioviruses had been separated into three antigenic types. In addition, a number of helpful diagnostic tests had been developed which had never before been available. These would go a long way toward increasing accuracy in measuring immunity to poliomyelitis, whether naturally acquired or artificially induced.

With all this going on the path might have looked easy—and yet, was it? Although the growing clamor for a vaccine had not yet reached a din, there were a few who regarded the caution with which progress was being made as procrastination. Knowledgeable workers who were especially identified in this field included at the time Drs. Howard A. Howe, Isabel Morgan, and David Bodian of Johns Hopkins University; Joseph L. Melnick and Dorothy M. Horstmann of Yale University; Gordon Brown of the University of Michigan; and Albert B. Sabin of the University of Cincinnati. The task was to determine what levels of antibody would have to be attained in chimpanzees and cynomolgus monkeys in order to insure their immunity and by what methods this immunity was to be challenged. The position taken in 1951 was expressed by Howe at the Second International Poliomyelitis Conference held at Copenhagen. He quoted Isabel Morgan's results on the immunization of primates with graded doses of virus with the objective of obtaining different levels of antibody which in turn could be an index of the degree of immunity. Howe reported that whereas low levels of antibody were unpredictable as a measure of protection against intracerebral challenge, with high levels, immunity was the rule. But he went on to say:

> However, experiments on chimpanzees have supplied valuable data from an animal which appears to react to the oral ingestion of poliomyelitis virus in a fashion similar, if not identical, to that of man.[2]

Here Howe was referring to work at Johns Hopkins and other laboratories indicating that chimpanzees were highly susceptible to exposure, and as in humans the commonest response to oral ingestion of poliovirus was an inapparent infection; sometimes with prolonged excretion of the virus from the intestinal tract and coincidentally with the development of protective antibody levels. At this time there had also been increasing evidence, from the results of poliovirus antibody surveys, of the high inapparent infection rate in most adult human populations. By means of such surveys in both juvenile and adult populations, the proportion of immune and nonimmune members in different populations could now be identified.

Oddly enough, at this same international conference there were no official papers delivered on preliminary vaccine studies, although among participants such efforts were discussed privately with more than consuming interest. Within a year, when once the floodgates were opened, the story was to become entirely different.

As far as killed (inactivated) poliovirus vaccine was concerned, some of the methods of fifteen years earlier were to be revived and gone over more thoroughly. These included exposure of the virus to formalin, as Brodie had done; and heating it to the critical temperature of inactivation, which had been tried years before by Landsteiner and Levaditi. Among newer methods was the use of ultraviolet light, which had been advocated by Milzer and Levenson. Also, high-speed electronic bombardment was tried unsuccessfully. The formalin method eventually proved to be the most satisfactory.

Of course, the techniques, not to speak of the principles, were far more sophisticated than they were in the days of Brodie and Kolmer. Now it was unnecessary—even contraindicated—to give the presumably inactivated virus in the form of a crude suspension of infected central nervous system tissue derived either from monkeys or mice. Not only could the vaccine be prepared in tissue culture, which resulted in a "purer" form of the virus, but the dose could be far more accurately measured.[3]

---

2. H. A. Howe: "Antibodies and immunity to poliomyelitis," in *Poliomyelitis; Papers and Discussions presented at the Second International Poliomyelitis Conference.* Philadelphia, Lippincott, 1952, p. 296.

3. This was thanks to the method devised by Dulbecco and Vogt for measuring the exact

In order to get on with the strategic and logistic aspects of the program of active immunization of man, in the spring of 1951 the NFIP had created a new group which went under the name of the Committee on Immunization.[4]

As far as I know the functions of this committee were never clearly outlined, but it was the impression of the majority of its members that it had been formed to deal broadly with the subject of immunization, and eventually would include a consideration of various poliovirus vaccines —their safety, efficacy, and their implementation.[5]

Regardless of the influence which the NFIP used in the guidance of its Immunization Committee in the first years, one feature seems certain: it was a propitious time for the formation of a cooperative group to tackle the problem, and the National Foundation was the logical organization to lead the way in this sort of development. If it had not, the U.S. Public Health Service would have promptly assumed this responsibility, or even WHO. The issues at stake were too important to have been left entirely in the hands of one or even two laboratories, as had been proved in the unfortunate vaccine trials of 1935.

It will not be my plan to review details covering the first discussions in which the NFIP's Immunization Committee indulged. At the start, in 1951, and for two and a half years thereafter, some members were not at all certain which methods of immunization should be tried, nor whether the killed or the live attenuated virus approach should be used. Needless to say there were sharp differences among this group of opinionated scientists. The discussions have been reported at some length in Benison's *Tom Rivers;*[6] they also have been described in Carter's book on Jonas Salk as "nervous brawling."[7]

I have chosen to review the principles with which the Immunization Committee was concerned in its first years, not the details of implementation. Many individuals would have considered it a mistake to dally for

number of virus particles in a given dose of virus that could be counted as individual foci (plaques) on agar plates containing infected tissue-culture cells. It was a method similar to that used when counting colonies of bacteria when spread upon an agar plate.

4. Members in this committee included: Drs. David Bodian, John F. Enders, Thomas Francis, Jr., William McD. Hammon, Howard A. Howe, John R. Paul, Andrew J. Rhodes (of Canada), Joseph E. Smadel, Albert B. Sabin, Jonas E. Salk, Thomas B. Turner, and Antonio Ciocco. Representing the National Foundation were Mr. Basil O'Connor, Drs. Thomas M. Rivers, Hart Van Riper, medical director, and Harry Weaver, director of research.

5. As regards the latter, the live poliovirus vaccine, this concept had become more than a pipedream in 1951. As a result of some trials which Koprowski and his collaborators had made at the Lederle Laboratories, a flood of speculation had been set off that an attenuated strain could be sufficiently tamed, so to speak, to make its use realistic.

6. S. Benison: *Tom Rivers; Reflections of a Life in Medicine and Science.* Boston, M.I.T. Press, 1967.

7. R. Carter: *Breakthrough; The Saga of Jonas Salk.* New York, Trident Press, 1967, p. 129.

more than a couple of years over this aspect, and yet in view of what eventually happened, i.e. the "Cutter incident," in late April 1955 (to be described in chap. 40) the degree of haste eventually exhibited by the foundation seems hardly to have been justified. At least it may be said that the NFIP program temporarily backfired.

Several questions were uppermost in the minds of the Immunization Committee members when it came to recommendations: Was the formalinized vaccine safe to use in preliminary experiments? Could it be made safer, even foolproof, when once it had gotten out of the hands of the experimenters and into the hands of manufacturers? Would it prove effective? If so, how effective? Would large-scale and statistically significant trials, which obviously would have to be made on enormous groups of children, be considered completely ethical?

Some of the NFIP committee members were experienced in testing vaccines in adult volunteers. During three and a half years of World War II, a number of them had served on various commissions of the Army Epidemiological Board (AEB). Consequently they were no novices when it came to trying new and improved methods of immunization, using both vaccines inactivated by formalin or attenuated vaccines, in influenza, mumps, viral encephalitis, and dengue, all of which can be serious threats to military personnel. But make no mistake, such trials were not put on lightly. None was authorized by the Army Epidemiological Board unless the members were convinced that the potential risks had been gone over painstakingly, and that as far as knowledge went there was a minimum of danger in the procedure. And as always, the investigators were aware that one must look critically at the other side of the coin, to the opposite policy of doing nothing, when hundreds, perhaps thousands, of illnesses (or even lives) of military personnel were threatened by potentially preventable diseases.

However, with the war over there came a sudden revulsion and with the adoption of the Articles of the Nuremberg Tribunal, criteria for the use of human subjects for medical trials came in for drastic revision. The world had been aroused by what was considered the misuse of the aims and principles of the medical profession especially by the Germans. Public opinion, the judges of this tribunal, and the pope—all made pronouncements in which the use of volunteers for experimental work was reviewed from legal, moral, and ethical standpoints. The traditional image of the *physician* was at stake. Was he to be transformed from a supposedly kindly, benevolent, and helpful figure into an archfiend who experimented on people?

If I seem to belabor the point here, it is only because during this particular postwar period, feelings ran high about using children, or any humans for that matter, for anything like an experiment.

In the preparation of a code of ethics for using human subjects for medical research, Dr. Andrew Ivy of the University of Illinois and his collaborators enunciated ten principles, all of which were accepted by the Nuremberg Tribunal.[8] But this did not lead to a clearing of the atmosphere by any manner of means. In this code, article 1 leads off with the statement:

> The voluntary consent of the human subject is absolutely essential. This means that the person involved should have legal capacity to give consent. . . .

And article 7 goes on to state:

> Proper preparations should be made and adequate facilities provided to protect the experimental subject against even remote possibilities of injury, disability, or death.

If either of these two articles had been followed to the letter during the early trials of either the inactivated or the attenuated poliovirus vaccines, not a single trial dose of these vaccines could have been administered, let alone the hundreds or tens of thousands which were actually given, because the children involved would have been considered "experimental subjects" who could not have granted consent; and obviously, there might have been a very slight risk of disability or death. The Code of Ethics posed a dilemma. Was it a dilemma which could be lightly brushed aside?

Numerous attempts have been made in recent years to clarify these issues. One such discussion was held as recently as 1964, "Moral Issues in Clinical Research," in which professors of medicine, law, and philosophy participated. It was decided on this occasion, in keeping with views expressed a decade or more before, that the Nuremberg code was inappropriate. This code was a document which explained why the war crimes involving human experimentation were unjustified, but it was not a document or a very good guide for clinical research when an urgent and reasonable humanitarian benefit was under consideration.

Within recent years the World Medical Association has also drawn up a revised code of ethics on human experimentation which has been endorsed by a large number of national medical societies, including the American Medical Association. This has cleared the atmosphere somewhat. Nevertheless, I should emphasize that lawyers, philosophers, and sociologists seldom have had the insight or exact knowledge (nor perhaps does anybody) to predict or define some of the aims which seem justified in human experimental programs in which medical science and the public health are concerned. Such probings have to be conducted on a basis

8. Panel Discussion: The moral issues in clinical research. Held on January 14, 1964 at Yale University. *Yale J. Biol. Med., 36*: 455–76, 1964.

of trial and error if one is to make any progress at all in these fields. The medical profession is the only group which should be relied upon to show the way here. To quote the words of a singularly well informed and ethical physician, "Medicine must *lead* in the search for this knowledge."[9]

But from 1950 on, sentiments were expressed by certain minorities both within and outside of the medical profession that neither the medical nor the public health profession should have any part in experimenting, in testing out a new product—even a new vaccine—if such tests were to be made on man. As late as 1966, Dr. Henry K. Beecher, a professor of research in anesthesia at Harvard wrote in the *New England Journal of Medicine* expounding such views. He laid down some guiding principles for clinical investigation in which the main one was that "The investigator has no right to choose martyrs for science."[10]

Yet, there has to be a first time that any reasonably safe new product or procedure is tried—either in an individual or on a larger scale. How many people realize that they owe their freedom from the fear of epidemic poliomyelitis to just these kinds of experimental trials? The inconceivable miracle wrought by the use of poliovaccines in the United States during the decade between 1955 and 1965 in reducing the yearly cases from some 20,000 or more to 100 or even fewer could never have been achieved had not the safety of the vaccines been tested in a series of experiments involving ever-increasing numbers of children. Was the NFIP's Immunization Committee to blame for dallying so long over such crucial questions when it had experience behind it and the vision of this controversy behind it, and before it that of "the more haste the less speed"? Was the experience of its members who had borne the brunt of trials with a variety of virus vaccines during wartime to be cast aside lightly? Yet the Immunization Committee was certainly not blameless. For one thing it was too big to arrive at unanimous decisions. It was not only a question of ethics which delayed them—far from it. Differences of opinion inevitably arose as to what kind of vaccine was best and what strains of poliovirus should be used; and the number of children on whom the new vaccine was to be tried—whether hundreds, thousands, or tens of thousands would be required. The greater the number, it would seem, the greater would be the risk; but also the greater the statistical adequacy on which a sound decision could be based.

In the meantime, acting on the advice of its other experts, the National Foundation was understandably anxious to get on with a vaccine; and, as

9. G. P. Berry: Search for a new Rosetta Stone. *Pharos., 30*: 7–11, 1967. Dr. George P. Berry, who is today an ex-dean of the Harvard Medical School, is an appropriate physician to speak for the medical profession on this subject.

10. H. K. Beecher: Some guiding principles for clinical investigation. *J. Amer. med. Ass., 195*: 157, 1966.

Harry Weaver, the director of research, is reported to have said in this connection: "to break a log jam."[11] In line with this, objective action was taken in the form of a realignment óf the organization's advisers and in the formation in the spring of 1953 of a new and smaller committee called the Vaccine Advisory Committee. In Carter's *Breakthrough,* Harry Weaver is quoted as saying:

> The immunization Committee was not able to function with the necessary dispatch. It could get entangled for months in technical debates. Furthermore, its members were virologists and the decisions on which we needed help were not exclusively virological. The Vaccine Advisory Committee with experienced public-health men . . . was a far more efficient group.

The Vaccine Advisory Committee[12] was certainly well qualified to deal with the problem of getting on with the inactivated vaccine. The two virologists on it, Smadel and Rivers, who had been associated with the NFIP's Immunization Committee from the start, were competent to handle most of the scientific problems, although unfortunately Smadel had at first to be frequently absent in Korea.[13] The Vaccine Advisory Committee had as its avowed purpose the expediting of an *inactivated* poliovirus vaccine, which up to this time had been on Jonas Salk's drawing board but now had been accepted as a product to be developed with all reasonable speed. There seemed to be little use to stand on ceremony from then on.

11. See n. 7, p. 176.

12. Members of the Vaccine Advisory Committee, which was formed in May 1953, with a listing of their current positions, follow: Dr. David Price of the Public Health Service; Dr. Thomas P. Murdock, a medical practitioner from Meriden, Conn. and a member of A.M.A. Board of Trustees; Thomas M. Rivers of the Rockefeller Hospital and Institute; Dr. Ernest L. Stebbins and Dr. Thomas B. Turner, of the Johns Hopkins School of Hygiene and dean of the Johns Hopkins Medical School respectively; Dr. Norman H. Topping, vice-president in charge of medical affairs at the University of Pennsylvania (later president of the University of Southern California); and Joseph E. Smadel of the National Institutes of Health.

13. As the Korean War was not terminated until July 1953, and Dr. Smadel held the important post of director of AFEB Commission on the Korean disease epidemic hemorrhagic fever, he was not able to give his undivided attention to the work of the Vaccine Committee, particularly at first.

CHAPTER 39

The Inactivated Poliovirus Vaccine, Salk Type

In January 1950 the National Foundation, aware that a vaccine was in the offing, announced that it was holding a meeting at which plans and developments for the future would be discussed. Members of its board of trustees were to be present. The speakers included two of the foundation's staff, Drs. Hart Van Riper and Harry Weaver, as well as two of the grantees of the foundation, Dr. Kenneth Maxcy of the Johns Hopkins School of Hygiene and Dr. Jonas Salk of the University of Pittsburgh. The meeting was an early intimation of the shape of things to come.

By this time the program of typing strains of poliovirus was well under way and progressing so satisfactorily that it was little wonder that the foundation decided that it could accomplish far more as a strategic leader in a cooperative endeavor than by leaving the plans up to one or more laboratories to work out individual programs.

Harry Weaver, the director of research, had gotten out a pamphlet, *The Research Story of Infantile Paralysis,* which indicated the way things were going. In referring to the Typing Program he said:

> A solution to these problems obviously calls for group planning and a pooling of ideas and resources. The National Foundation for Infantile Paralysis invited the workers interested in this problem to evolve a master plan which would permit a cheaper and quicker solution than is possible by the individual approach. Because of the unselfish efforts of this group, a large-scale cooperative study will soon be under way.[1]

This program, upon which the foundation was to spend large sums, proved eminently successful, and understandably the result contributed to Weaver's confidence. But Harry Weaver had already begun to tread on shaky ground; some principles and generalizations he had enunciated sometimes ran counter to those dictated by scientific tradition. If he was assuming that all grantees might be willing and ready to rally round the foundation and pool their talents and ideas just because they happened to receive financial support from this particular source, he was de-

---

1. H. M. Weaver: *The Research Story of Infantile Paralysis.* New York, the National Foundation for Infantile Paralysis, Publication No. 42, Dec. 1948, p. 17.

cidedly in error. As one grantee expressed it, rightly or wrongly: "We are beginning to look like a troupe of trained seals." The pooling of ideas from the start was rational and eminently satisfactory under some circumstances, but not under others. For example, a pioneer who has achieved something of real merit and promise, who sees clearly the implications of his discovery, should be allowed a brief period in which to develop and exploit his own concepts before the inevitable rush of other scientific and technical rivals (or even administrators) who are apt to leap aboard the bandwagon and take over.

These are controversial matters, and different individuals entertain entirely different views about them, particularly in our changing times. It is not admissible for a physician to take out a patent for his own personal gain on a medical discovery from which mankind stands to benefit, but he should at least be allowed a certain amount of time to launch his discovery. This is more satisfying in the long run than any buildup of the image of the discoverer after the work of exploitation has been completed by others.

As an example, take the discovery of penicillin. The antibacterial action of the mold *Penicillium notatum* had been observed by Fleming in the early 1930s. During the years 1939–41 Howard Florey, with the help of Chain, a biochemist, recognized the therapeutic potential of penicillin and carried this important work forward under a small grant from the Rockefeller Foundation. Being wise and hardheaded scientists, these men succeeded in working out ways of exploiting *their* discovery without interference from others or premature publicity.[2]

But to get back to the foundation's Typing Program, which was begun in 1948, here the extraordinary ability of the young Jonas Salk had immediately become manifest. In the words of Dr. Herbert A. Wenner: "Salk served as a spearhead in this venture. . . . Credit must go to Salk for discharging the program so effectively." But he adds: "Weaver played a considerable role in coordinating, expediting (among the four laboratories) and seeing to it that we were financially able to get the job done."

Salk was also peculiarly equipped to conduct an experimental program that had to do with artificial immunization of large numbers of individuals. In World War II he had received training along these lines as a participant in the program of the Commission on Influenza of the Armed Forces Epidemiological Board (AFEB).[3] This board still remembered what

2. K. B. Raper: Researches in the development of penicillin, chap. 53 in *Advances in Military Medicine.* Boston, Little, Brown, 1948, vol. 2, pp. 723–27.

3. This board, organized in January 1941, in the Preventive Medicine Division of the Office of the Surgeon General of the U.S. Army, originally had the name, Board for the Investigation and Control of Influenza and other Epidemic Diseases in the Army. This name was soon shortened to the Army Epidemiological Board and eventually to the Armed Forces Epidemiological Board.

had happened during World War I in the disastrous influenza pandemic of 1918. Members of the Preventive Medicine Division of the U.S. Army, particularly Col. (later Brig. Gen.) J. S. Simmons, MC (Medical Corps), were determined to do everything in their power to prevent such a catastrophe from occurring again.[4]

Even though influenza virus had only been discovered in 1933, experiments in artificial immunization were already under way in the mid-1930s. The emergency posed by wartime conditions was enough to give a considerable boost to mass immunization experiments, and the Commission on Influenza of the AFEB responded accordingly. Extensive efforts were spent not only to improve technical methods in the preparation of the vaccines but also to streamline logistics of administration and to devise accurate measurements of effectiveness.

The influenza vaccine trials directed by Thomas Francis, Jr. had been going on for some time before Jonas Salk became a full participant in the work of the Influenza Commission. Development of an effective vaccine was complicated because the influenza virus family, besides being divided into two main groups, A and B, is further subdivided into substrains (serotypes) both old and new, which, to say the least, have mercurial properties. Because of periodic major shifts in antigenic composition, the vaccine has to be modified according to the composition of currently prevalent strains, whose "antigenic drift" is in turn dictated by the changes inherent in the viruses of a particular year. For ten years Jonas Salk was actively engaged with Dr. Francis in a series of extensive trials designed to test the efficacy of various influenza vaccines in U.S. Army troops. Luckily vaccines made of formalin-inactivated influenza virus did not have the potentiality of causing serious disease, as for instance, the strains contained in a poliovirus vaccine might have.

In earlier years Francis, while on the staff of the Hospital of the Rockefeller Institute, had been an ardent student of experimental influenza and its recently discovered virus. His contributions were enough to put him in the front rank of workers in this field in the United States, and were certainly reason enough that he should be chosen in early 1941 as director of the Commission on Influenza of the Army Epidemiological Board (AEB) when it seemed as though the United States would be inevitably drawn into the world conflict.

The president of the AEB at this time was Prof. Francis G. Blake, who had been Tommy Francis' former teacher at the Yale University Medical School. Francis had also served under Blake as chief resident in medicine at the New Haven Hospital. Dr. Blake was the kind of chief whom the

4. S. Bayne-Jones: *The Evolution of Preventive Medicine in the United States Army 1607–1939*. Office of the Surgeon General, Dept. of the Army, Washington, D.C., Gov't. Printing Office, 1968, pp. 152–53.

young house officer looked up to with complete loyalty and trust. So when some thirteen years later Dr. Francis was elected to lead the army's Commission on Influenza, the happy relationship with his old chief could be renewed. As long as Dr. Blake was at the helm (and with General Simmons behind him) there was assurance that the assignment could be carried out with a minimum of military red tape.

Into this critical situation Jonas Salk was precipitated. He proved to be a keen participant and after two years, in 1944, became a full-fledged member of the Commission on Influenza.

Because influenza vaccine trials were carried out under conditions of military jurisdiction, both vaccinees and control groups could be followed closely. Here was a method of ascertaining what actually happened in the field, and whether the attack rate of clinical influenza was reduced as a result of vaccination. In addition, frequent serum surveys, spaced at intervals up to a year, could be made on the vaccinees to determine what levels of antibodies had been achieved and how well they persisted. In the ten-year period of apprenticeship under the best of leadership, Salk soon displayed the ability and resourcefulness of an independent research worker. He became expert in the technicalities of vaccine production and in the evaluation of the efficacy of various vaccines. This experience alone would have been more than enough to qualify him as an ideal person to pursue a similar program to test a vaccine against poliomyelitis. But if the influenza experience was not enough, Salk soon emerged into a position of leadership in the Poliovirus Typing Program during the years 1948–51. The foundation was quick to discover that here was a keen young man who knew his business and was independent in forwarding his own ideas —one who could outline a program of experimental work and carry it through in spite of formidable difficulties—and lastly, was a man with whom the foundation could work. In practically every way he was the right person to lead the "vaccination program," as it was beginning to take shape by 1950.

At this point in his career Jonas Salk (see fig. 56) was a slight man who radiated a sort of restless eagerness and energy. He had been born in New York City in 1914, was educated in local high schools, and attended the College of the City of New York and New York University Medical College. Here, at the end of his first year he did the unusual thing by taking a year off to study biochemistry under a student fellowship. It was a move which indicated a growing inclination to follow an academic career for which he must have already begun to sense his own capabilities. In any event, the year taken out of his formal course did not seem to have set him back as far as age was concerned. He reentered his regular medical course as a second year student and graduated as an M.D. in 1939 at the age of twenty-four. The following year he joined NYU's Department of Bacteri-

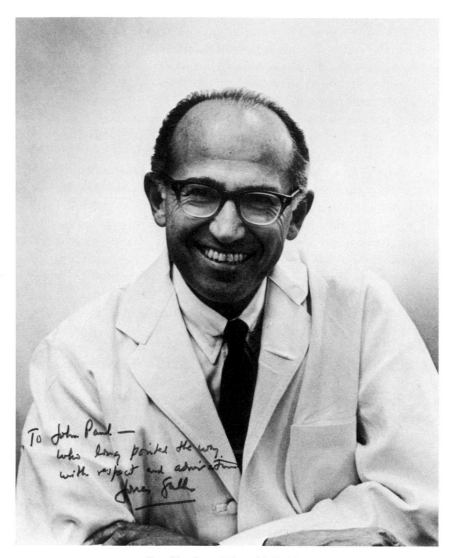

Fig. 56.   Jonas Edward Salk, M.D.

ology under Dr. Thomas Francis, Jr. and went on to intern at New York's
Mt. Sinai Hospital.

Meanwhile Dr. Francis had already moved from New York University's
Department of Bacteriology to Ann Arbor, to become chairman of the
Department of Epidemiology at the University of Michigan's new School
of Public Health.

After five years of apprenticeship under Francis, Salk was ready to branch
out on his own. When an offer came in 1947 to become an associate professor at the University of Pittsburgh, he accepted, for it gave him the
opportunity for independence which he knew by that time he should have.

In the meantime, with World War II over, and for the next seven years, several investigators, including grantees of the foundation and even future members of its Immunization Committee, had begun to make renewed and cautious experimental attempts to immunize against poliomyelitis. Factors already mentioned that contributed mightily to these efforts were the advances in tissue culture made possible in part by the availability of antibiotics; the separation of the poliovirus family into its three respective types; and of course, the discovery by 1952 that viremia occurs with regularity in the early stages of poliovirus infection, indicating that even low levels of antibody were sufficient to protect. Hopes were running high, and the opinion was widespread that it might not be so difficult to prevent poliomyelitis after all.

And so it was, that investigators began to reassess the possibilities of active immunization of man with either an attenuated or an inactivated poliovirus vaccine. The human experiment performed by Koprowski's group with an attenuated virus and those few trials by Dr. Howard Howe using an inactivated poliovirus vaccine[5] were the only ones that had been published by 1952. Yet Salk was definitely out in front, and also definitely in favor of a killed virus vaccine. Not only was he experienced in the use of a formalin-inactivated vaccine as a result of his role in the army influenza immunization program, but he had also become thoroughly familiar with the problems of designing controlled trials to evaluate effectiveness. Salk was the first one to have the courage to utilize large numbers of volunteers (more than 100) in his early poliovirus vaccine experiments. Some might have called it brashness, but Salk's trials, which were published in March 1953, marked a bold and prodigious step. To justify it he said:

> In extending to man studies on vaccination performed in laboratory animals, tests on more than a few individuals had to be anticipated. The first persons to participate in these studies were patients paralyzed in recent years by a poliomyelitis infection and who were in residence at the D. T. Watson Home for Crippled Children, Leetsdale, Pa.[6]

The kind of patients Salk used made it evident that he was running a minimal risk. Salk was to continue his investigations both at the Watson Home and at the Polk State School in Polk, Pennsylvania, where he tried his vaccine on other than convalescent poliomyelitis patients.

In these early trials at the two institutions, 98 and 63 subjects, respec-

---

5. H. A. Howe: Antibody response of chimpanzees and human beings to formalin-inactivated trivalent poliomyelitis vaccine. *Amer. J. Hyg.,* 56: 265, 1952.

6. J. E. Salk (with the collaboration of B. L. Bennett, L. J. Lewis, E. N. Ward, and J. S. Youngner): Studies in human subjects on active immunization against poliomyelitis. I. A preliminary report of experiments in progress. *J. Amer. med. Ass., 151:* 1081–98, 1953.

tively, were involved. Different kinds of vaccines were administered to various groups ranging in age from 4 to 40 years. Had the experiments gone wrong at this point there might well have been a tremendous outcry. Some would have called it unnecessarily hasty to use so many subjects all at once. Some would have said that Salk, having received his training in the trial use of vaccines in "captive" military populations, was not the man to be trying his experiments on juvenile or adult civilians, were they crippled or otherwise. And others would have called it a crime to subject helpless children and adults to this sort of experimentation. But fortunately the trials came out all right. Salk had achieved an early success and was now confident and ready to move forward quickly. At the conclusion of his paper, he said:

> Although the results obtained in these studies can be regarded as encouraging, they should *not* be interpreted to indicate that a practical vaccine is now at hand. However, it does appear that at least one course of further investigation is clear.

Salk had chosen the right moment to conduct his immunization tests, considering the technical and administrative improvements since the early 1940s and the financial support that was now available. It is, however, not accurate to call him the discoverer of the formalinized poliovirus vaccine, since a similar approach had been used by Brodie in 1935; it is more correct to say that Salk perfected its use for mass immunization in man and cleared the way for its wholesale adoption. Besides having taken advantage of the advances in tissue culture and of the Typing Program, he owed much to methods introduced by Jerome Syverton and his team at the University of Minnesota. This group had discovered that all three types of poliovirus could be propagated in tissue cultures containing the cells of monkey testes and that the various strains could also be grown in a continuous line of human cancer cells, so-called HeLa cells. Although HeLa cells could not be used for purposes of vaccine production, they were enormously valuable for the serologic tests which were so essential for measuring effectiveness by means of serial antibody determinations on sera taken before and after administration of the vaccine. Credit must also go to Dr. Raymond Parker at the Connaught Laboratory in Toronto, Canada for solving in 1952 the problem of producing poliovirus in large quantities in tissue culture, and to Dr. Andrew Rhodes of Toronto, a long-time investigator of poliovirus infection and incidentally one of its soundest students, who was in the forefront of this trial. The choice of the Connaught Laboratory as the first to produce virus-containing tissue cultures on the large scale that was needed was a happy one.

All these advances were grist for Jonas Salk's mill, and when he reported his results at a meeting of the National Foundation's Immunization Committee held at Hershey, Pennsylvania on January 23, 1953, members of the group were quick to recognize that he had scored a major triumph. I was prompted to write to him five days later to express my own feeling and proffered him some unsolicited advice:

Congratulations on your most excellent studies and tests with the formalinized poliomyelitis vaccines in children. I was sorry indeed not to be in Hershey, Pennsylvania, last week to hear it but Joe Melnick has given me as good a report as possible and you can understand how tremendously interested we are in this work.

It seems to be far and away the first significant work in experimental vaccination done as yet. Consequently, I want to add my voice to those of others, not only in praise of the well planned and carried out experiments, but particularly for the forthright stand taken as to the future. You must not and no doubt will not be railroaded into doing anything that you yourself have not planned or desired.[7]

Salk replied with kind words to this letter, adding at the end: "Your wise words of caution will be with me when we move into the future." The only reason for quoting this correspondence is to indicate that already there was a certain uneasiness in the wind that the vaccine trials were about to be "taken over."

At the Hershey meeting in January 1953, one of the participants was Dr. Joseph Smadel, at that time still scientific director of the Department of Virus and Rickettsial Research at the Walter Reed Army Medical Center in Washington. Smadel, who was always ready to come to the point and incidentally to deliver his pronouncements in colorful language, is allegedly reported to have said: "What are you waiting for? Why don't you get busy and put on a proper field trial?" Other members favored this suggestion, and Harry Weaver proved to be an ardent backer. Though Rivers was not present at the meeting, later he also threw in his support. Nevertheless, the decision was not unanimous, for others of the committee, including Enders and Sabin, were not so enthusiastic. When the vote came, it was enough to give the green light for a large field trial of the Salk-type vaccine. The size of the trial was not specified.

Smadel's remarks could have been interpreted in various ways. The group of investigators comprising the NFIP Committee on Immunization believed that progress in the laboratory and in the field would proceed in the usual manner—without undue haste, without the use of huge numbers of vaccinees, and especially without wide publicity. On the other hand, the administrators at the foundation, including Dr. Rivers, were anxious

7. Letters from: John R. Paul to Jonas E. Salk, written Jan. 28, 1953; and a reply, from Salk, Feb. 2, 1953.

to push ahead speedily, and also bring in the public. The press was hardly anxious to be caught napping on such a hot subject. A premature news release would be vastly superior in its eyes to one that brought up the rear.

Salk's pioneer and promising results were published in the *Journal of the American Medical Association* in late March 1953. In the following week this journal backed him up with a highly favorable editorial; and in the same issue Rivers published a letter which spoke of a meeting attended by many prominent medical and lay people alike, at which Salk had presented some of his results. Dr. Rivers was obviously enthusiastic; but while he regarded them "as encouraging, they should not be interpreted that a practical vaccine is now at hand."

In the subsequent months Salk continued to administer his vaccine to children until the total number had reached approximately 5,000. More to the point, he had had his confidence bolstered and his resolve strengthened to proceed with determined action. One of the first moves by the foundation was to form, in April 1953, the Vaccine Advisory Committee to deal solely with plans for the coming vaccine. Later on, the foundation would attend to the downgrading of its Immunization Committee. Such matters have been discussed in Carter's book;[8] and somewhat more dispassionately in statements made by Rivers, which have been transcribed by Benison.[9]

The NFIP's Vaccine Advisory Committee was an executive committee that could act promptly and could get on with the work of promoting "Dr. Salk's vaccine."[10] It was indeed an excellent committee for doing just that. On the other hand was the question: With the weight of the foundation having been thrown solidly in favor of Salk's *inactivated* vaccine in the name of speed and efficiency, would this deny serious consideration of an *attenuated* vaccine and prevent recognition of its potential? From one point of view it was eminently reasonable that the foundation should deal with one thing at a time. The inactivated vaccine project was certainly big enough and by this time so far advanced that there could be no turning back. Furthermore, the attenuated poliovirus vaccine was still in its infancy, and it would have been inadvisable to postpone the inactivated vaccine until the other approach had produced more solid evidence of its safety and effectiveness. But whether it was wise for the foundation to have discouraged consideration of the live (attenuated) virus vaccine at this particular point, or to have excluded the idea of a choice between the two approaches to active immunization, is a question that has continued to be argued to this very day.

    8. R. Carter: *Breakthrough; The Saga of Jonas Salk.* New York, Trident Press, 1966.
    9. S. Benison: *Tom Rivers; Reflections on a Life of Medicine and Science.* Boston, M.I.T. Press, 1967.
    10. "Dr. Salk's vaccine" was the original term, which was presently supplanted by the "Salk-type vaccine."

The year 1953 was a busy one as far as a number of members of the foundation's Immunization Committee was concerned. For one thing, the Korean War was still on. Hostilities did not cease until July. Accordingly, the interest and energies of several members of the committee, including Dr. Smadel and myself, had been occupied for some months with Army Epidemiological Board problems both in the laboratory and in the field, even in the war zone.

No sooner was the Korean War over than another obligation was in sight, for in mid-September 1953 the World Health Organization's Expert Committee on Poliomyelitis[11] was scheduled to meet in Rome. Belated as this first meeting was for dealing with poliomyelitis as a world problem, it and each of the four subsequent week-long meetings of the WHO Poliomyelitis Committee represented significant landmarks in the history of the disease. It is fair to say that at least the documents which were produced ranked with the publications of the papers and discussions presented at the first to fifth international poliomyelitis conferences, sponsored by the National Foundation. Although the WHO Expert Committee on Poliomyelitis was late in getting under way, for it only began in 1952, it held a series of meetings which in the eyes of the world had a truly authoritative ring, and reports of the discussions received the widest kind of international circulation. The reason they carried such weight was that it was immediately recognized that WHO opinions were not personal ones, but had been hammered out around a table by an international committee composed of scientists who represented entirely different backgrounds—scientific, political, and academic. It was an example of an international agency being able to settle its differences on the basis of a common aim which luckily had a worldwide appeal. No matter what different political ideologies were entertained by individual committee members, when the subject of the control of infantile paralysis was brought up, it received enough endorsement to make most kinds of group judgment possible. The members of the WHO committee quite naturally expected that these excellent vaccination experiments would proceed in the way scientific experiments were usually conducted, that undue haste would be avoided and most of all, that fanfare of publicity would be kept to a minimum. Every one of the members of the WHO committee was aware that the National Foundation was planning a field trial that would involve some hundreds, perhaps thousands, of children, but the last thing they wanted to do was to drop a broad hint that a vaccine was so imminent.

11. Members of WHO's Expert Committee on Poliomyelitis exclusive of the Secretariat Members were: Dr. H. Bernkopf, Hebrew University, Jerusalem, Israel; T. Francis, Jr., Univ. of Michigan, U.S.A.; S. Gard, Karolinska Institutet, Sweden (vice-chairman); J. H. S. Gear, So. African Institute for Medical Research, Union of South Africa; P. Lépine, Institute Pasteur, Paris; F. O. MacCallum, Public Health Laboratory Service, England; J. R. Paul, Yale University, U.S.A. (chairman); A. J. Rhodes, director, Research Institute, Hospital for Sick Children, Toronto, Canada (Rapporteur).

It is significant that in the committee's report to the World Health Organization, the statement about vaccination against poliomyelitis contains the following, released in September 1953 but unfortunately not published till six months later. In referring to experiments by Salk and others, it said:

> Nevertheless, the committee points out that, however promising these results may be, vaccination procedures against poliomyelitis are still in an experimental stage and that "poliomyelitis vaccines" of unquestionable value are not yet available for general use. It is highly desirable, therefore, that further studies of methods of immunization be carefully pursued, and carried out under proper scientific supervision. Mass immunization should not be generally adopted until such times as scientific data are available on the innocuity and efficacy of the vaccines, and information on the level and duration of induced immunity should be sought.[12]

It is regrettable that publication of this report was held up for six months, and released when the moment was inopportune and it was too late for it to have direct influence. Dr. Rivers, of the foundation's Vaccine Advisory Committee, also had already expressed a fear that even carefully controlled publicity might create a public demand for the vaccine, but his voice was lost in the public clamor.

By this time activities of the Vaccine Advisory Committee were going full speed ahead. Once administrative supervision in the matter of field trials had been assumed, it was easy to see the direction matters would take. This course and the arguments to back it up seemed altogether reasonable to the NFIP and to others: that Salk's trials created a situation that was far too big, far too important, to be handled in a single laboratory, and by one man. This did not mean that Jonas Salk was going to be eliminated—far from it. But nevertheless the vaccine had been "taken over." So even by midsummer of 1953, the foundation plans were shaping up for an early field trial. Harry Weaver had already resigned as director of research, but before doing so had appointed Dr. Joseph Bell, an experienced Public Health Service epidemiologist from the National Institutes of Health, to direct the contemplated field trial. Bell immediately found fault with the proposed addition of an adjuvant, which Salk had in mind for increasing the immunizing power of the vaccine. Bell maintained that an adjuvant would lead to local irritation and as a result complications might arise, particularly if multiple inoculations were planned. He also had certain recommendations in the way of control inoculations which

12. Expert Committee on Poliomyelitis. *1st Report*. World Health Organization, Tech. Rep. Series, No. 81, Geneva (April) 1954, p. 29. Among other features this report contains an excellent current bibliography, not limited entirely to literature that emanated from the United States.

were argued back and forth; the upshot of these discussions and arguments was that Dr. Bell submitted his resignation at the end of October 1953.

Sensing the direction in which things were moving and the foundation's complete preoccupation with the killed virus vaccine, questions had already been raised by members of the NFIP's Immunization Committee in early October 1953 whether it might abandon NFIP support and turn to the National Institutes of Health as a source of government support, at least for a certain portion of the research on poliomyelitis. This would aid a number of laboratories that were engaged in immunization work, particularly those that were trying to develop attenuated strains of poliovirus to be used as a vaccine. These queries were not raised with the intention of obstructing the Salk vaccine program—far from it. But they contained the idea that work on the two programs might proceed simultaneously, although one of them was nearly completed, and the other one had just started. I mention this because it did not seem that the source of support was as important as the ability of the men who were to engage in doing their share on the vaccine project. However, the suggestion to involve the NIH never went beyond the discussion stage.

Although the hour was by now already late to inform the Immunization Committee of what had been going on, Dr. H. W. Kumm, the foundation's newly appointed director of research in place of Harry Weaver, announced that a meeting was to be held on October 24, 1953 at the Henry Ford Hospital in Detroit, and that Jonas Salk would present his most recent studies on the use of an inactivated vaccine. He wrote:

> It is intended to acquaint members of the Immunization Committee with the present status of the program for active immunization and to invite their collaboration in this very important undertaking.[13]

Jonas Salk came to my hotel room on the evening before this meeting. He was aware that our immunization group was going to be disturbed on the morrow and was anxious to find out how certain members would react.

For the foundation was on thin ice here, and it was at this meeting that a serious confrontation took place. The trial with the Salk vaccine was by this time much further along than many of the Immunization Committee members realized. And it was immediately made apparent to the members that they were to have a passive, not active, future participation in the plans. I believe that this meeting, more than any other single factor, was responsible for the belief and the accusation that the foundation had been secretive about its plans and had withheld information from its own scientific advisers. This interpretation, whether true or false, exists in various forms to this day. At the beginning of the meeting Albert Sabin and

13. Letter from H. W. Kumm to J. R. Paul, Sept. 18, 1953.

Joseph Melnick both presented individual work on attenuated strains of poliovirus with the idea that this approach might also be considered for developing a vaccine of an entirely different and more lasting nature. Live virus vaccine trials concerned with other infections had been in progress under the aegis of the Neurotropic Virus Commission (AEB) during World War II and the years immediately following it. No matter how one looked at the results with formalin-inactivated vaccines against viral neurotropic diseases, the technical and logistic problems, particularly the necessity for repeated doses, loomed large. But when the question was asked whether a choice was going to be available as to the kind of immunization or the approach to be used against poliomyelitis, Mr. O'Connor remarked sharply: "That's not the function of this Committee," a statement that was taken up and enlarged upon by Hart Van Riper. As far as the Immunization Committee was concerned, it was a pertinent question, and it amounted to a realization that henceforth its deliberations on such matters were no longer necessary. Dr. Kumm's invitation to this meeting should have alerted the participants as to what was in store for them. For the wording had been "to collaborate." The foundation had already thrown in its lot with the inactivated vaccine and its newly appointed Vaccine Advisory Committee. The subsequent discussion that went on at great length was about technical aspects of the Salk-type vaccine, including which poliovirus strains were to be used. It was difficult even to suggest or to discuss significant changes in a program that had been decided upon by another committee. At this point it might have been better for the Immunization Committee to resign, and it might also have saved the foundation some future embarrassment. But such an action would have been ascribed to pique, and this was not what the cause of poliomyelitis deserved. After all, the main objective was to get on with the problem by the best means that any one of the interested parties could devise. And yet the breach that was to develop as a result of this meeting has remained for some members of the Immunization Committee an open and sore wound. But it was not inevitable that such differences of opinion were to last so long or were to be brought up time and again later.

Thirteen years after these confrontations, echoes of the controversy were sounded in an address made by Dr. James A. Shannon, director of the National Institutes of Health, in Oklahoma City in October 1966. He said:

> As I will point out later, the decision of the Foundation to throw its resources behind the development of an inactivated vaccine markedly increased the difficulties and greatly protracted the time required to develop the generally accepted polio vaccine we have today.[14]

14. J. A. Shannon: NIH—Present and potential contribution to application of biomedical knowledge. Remarks presented at the Conference on Research in the Service of Man, Okla-

Nevertheless, Mr. O'Connor did not look at the problem from this point of view, either in 1953 or in 1966. In the latter instance he took up cudgels in defense and tried to show the error of Dr. Shannon's remarks.[15] I will not attempt at this point to give detailed pros and cons of these arguments, nor could I. Such an effort would be detrimental to the purposes of this account, and besides, there are much more important things to be considered in the few remaining chapters. Decks had been cleared for action on a vaccine, and if in the process some individuals had been hurt and some wrong decisions had been made, that was just too bad.

homa City, Oct. 25, 1966. *Committee Print for the Com. on Govt. Operations, U.S. Senate,* U.S. Govt. Printing Office, Washington, D.C., 1967, p. 80.

15. A letter from S. Benison to Robert Greene, exec. secy., Committee on Science and Public Policy, National Academy Sciences, Washington, D.C., Dec. 1966, presented the foundation's reply. It was circulated to the deans of various U.S. medical schools by Mr. O'Connor.

CHAPTER 40

Evaluation of the 1954 Field Trial
Triumph and Aftermath

By December 1953, plans laid by the foundation's Vaccine Advisory Committee for a mass field trial on the Salk-type vaccine had progressed to the launching stage. The huge project was to be conducted as a scientifically and statistically significant trial. Otherwise it would not have been worth all the expense and all the effort that had to go into it. The underlying idea in making the evaluation trial so large was that this seemed to be the only way to determine whether the vaccine was really safe and effective. Large numbers of vaccinees and control children would be necessary to satisfy the demands of statistical adequacy. Nothing like it, at least nothing like a trial of such magnitude, had ever been contemplated, let alone implemented. To direct such a massive project was going to require substantial organization and a man of considerable knowledge, stature, and ability.

Dr. Thomas Francis, Jr., who had been abroad on sabbatical leave from the University of Michigan since the summer before, has recounted to me how he came to be saddled with this tremendous task.[1] It was about Thanksgiving time 1953, when he was visiting friends in London, that he received a telephone call from Dr. Van Riper in New York asking him whether he would consider the assignment as director of the National Foundation's field trial of the Salk-type vaccine. This was shortly after Dr. Joseph Bell's resignation from this difficult position.

After a bit of soul-searching and a number of conferences including a session with Professor Bradford Hill, the eminent biostatistician at the London School of Tropical Medicine and Hygiene, Dr. Francis came to New York around Christmas and there laid down in no uncertain manner the only terms under which he would accept such a challenging assignment. These included the crucial point that an equal or greater number of children than were to be vaccinated should receive an injection of an inert solution, i.e. should act as placebo controls. The two groups would then be followed in exactly the same manner. He also insisted, emphat-

---

1. I am much indebted to the late Dr. Thomas Francis, Jr. for his contributions to this account, which were so freely given to me, particularly for his verbal description of events during the 1954 Field Trial.

ically, on a policy of noninterference by the foundation. Only when all of these conditions were agreed to did he accept. Thus the Poliomyelitis Vaccine Evaluation Center was quickly established at his home base, the University of Michigan, Ann Arbor, Michigan.

In late February 1954 Dr. Francis assembled a small group of individuals experienced in neutralization tests with polioviruses, at a meeting held in Baltimore, to undertake preliminary planning of the laboratory studies, particularly the evaluation of antibody responses, needed in connection with the field trial. Here Dr. Francis, who had been apprised of the uneasiness among members of the foundation's Immunization Committee in recent weeks, was dealing with a delicate situation. But the participants at the February meeting, most of whom represented the laboratories where the major work on poliomyelitis serology was being done in the United States, gave their enthusiastic support to this phase of the work of the field trial. As a matter of fact Dr. Francis, in his report of the meeting, ended on a cheerful note:

> It is well to comment that the group looked upon the problems involved in a positive manner, recognized the limitations of the different laboratories with respect to the size of the study but were quite willing to undertake participation in the work.[2]

Dr. Francis went on to describe the two groups of controls to be included in the trial, one *injected* (placebo), and the other *observed*. His plans at that time were to inoculate 600,000 to 700,000 children in the first, second, and third school grades in widely scattered parts of the country; they would receive alternately either vaccine or placebo control material, under code. For the observed control study, approximately 400,000 second grade school children would receive the vaccine, and those in the first and third grades would act as observed controls.[3] It was anticipated that the vaccination trial would begin in the off season for poliomyelitis, i.e. in the latter part of March 1954, and would be concluded early in June. The collection and testing of an adequate number of matched samples of sera from vaccinees and control children was a mammoth task, for it was estimated that only 10 to 20 percent of the children in the age group selected would lack antibody to polioviruses before vaccination. It was hoped that in this small fraction, the postvaccinal sera would show rises to the desired antibody levels. On this, success or failure of the great experiment partially rested.

2. T. Francis, Jr.: Summary of Meeting with Advisory Group of Virologists in relation to Poliomyelitis Vaccination Program. Baltimore, Md., Feb. 27, 1954.

3. In the final report of the *Evaluation of the 1954 Field Trial of Poliomyelitis Vaccine* (Ann Arbor, Michigan, Edwards Brothers, 1957, pp. 1–563), it is stated that the results of the vaccine Evaluation Program had involved 1,829,916 children in 211 areas of 44 states. These included the placebo controls and the observed controls.

Of course, Salk himself had performed similar tests on vaccinees on innumerable occasions, but never had antibody tests been made on such a tremendous scale. Children representative of most of the states of the Union and all walks of life, from urban and rural communities and different hygienic and socioeconomic strata, were to be tested. The work involved was no light task for some laboratories.[4] Fortunately, however, the serologic studies were regarded by the National Foundation as extra undertakings by most of their grantee laboratories, and the NFIP provided additional financial support for them.

Over and above the task of testing matched serum samples was the much larger problem facing the Poliomyelitis Vaccine Evaluation Center of determining how the approximately 400,000 second grade vaccinated children would fare with regard to the acquisition of poliomyelitis during the summer of 1954, and whether a degree of protection amounting to 25, 50, or even 75 percent would be achieved over the poliomyelitis rate in the observed controls within the same area. The success of the trial could not have been achieved without the excellent planning and carefully worked out controlled conditions under which it was conducted. As it was, it did not escape criticism. But probably never in the history of medicine has a new public health measure been tested on such a wide scale and so thoroughly. There were many risks in vaccinating so many, but, as events turned out, the trial succeeded. It was worth the tremendous effort involved.

To aid in this huge operation, which required the services of laboratory workers, fieldworkers, and statisticians, Dr. Francis enlisted Robert F. Korns, epidemiologist of the New York State Health Department, as his deputy director and employed an army of other workers to make up a large staff. Two technical assistants who were well qualified to deal with population problems were recruited from the U.S. Bureau of the Census.

The actual technical and administrative details of the trial will not be gone into, but a word should be said as to where and under what circumstances the supplies of inactivated vaccine were produced. The production of live poliovirus antigen in high concentration was entrusted to the Connaught Laboratories of the University of Toronto. This Canadian institute was familiar with the use of monkey kidney tissue-culture techniques on a mass scale. A group of American manufacturers with extensive experience in the preparation of vaccines was then recruited to undertake the *inactivation* of these large amounts of poliovirus and the actual production of the vaccine. Two manufacturers agreed to participate in this phase of the program on a nonprofit basis. The ultimate product was subjected

4. Dr. Joseph L. Melnick deserves the entire credit for performing this task on the quota of tests allotted by the Evaluation Center to the Yale Poliomyelitis Study Unit.

to stringent testing procedures to see whether it fulfilled certain criteria, and especially whether it contained any living poliovirus which might have managed to escape the formalin inactivation process. The testing for sterility was performed by each of three laboratories: the producer; the Public Health Service, represented by the Laboratory of Biologics Standards of the National Institutes of Health; and Dr. Salk's laboratory. In the wake of this testing, records were gone over at the foundation's headquarters by Drs. Thomas Rivers and Theodore Boyd, and any lots that looked suspicious were thrown out. It was a colossal task.

During the next seven or eight months the nation waited expectantly to see what results would be forthcoming in the widely heralded field trial. Inevitably as it drew to a close, interest of the public press mounted accordingly. Dr. Francis has told me how repeated attempts were made by several news agencies to obtain a release, a preview of results, before he or anyone else was ready, even before the comparative data on vaccinees and controls had been assembled. One news agency is reported to have announced some time in early February or March 1955 that it had learned from an unimpeachable source that the vaccine had proved 100 percent effective. Immediately thereafter other newspapers began to storm Dr. Francis' office by telephone for a verification or a denial. Accordingly, with a reporter on the wire Dr. Francis' words were: "I have absolutely nothing to say. If I said 'Yes, it is true'; or if I said 'No, it is not true,' my statement would be taken as if I had something to say, but to tell you the honest truth I *really* have nothing to say. If you are so anxious for news at this point, I advise you to go back to that unimpeachable source from whence the rumor originally came."

Clearly the field trial had been taken out of its proper setting as a scientific experiment of extremely difficult and great magnitude and emerged as a dramatic spectacle. This was inevitable, in view of the nature of the trial, for by this time a far larger audience than the medical profession had been aroused. More than 1,800,000 children throughout the length and breadth of the land had participated in the great "experiment," and all were anxious and eager about the results.

Describing the day of the news release, April 12, 1955, Dr. Francis had occasion some years later to say:

> It may be worthwhile to visualize the circumstances which prompted the undertaking. Just think: After years of theoretical consideration, of investigating and speculating, here was a vaccine which was a natural development of accumulated technical advances and experimental demonstrations that antibody is directly correlated with protection against poliomyelitis. Here was substantial evidence that children receiving the material developed significant levels of antibody

without harmful effect. Here was an agency, headed by a forceful imaginative administrator, possessing the financial resources, the staff, the nationwide organization, the public support, and the desire to subject the material to a critical test of effectiveness. . . . This was the situation in December 1953, when the proposal was made that the evaluation be conducted at the University of Michigan.[5]

This revealing and realistic statement contained evidence that Dr. Francis was a man who not only combined the talents of physician, microbiologist, and epidemiologist, who had been brought up in the strictest of scientific ideals and traditions, but could work satisfactorily with the foundation in spite of its publicity people; and not only could he work successfully but also effectively.

A word about Dr. Francis at this point is in order. Although he had only come into the poliovirus field since World War II, he deserves a high place in the history of the disease.

Thomas Francis, Jr. (see fig. 57) was born in 1900. He was educated at Allegheny College and at the Yale University School of Medicine, from which he graduated in 1925. At Yale he had come under the guidance of Francis G. Blake and James D. Trask[6] as a student and intern on the medical service of the New Haven Hospital. Both of these teachers had a consuming interest in acute bacterial respiratory disease in those previral days, and Dr. Francis absorbed much of their enthusiasm for the subject.

Dr. Blake soon recognized Francis as a young man who gave promise of being an independent worker; as such he recommended him as a suitable candidate for a place on Dr. Rufus Cole's staff at the Hospital of the Rockefeller Institute, where he himself had served six years earlier. It was evidently a lucky and successful choice, for Dr. Francis spent the next ten years under the wing of the institute, where he had the opportunity of coming in contact with senior scientists besides Dr. R. I. Cole, such as T. M. Rivers, O. T. Avery, and junior ones, such as W. S. Tillett, Colin McLeod, and others. These men were avid students of infectious disease who had much to contribute in the way of keen observations and searching theory on just the kinds of subjects in which the young Dr. Francis was interested. But of all the men to whom he looked with a combination of respect and affection, Francis Blake and Rufus Cole[7] topped the list.

It was at the Rockefeller Institute that work on the newly discovered influenza virus and on experimental influenza was begun in 1934. The dis-

5. See "Introduction" in n. 3, p. xxvii. The report mentioned in n. 3 was more complete than the abbreviated edition available on April 12, 1955.

6. See accounts of the careers of both F. G. Blake and J. D. Trask in chapter 20.

7. It may be recalled that Rufus Cole had been the director of the Hospital of the Rockefeller Institute in 1911–12 when the team of Peabody, Draper, and Dochez engaged in their study on poliomyelitis (see chap. 12).

covery in England by Smith, Andrewes, and Laidlaw that influenza virus could be isolated in the ferret—of all animals—had been made a year earlier, and Francis was quick to take advantage of it. He proceeded to make what was probably the first isolation of influenza virus on this side of the

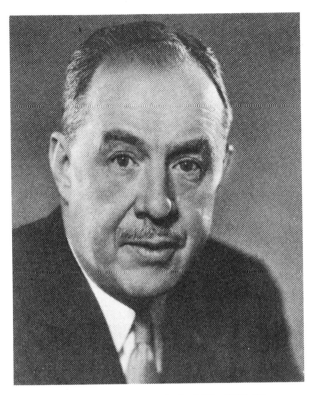

FIG. 57. Thomas Francis, Jr., M.D. (1900–69).

Atlantic, the PR-8 strain. Together with his colleague Dr. Stuart-Harris of England, who was a fellow at the institute, this team was to make many contributions in the field of experimental influenza. The work precipitated Francis promptly into a position of authority on influenza in the United States much as Flexner had found himself in the position of being the first American authority on poliovirus twenty-five years earlier at the same institution. The difference was that Flexner soon went off on several unrewarding tangents, pursuing his own theories, while Francis' position of leadership in the influenza field was steadfastly maintained by his ability to keep in step with his own solid judgments and those of his colleagues.

It was inevitable that the services of Thomas Francis, Jr. should have been sought in the 1930s for a chair in a prominent American medical school. His qualifications were such that he could have had a professorship in any one of the fields in which he was active, i.e. microbiology, internal medicine, and epidemiology. He had shown remarkable talents in all three. So it was no surprise when he became professor of bacteriology at New York University's College of Medicine, with a supplementary appointment as visiting physician at New York City's Bellevue and Willard Parker Hospitals. The story of his three-year stay at NYU and the part which he played in training Jonas Salk in the knowledge and techniques of influenza vaccination at both NYU and the University of Michigan has already been recounted. Throughout his long career at the University of Michigan Dr. Francis has subsequently occupied countless important academic and scientific governmental positions in American medicine. He was for many years the director of the Influenza Commission of the Army Epidemiological Board; later he followed in the footsteps of his former teacher at Yale, Dr. Francis Blake, by serving for two years as president of this board, 1958–60. Not only was Dr. Francis a distinguished figure in American medicine, but more than being distinguished he combined friendly qualities and an excellent sense of humor, while at the same time being a tough though resilient opponent. He was an amateur boxer at college, and he had never gotten over being combative on occasions.

But to return to the outcome of the story of the evaluation of the field trial of 1954, for a time it seemed appropriate that news of the outcome should be made public at a meeting of an important scientific society. The annual meeting of the National Academy of Sciences was suggested. There the report might have had at least a slim chance of being discussed dispassionately. But gradually the forces of publicity and sensationalism took over, and since the Evaluation Center had been established at the University of Michigan it seemed as if the university wished to capitalize on the project, which by this time had become one of great national interest. Furthermore the University of Michigan had an appropriately large hall to accommodate the army of newsmen that was expected to be on hand to hear the momentous news. A full-dress meeting was therefore set to be held in Ann Arbor on April 12, 1955, which incidentally turned out to be the tenth anniversary of President Franklin D. Roosevelt's death.

In the abbreviated report that Dr. Francis gave at this meeting, the success of the product developed and tested by Dr. Salk as an effective vaccine for the prevention of poliomyelitis was unequivocally stated. Francis stressed that the report was not a preliminary communication, but a summary of objective analyses of valid data from records which were essentially complete. No one can say that it was not a prodigious triumph.

Yet the circumstances under which the report was released proved to be a temporary disaster for the reputation of American science. Perhaps this was unimportant, all things considered. One witness described the performance as being set to the tune of "the rockets red glare and flashbulbs bursting in air." The information that had been gathered so painstakingly at the Evaluation Center, and at such an expense of time, money, and energy, did not deserve to be so cheapened by the outburst that ensued. One lame excuse was that it was "the American way of doing things." In any event the triumphant manner in which the news was announced to a waiting public was almost bound to have a backlash. And when one came just fifteen days later it was a major tragedy.

In reviewing the events of April 12, 1958 in retrospect, one Swedish scientist, Dr. Sven Gard of Stockholm, a man who occupies a high place in the annals of poliomyelitis research today, was to take those severely to task for the way the news on the Salk-type vaccine had been handled—and released. He indicated that such a sensational finding in the field of medicine is something which concerns all human beings and should be treated accordingly. A stage show giving a distorted or one-sided presentation of such news may cause great harm. And at the same time he also criticized Salk for his claim that the estimated speed of formaldehyde inactivation of poliomyelitis virus was not what his calculations had shown it to be.[8]

No one can deny that it is an extremely difficult question whether to release an urgently needed prophylactic agent before it is completely ready, in an effort to control safely a preventable disease such as paralytic poliomyelitis. But once it has been released (if "it works") a wave of popular feeling is likely to sweep the country in the belief that "Now, *at last*, we have a vaccine!" This tide is well-nigh irresistible.

A few days prior to the meeting of April 12, the National Institutes of Health had asked a small group of physicians, immunologists, and public health workers who had been in close touch with the progress of the inactivated vaccine to be on hand at Ann Arbor so that they could make the decision as to whether or not this vaccine should be licensed by the Public Health Service.

Considering the circumstances and the presence of an army of newsmen anxious to get their stories filed in time for the evening papers, the meeting of the Licensing Committee can be said to have been held amid tumultuous surroundings. Indeed in the atmosphere of triumph which prevailed it is doubtful whether the committee could have viewed the results of the field trial dispassionately. And it is doubtful whether any group would have had the fortitude to hold out for long against the tremendous pressure to release the vaccine for general use. To make matters more difficult for the committee, the abbreviated report had been under wraps until the very morning of its presentation. Although the data and results in the Francis report had been explained by the speakers at the morning meet-

---

8. S. Gard: Aspects on production and control of formol-treated poliovirus vaccines. *Europ. Assn. Poliomyelitis, IV Symposium,* 1956, pp. 22–25.

ing, none of the members of the Licensing Committee had had the opportunity of perusing it, let alone reviewing it, except for hasty glimpses during a crowded and noisy lunch hour.

The data in the summary Francis report indicated that the vaccine had been given to 200,745 children without causing any serious accidents or reactions. It contained the following statement:

> Thus, extensive examination of available data has yielded no evidence that cases of poliomyelitis attributable to the inoculation of vaccine occurred during the 1954 Field Trial.[9]

Added to this remarkable record of safety were indications that the rate of poliomyelitis cases had been reduced by more than 50 percent among children to whom the complete course of vaccination had been given. But what was not made clear, at least to some members of the Licensing Committee, was that in anticipation that the vaccine would be licensed, a larger group of manufacturers, i.e. other than the firms which had been supplying the needs of the field trial, would be producing the vaccine subsequently—for public consumption. Such a step was inherent in any shift from a limited research operation to mass production. The committee was not in a position to ascertain on the spot, whether mechanisms for adequate evaluation of the capabilities of certain drug companies to make the vaccine had been set up, nor could its members foresee the pressure that the manufacturers would be under. These were difficult problems, and more time was required to deal with them satisfactorily. To drug companies, however, speed was of the essence. It was a tremendous advantage to be first in the market with a new and highly desirable product, for it put the name of the manufacturer out in front.

But to get back to the Licensing Committee, it was far past the appropriate time for a deliberative body to have been brought on the scene. With all the clamor for a favorable decision going on and with the office of the surgeon general of the Public Health Service constantly telephoning from Washington during the meeting to ask whether a favorable decision had been reached yet, the committee obviously operated under duress. And so, after a few hours of discussion the members finally decided to license the Salk-type vaccine. The decision was reached almost entirely on the evidence so painstakingly gathered by the Evaluation Center, that more than 200,000 children had been vaccinated without serious accident and that the protective rate had proved to be more than 50 percent. No other potentially dangerous product in the history of public health procedure had ever undergone such an extensive and rigid test,[10] and the matter of safety

9. See n. 3, p. 255.

10. These experiences were supplemented in 1954 by trials in Canada and Finland. In Canada 8,051 children had received a complete course of vaccination without serious reaction, and

of the vaccine for general use seemed to have been settled. The crucial period however was to come when the manufacture of the poliovirus vaccine had passed beyond the experimental and into the production stage —even beyond and out of the hands of the Vaccine Advisory Committee and the Evaluation Center, to the point when it landed in the hurly-burly of the market place.

The successful progress of the nationwide vaccination program was rudely shattered some fifteen days after the Ann Arbor meeting with the alarming announcement that several children who had been vaccinated with the Salk-type vaccine had come down with poliomyelitis! By that time about 400,000 inoculations had already been given. Had it not been for the alertness of Dr. Alexander Langmuir's staff at the Public Health Service's Communicable Disease Center (CDC) in Atlanta, Georgia, another few days might have elapsed before the ugly situation was detected. As it was, evidence from both epidemiological and laboratory aspects soon established that certain lots of vaccine had contained live poliovirus. The situation was alarming because during the latter part of April and most of May 1955, no one knew exactly what to expect. Had several of the manufacturers turned out lots that would prove to be contaminated, or had only one? Should the whole program of vaccination be called off, or perhaps postponed indefinitely? These were matters for the surgeon general of the Public Health Service, Dr. Leonard Scheele, to decide. The triumphant announcement made on April 12, 1955 had been followed by a serious setback. For a short space it seemed that the old tragedies which had beset the efforts of Brodie and Kolmer in 1935 were upon us once more. Indeed this was a fear that lasted for many weeks.

On April 29, the responsible persons, including the Licensing Committee, were summoned to Washington, where they could do little but wait and watch for further developments. The vaccine-associated cases seemed to be limited to the states of California and Idaho, where certain lots of vaccine, manufactured by Cutter Laboratories of Berkeley, California, had been and were being used. On April 27, the state health officer of California had ordered that vaccine manufactured by the Cutter Laboratories be withdrawn from use. For some weeks it was uncertain whether other lots from other drug firms would also prove guilty of containing some live poliovirus. During a brief period the confidence of the nation was sadly shaken. But it was too soon, and it would have proved too precipitous an action to have called off the whole vaccination program immediately.

The confusion and uneasiness lasted throughout the entire month of

---

in Finland 9,482. However, as regards evaluating the efficacy of the product in these two countries it was clear that the data were inadequate for a significant conclusion (see n. 3, pp. 327–31).

May and well into June 1955, during which the vaccination program was temporarily interrupted. Innumerable meetings were held, and accusations of bungling and mismanagement on the part of scientific authorities and of public health officials were made. There even arose a clamor at this time in the public press as to why vaccination programs in Canada and Denmark, which had been inaugurated immediately upon the release of the evaluation report, had gone so well, whereas the one in the United States had been "bungled."

The Canadians had previously had ample experience in making the Salk-type vaccine and after the news release on April 12 had started a program to vaccinate 860,000 children between April and June 1955.

Denmark also had been quick to seize upon the latest developments and techniques of vaccine production which had been expounded in Salk's publications as early as March 1953. Two representatives of their State Serum Institute, the husband and wife team of Preben and Herdis von Magnus, had visited Salk's laboratory in the fall of 1953, in response to his invitation. They obtained from him a wealth of important information that enabled the Danish Serum Institute to be more in advance of any institution in Europe in its efforts to prepare and administer its own inactivated vaccine on a large scale. The procedures followed by the Danes were somewhat different from those used in the United States in 1955. One practice was dictated partially by the limited supply of vaccine available; this was the use of intracutaneous inoculation, a method which, while not quite so effective, allowed much smaller doses to be given than those used for intramuscular inoculation in the American field trial. As a result, a greater number of children might be protected. In any event the success of the Canadian and Danish programs made it advisable to invite responsible representatives of these two countries to attend a Washington meeting on May 20, 1955, to tell of their programs.

It was at this meeting, held under the auspices of the Department of Health, Education, and Welfare, that considerable clearing of the atmosphere was achieved. With both Rivers and O'Connor in attendance, one could not help contrasting its tone with a meeting held twenty years earlier (1935), when the disastrous but numerically smaller, tragic results of the ill-fated Brodie-Park and Kolmer vaccines had been reviewed. It might be said, of course, that the situations were in no way comparable, for the Brodie-Kolmer vaccines had been launched in the face of colossal ignorance, whereas the Salk-type vaccine had been promoted under circumstances which from the start almost guaranteed success. And yet one cannot help feeling a twinge of sympathy for the two figures of 1935 who were so alone in the midst of their disgrace, in contrast to the powerful forces of the National Foundation, the U.S. Public Health Service, and innumerable advisory committees—including the Licensing Committee—that stood back of the Salk-type vaccine.

At the Washington meeting of May 20, further steps were taken to determine, if possible, just what had happened. By this time attention had been concentrated on the vaccine lots manufactured by only one drug firm. These lots had suffered from deficiencies of control, which had resulted in a failure to detect living virus in the supposedly inactivated product. One favorable feature, however, that emerged at the meeting was recognition of the way that Dr. Langmuir of the Public Health Service's Communicable Disease Center (CDC) had been so prompt in alerting the nation to the so-called Cutter incident. In recognition of this, a vote of confidence was made which went far to creating at the CDC a permanent surveillance unit which was soon to deal with various diseases in this country by techniques which were eventually copied throughout the world.

It was also at this meeting that a prompt course of action was determined, and Dr. Scheele, the surgeon general of the Public Health Service, appointed a small committee of competent individuals, the Technical Advisory Committee. Various members were subsequently dispatched to the pharmaceutical plants that were at that time engaged in making the vaccine with the mandate of finding out what, if anything, had gone wrong. After a thorough search, they were able to report that deficiencies probably had been limited to only one laboratory.

Meanwhile the incident was proving serious enough to cause much anxiety among the individuals that had been in any way responsible. A later review of this unfortunate episode revealed the following:

> A total of 204 vaccine-associated cases occurred. Of these, 79 were among vaccinated children, 105 among family contacts of vaccinated children, and 20 among community contacts. Approximately three-fourths of the cases were paralytic. There were 11 deaths, making a case-fatality rate of 5%.
>
> Isolation of poliovirus was reported in association with about half of the paralytic cases and one-third of the non-paralytic cases. Type 1 virus was identified in all but two of these instances, and type 2 and 3 viruses were found only once.
>
> Laboratory tests performed on the 17 lots of vaccine distributed by the laboratory in question resulted in isolation of poliovirus from seven lots.[11]

In looking for a possible explanation of the disaster the advisability of using the highly virulent Mahoney Type I strain in the vaccine was ques-

---

11. Extract from: *Poliomyelitis Vaccination; A Preliminary Review.* WHO Tech. Report Series, No. 101, Geneva, 1956, p. 5. This summary was included in a report by an international group convened at Stockholm, November 21–25, 1955. It has been taken from an article by A. D. Langmuir, N. Nathanson, and W. J. Hall: The surveillance of poliomyelitis in the United States in 1955. These authors had given a similar report at a meeting of the Amer. Public Hlth Ass. in the United States on November 15, 1955.

tioned. The Danes had used a less virulent strain. Indeed it was on this very point that three members of the Immunization Committee testified at a congressional hearing held on June 22–23, 1955, that it was dangerous to proceed with a vaccine that contained the Mahoney strain of poliovirus. They urged postponement of the whole program until that situation could be rectified.[12] They were overruled, however, when members of an advisory group that had been chosen by the National Academy of Sciences (and who were giving evidence before the Congressional Committee of Interstate and Foreign Commerce) voted eight to three to go ahead with the vaccination program. It was indicative nonetheless of the country's mood in the spring of 1955, that Congress should have demanded a hearing on the matter.

These complicated problems were not to be resolved for at least another five months, although by this time overall favorable results were beginning to come in from the increasingly large-scale and successful use of the Salk-type vaccine.

In the United States, from April 12 to May 7, approximately 4 million doses of poliomyelitis vaccine manufactured by five different commercial laboratories had been administered to children without anything untoward happening other than the single Cutter incident. Dr. Langmuir was able to report in November that the decline in attack rates for naturally acquired paralytic cases had been from two to more than five times greater among vaccinated children than among the unvaccinated in the same age groups.[13]

Also, Canada, Denmark, France, Germany, and South Africa had begun to manufacture and administer the inactivated vaccine by mid-1955.

And yet during the remaining months of 1955, the haunting fear existed in the United States and elsewhere: Would such a tragedy happen again? There was a sigh of relief from those who had the responsibility in this matter when the year drew to a close without another accident. Once the painful episode of the Cutter incident had subsided, the triumph of the Salk-type vaccine became even more manifest. With each succeeding year in areas where it was used efficiently rates of paralytic poliomyelitis declined remarkably. In the United States they fell from 13.9 per 100,000 in 1954 to 0.5 in 1961 (see figs. 58 and 59). Not only was the incidence reduced but also the epidemiological picture was altered so that outbreaks appeared largely in localized urban unvaccinated groups, i.e. in children in the lower socioeconomic strata, living in crowded substandard areas.

The recommendations for administering the Salk-type vaccine underwent substantial evolutionary changes, for, as had been predicted, it was found that the immunity of some children had to be repeatedly rein-

12. *Testimony of Hearings on Poliomyelitis Vaccine.* House of Representatives: Interstate and Foreign Commerce Committee. 84th Congress, June 22–23, 1955.

13. See n. 11, p. 6.

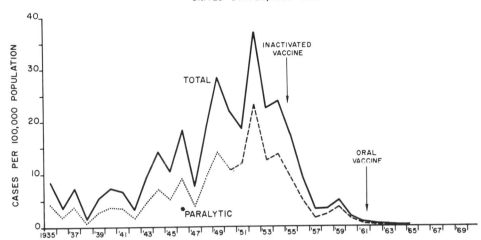

FIG. 58. Thirty years of rates of poliomyelitis in the United States. Data from Poliomyelitis Surveillance Reports, U.S. Public Health Service, Atlanta, Ga.

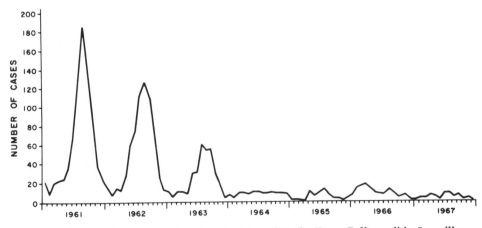

FIG. 59. Poliomyelitis rates in the United States 1961–67. From Poliomyelitis Surveillance Reports, U.S. Public Health Service, Atlanta, Ga.

forced.[14] From the usual course of four inoculations (one given a full year after the primary course of three), the practice was soon established of recommending an annual "Salk shot." The duration and persistence of immunity following immunization with inactivated vaccines was indeed a complicated business. It depended on such variables as the potency of anti-

14. Department of Health, Education, & Welfare: *Technical report on the Salk poliomyelitis vaccine.* Washington, June 1955; also *Minimum Requirements: Poliomyelitis Vaccine.* Nat. Institutes of Health, Washington, D.C., April 1955 (with amendments May, Sept., and Nov., 1955).

genic material in the vaccine, the number of doses administered, and the previous experience of the child (or adult) with natural poliovirus infection.

A review of the situation in 1960, five years after the first introduction of the inactivated vaccine, indicated that its efficacy had increased as the antigenic potency of the product had improved.[15] Thus after three doses, effectiveness had reached over 90 percent in ages 0–14, and 82 percent in ages 15–39 years; but for persons vaccinated four times the estimate was 96 percent and 86 percent for these two age groups respectively. The spectacular decline in incidence that had taken place first in the United States, Canada, and Denmark had spread to many parts of the world by 1960. Indeed by that date, the only failure to obtain satisfactory protection on a national basis when the population had been adequately covered appeared to have been experienced by Hungary and possibly Israel. But effectiveness of the vaccine in stopping epidemics already under way or just starting had not been evident.

In spite of such a remarkable record it was inevitable that improvements in the very principles and the methods of immunization should still be sought. It was now manifest that the Salk-type vaccine had its limitations as far as the ultimate control of poliomyelitis as a *world* problem was concerned. For instance, in remote rural areas and where primitive public health facilities existed, a major drawback was the difficulty in reaching a large enough segment of the population, particularly the highly susceptible preschool children, who must receive four or more doses in order to be adequately protected. While intensive vaccination campaigns with the Salk-type vaccine might be feasible in small, economically advanced countries such as Sweden, this was not the case for developing countries, either small or large. In Sweden, which was once a country with a most evil reputation regarding poliomyelitis, since 1962 the disease has virtually ceased to exist as a result of the use of the inactivated vaccine.[16] In developing countries, on the other hand, logistic problems of adequate distribution and administration have remained almost insurmountable for the use of the Salk-type vaccine.

Another approach to the solution of the poliomyelitis problem on a national and international scale was by this time gaining force. This trend will be recounted in the next and final chapters.

15. *W.H.O. Expert Committee Report on Poliomyelitis.* Third Report. Tech. Rep. Series, No. 203. Geneva, 1960.

16. In Sweden, where a potent inactivated vaccine has been used, not only has there been a spectacular decline in incidence of paralytic cases in vaccinees but in nonvaccinated persons as well. In this country also since 1962 poliovirus strains have rarely been found in routine tests on 6,000 to 10,000 stool samples or by systematic examination of sewage.

S. Gard: Poliomyelitis: present and future, killed virus vaccine. *Internatl. Conf. on Vaccines against Viral and Rickettsial Diseases of Man.* Pan Amer. Hlth Organization, World Hlth Organization, Washington, D.C., Oct. 1966, p. 22.

CHAPTER 41

The Attenuated Poliovirus Vaccine, Sabin Type

Apart from the activity that took place in the mid-1950s in connection with the inactivated vaccine, a renewed and growing interest in live virus immunization against poliomyelitis had begun to take shape. As early as October 1950, Burnet, in the third of his series of Herter lectures given at the Johns Hopkins Medical School, had occasion to say: "I feel confident that sooner or later it will become necessary to use living virus vaccine given by mouth in infancy, perhaps under cover of gamma globulin passive protection."[1]

The principle was not new. Such vaccines had been used in the veterinary field for some time, and in man a live virus vaccine had been in effect for the prevention of smallpox for 150 years, and of yellow fever, for nearly 20 years.

Immunization by modified (attenuated) polioviruses that still retained the power to produce infection had been suggested as a possibility since the 1920s, and such an approach has been frequently discussed in this history. Early investigators who had considered it included Flexner and Amoss, and later even John Kolmer had a live virus vaccine in mind in 1935 when he thought (erroneously) that the highly neurotropic MV strain had lost its pathogenicity for man as a result of repeated intracerebral monkey passage. Kolmer had no proof whatever that this was true and indeed did not have the courage of his convictions because he was unwilling to take the chance of administrating the MV virus to children without its being "partially inactivated." So in preparing his vaccine, he subjected the virus to sodium ricineolate. As we have seen in chapter 24, even this treatment proved inadequate.

During the mid-1940s Max Theiler, who was responsible for developing the yellow fever vaccine, sought to do the same thing for poliomyelitis. He reported at an NFIP meeting on immunization in 1946 that he had produced a special strain of Lansing poliovirus that had lost its paralytogenic power for the monkey after continuous passage through mice and yet had retained its ability to immunize monkeys. But Theiler, having introduced the idea of attenuated strains of poliovirus, did not pursue this lead, feeling that others more interested in poliomyelitis than he was would carry on with it.

1. F. M. Burnet: Lecture III. The ecological approach to the common virus diseases of today. *Bull. Johns Hopk. Hosp., 88*: 157–79, 1951.

It remained for Hilary Koprowski and his colleagues to pick up the trail some five years later, in 1951. He reported at a meeting of the foundation's Immunization Committee that he had taken the bold step of feeding 20 volunteers a strain of poliovirus that had been modified through adaptation to cotton rats! The principle was more or less similar to Theiler's, but the Lederle group had gone infinitely further than the immunization of monkeys and had proceeded to immunize man! Koprowski stated, and subsequently published, that not only had the volunteers suffered no harm but

> Following oral administration of the virus, most of the volunteers manifested a carrier state demonstrated by excretion of virus in their stools, and all of the non-immune volunteers promptly developed antibodies in their blood.[2]

The announcement was of such consequence that members of the Immunization Committee were caught off balance in an attitude of complete incredulity, but only for a moment; then they all began talking at once. In the coffee break that followed, Koprowski, who was never one lacking in bravura, was plied with all kinds of queries; for those present realized that a forward step had been taken in a path which led directly down the road to a live poliovirus vaccine that might eventually be suitable for universal use in man.

Within the next year tissue-culture methods began to supplant rodent adaptation for altering the properties of a virus and rendering it avirulent. In 1952 Enders, Weller, and Robbins had been the first to show that tissue-culture passage of a strain of virulent Type I poliovirus was followed by a marked reduction in its paralytogenic activity in primates.[3] As a result of this finding the idea of an attenuated poliovirus vaccine received a great boost.

In the four or five years that followed, Herald Cox and his associates at the Lederle Laboratories and Koprowski, who was shortly to sever his connection with that company, took the lead in the live poliovirus vaccine field. With Roca-Garcia they had even succeeded in attenuating one of their strains (a Type II) by adapting it to grow in chick embryos, which was indeed a unique achievement.[4] Soon other investigators became involved in this problem, and although Koprowski remained one of the

---

2. H. Koprowski, G. A. Jervis, and T. W. Norton: Immune responses in human volunteers upon oral administration of a rodent-adapted strain of poliomyelitis virus. *Amer. J. Hyg., 55:* 108–26, 1952.

3. J. F. Enders, T. H. Weller, and F. C. Robbins: Alterations in pathogenicity for monkeys of Brunhilde strain of poliomyelitis virus following cultivation in human tissues. *Fed. Proc. 11:* 467, 1952.

4. M. Roca-Garcia, H. Koprowski, G. A. Jervis, T. W. Norton, T. L. Nelson, and H. R. Cox: Immunization of humans with chick embryo-adapted strain of MEF[1] poliovirus. *J. Immunol., 77:* 123–31, 1956.

leaders, he was later to lament the fact that the vaccine against poliomyelitis, which he had "discovered," should later bear the name of the Sabin vaccine.

At the Detroit meeting of the Immunization Committee in October 1953, when the foundation had already made plans to move full speed ahead on the inactivated Salk-type vaccine, both Dr. Sabin and Dr. Melnick told of their results in the development of attenuated strains by means of tissue-culture passage. But, as already recounted in chapter 39, this promising approach was hardly greeted with much enthusiasm by National Foundation authorities. Yet at the same time Sabin reported that he had gone far toward modifying virus virulence by serial passage in cynomolgus monkey kidney tissue cultures and had been able to segregate avirulent variants:

> The results further indicated that one was now dealing with a mixture of particles, some virulent and some avirulent. An attempt to separate the avirulent from the virulent was made utilizing the terminal dilution technique on the assumption that if the avirulent particles were present in very much larger numbers the progeny of single or small numbers of particles at the terminal dilution might consist entirely of avirulent particles.[5]

In Sabin's experiments not one of the 28 monkeys that had been fed attenuated viruses failed to resist subsequent challenge with virulent strains. They were inoculated intracerebrally with 10 to 10 million infecting doses, but none developed paralysis or exhibited any lesions in the central nervous system. In these and later experiments most monkeys and chimpanzees developed inapparent infection with resulting antibody production, and they also continued to excrete the attenuated viruses in their feces for longer or shorter periods of time. At the moment, foundation authorities paid little attention to these findings. They had other fish to fry —the launching of the inactivated Salk-type vaccine.

Not until a year later, in the late fall of 1954, was consideration given to the thought that the Immunization Committee might, after all, have been treated shabbily, and members should be allowed to air their views once more on various matters. And so, in a conciliatory vein, Dr. Hart Van Riper wrote the following cordial letter to members of the disgruntled Immunization Committee:

> Recent developments would seem to warrant a full discussion of where we stand today in the field of immunization, problems that remain unresolved and what changes in emphasis, if any, in the research

5. Extract from remarks by A. B. Sabin: "Experimental production and properties of avirulent strains of poliomyelitis virus." Presented at the meeting of the NFIP's Committee on Immunization, Oct. 24, 1953, Detroit, Michigan.

program should be presented to the Advisory Committees of the National Foundation.[6]

To understand the atmosphere in which this change of heart was taking place, it is important to appreciate that although no actual information' had been forthcoming from the Francis field trial as yet, a substantial number of those who had been following events of the past two or three years, and particularly those of the last three or four months, were convinced that the inactivated poliovirus vaccine developed by Salk, expedited by the Vaccine Advisory Committee, and currently being put to the test under Francis, would prove successful. How effective it would be remained to be determined.

Yet this was only one solution to the problem of immunization against poliomyelitis, and the possibility of another remained very much to the fore. Whether the totally new live virus approach would prove feasible, it was still too early to say; but it is important to realize that the sentiment in favor of a live vaccine was beginning to be expressed even at this early date. If the foundation was the philanthropic organization it claimed to be, it was logical to assume that it would maintain a generous attitude toward all forms of immunization until a long-term decision had been made as to which was the best method. Obviously·this would require several years.

In my reply to Dr. Van Riper's cordial invitation and his subsequent request for items to be discussed, I said:

> Among subjects which I would like to propose for the Agenda, are some which are not *scientific* problems but policy problems. They would include:—
>
> i) What is the function of the Immunization Committee?
>
> ii) How can a scheme or an organization be worked out, in which the various laboratories, who are interested in working on "immunization of *humans* against poliomyelitis," be welded into a group, so that various segments of this problem can perhaps be designated to special groups of grantees (and non-grantees) possibly in the way in which the typing program was carried out.
>
> I am quite conscious that this plan introduces certain difficult and delicate problems, for it may not be fitting for grantees of the Foundation to be attempting to write their own tickets. On the other hand, such drawbacks are not as great as those which come to pass when those of us (who are devoting so much time, energy—and your money to this subject,) develop a feeling that we have no part in the planning of our campaign in this direction.[7]

6. Letter from H. E. Van Riper to J. R. Paul, Nov. 16, 1954.
7. Letter from J. R. Paul to H. E. Van Riper, Nov. 17, 1954.

Commenting on this communication, Dr. Sabin sent a reply which stated: "I am in full agreement with all the [pertinent] sentiments. . . ."[8]

At the meeting in December 1954, Sabin, who had been making real progress with his attenuated strains, was given a free hand. Already there were few doubts in his mind that eventually the live virus vaccine would turn out to be the most effective method.

It is high time that we examined the career and personality of this remarkable man—Albert B. Sabin, whom we have had occasion to mention many times in this history. The reader must already have an impression of him as an able, tireless, and articulate medical scientist, who did not stand on ceremony and seldom dealt delicately with situations which from his point of view required direct, immediate, and strong action. Albert Sabin could be more than generous on occasions, and equally egotistic and possessive on others. It was in controversial situations with his reputation at stake that he really came into his own. Often he was misjudged by an audience whose members did not appreciate that perhaps he was much more familiar with the background or the actual facts of the case than they were. Naturally, they regarded him as an obstinate fellow. Yet in my estimation no man has ever contributed so much effective information— and so continuously over so many years—to so many aspects of poliomyelitis, as Sabin. He possessed not only an uncanny sense for nosing out the fallacies contained in old ideas but also an ability to correct his own mistakes. His was a fierce joy when he turned up a new observation and put it to his own good use.

Albert Sabin (see fig. 60) was born in Poland in 1906 and came to this country when he was fifteen years old. He attended New York University and started out his professional education as a dental student in that same university but soon shifted to its College of Medicine. This move was said to have been prompted by his reading of Paul de Kruif's *Microbe Hunters,* a book that made such an impression on the young Sabin that for the next decade he could think of little else than the challenge of unsolved problems in infectious disease. In any event, when he had barely finished medical school he had already begun a lifetime interest in the virus of poliomyelitis. In the year of his graduation he accepted a position as a research assistant in the Department of Bacteriology at NYU's College of Medicine under W. H. Park. And it was here, in the epidemic year of 1931, that he was initially exposed to all the urgencies and pressures of an extensive poliomyelitis epidemic for which nobody had satisfactory answers. In the course of this experience he first felt that surge of confidence which would enable him eventually to meet the challenge of poliomyelitis, in spite of overwhelming odds.

8. Letter from A. B. Sabin to J. R. Paul, Nov. 29, 1954.

The 1931 epidemic enlisted the energies of Aycock and Kramer of the Harvard Infantile Paralysis Commission in Boston; Trask and Paul in New Haven; and in New York, Park and his associates at the city health laboratories, Simon Flexner at the Rockefeller Institute, Jungeblut at

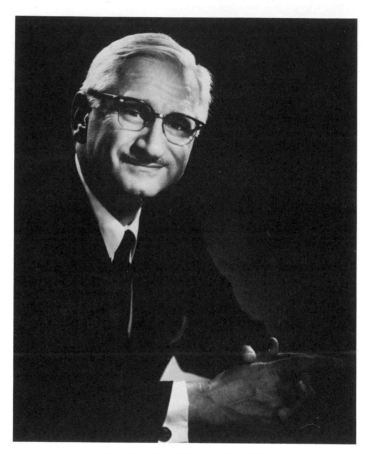

Fig. 60.   Albert Bruce Sabin, M.D.

Columbia University's College of Physicians and Surgeons, and Lawrence Smith of the Cornell University Medical College. And yet, with all this expertise set in motion the epidemic ran its course completely unimpeded by any of the futile efforts of the then current authorities. This did not deter the young Dr. Sabin, who wrote and presented his first paper on the virus of poliomyelitis that fall and which incidentally, I happened to hear. His ambition had been stirred by the summer's experience. And it was at this time that Dr. W. H. Park first recognized that here was no ordinary young man.

Sabin took his residency training at Bellevue Hospital in New York

(1932–34) and then spent some months abroad on a fellowship at the Lister Institute in London. On his return in 1934, he received an appointment at the Rockefeller Institute, where he worked with Peter Olitsky. Between the two of them, with the assistance of Herald Cox, they made some truly remarkable observations on poliovirus. These included the experiments of Sabin and Olitsky in which they succeeded in growing the MV strain in human embryonic nervous tissue. Six months later they reported the presence of lesions in the olfactory bulbs of monkeys that had been experimentally infected by the nasal route.

By 1939, after five years at the Rockefeller Institute, Dr. Sabin was more than qualified to head a university department in a number of different fields. When the choice came, he joined the Children's Hospital Research Foundation of Cincinnati as an associate professor of pediatrics in the College of Medicine of the University of Cincinnati. The Research Foundation consisted of a newly established, vigorous small group headed by the pediatrician Dr. A. Graeme Mitchell, who was succeeded by Dr. Ashley Weech. Twenty years later Sabin became a Distinguished Service Professor of this university.

During the early years at Cincinnati and even before, Sabin began to recognize and identify the special characteristics that poliovirus infections exhibited. By this time he had contrived to study a number of other viruses that invaded the central nervous system, and this gave him a certain advantage over the rest of the field of "poliovirologists." With his associate Robert Ward, he conducted studies on the neuropathology of poliomyelitis, its pathogenesis and natural history; also as to how it differed from other neurotropic virus infections, especially neuropathologically. These investigations were carried out with a speed and determination that few scientists other than Sabin could have mustered. This was where his strength lay. In the period 1939–42, before he entered the Medical Corps to serve in World War II, he came to the conclusion that if virulent poliovirus entered by way of the mouth to initiate an infection in the alimentary tract that usually remained inapparent, then an orally administered attenuated poliovirus vaccine that caused an inapparent infection might be as effective as an injected inactivated vaccine in inducing immunity.

With World War II imminent, Sabin became a charter—and I may say a vigorous—member of the Army Epidemiological Board's Commission on Neurotropic Virus Diseases in the early months of 1941. When the United States finally entered the war, Sabin was able as a major on active duty in the Medical Corps, to continue his association with the commission and utilize to the full his talents for the investigation of viral infections. This military interlude allowed him to take a recess of at least three years from benchwork on poliomyelitis and to turn his attention to other virus infections that in wartime were of a more pressing nature. Incidentally it was during this "holiday from polio" that Major Sabin took a long hard look at this disease and rearranged his ideas accordingly.[9]

He was dealing at this time with military diseases of viral nature—sandfly fever and hepatitis in the Middle East and Mediterranean area. Only gradually did poliomyelitis come to be recognized as an occasional menace to the military that it eventually became. In due time (1943–45), on the other side of the world, the prominent viral infections were hepatitis, which by this time had become a universal military plague; dengue in the South Pacific and in the Philippines; and, the most serious of them all, Japanese encephalitis,[10] which soon raised its ugly head on Okinawa. By 1945 members of the commission including Sabin also worked in association with a team from Commodore Rivers' Naval Medical Research Unit No. 2 (NAMRU-2), which had established its base laboratory on the island of Guam. The story is too long to tell here.

During this wartime period Major (soon to become Lieutenant Colonel) Sabin and others of the Army Epidemiological Board on the commissions used human subjects (volunteers) in investigations for which no animal hosts were available. All of the exacting precautions that this form of clinical research entails were worked out, and all of the anxieties that go with it were shared by the commission investigators. The experiences with two viral infections, sand-fly fever and particularly dengue, both relatively mild diseases in comparison to poliomyelitis, proved of infinite value to Colonel Sabin, who within the next decade was to test his live attenuated poliovirus strains in human subjects. Salk had profited in similar fashion from his work with influenza vaccines among military personnel.

But this was not the only experience that Sabin gained in the management of immunization programs. During the postwar years various problems regarding the control of Japanese encephalitis arose, and in the course of dealing with these he took advantage of military and international facilities to make serological surveys in Okinawa, Japan, China, and Korea and to institute some immunization campaigns in Japan.[11]

Thus in cooperation with fellow members of the Neurotropic Virus Commission, notably Dr. W. McD. Hammon, a project was launched to

9. A. B. Sabin: Studies on the natural history of poliomyelitis. *J. Mt. Sinai Hosp., 11*: 185–206, 1944.

10. Although U.S. military authorities had been constantly aware of the dangers of Japanese encephalitis, its Commission on Neurotropic Virus Diseases was further warned in 1944. This time the information came from A. Smorodintsev and V. D. Soloviev, Russian virologists, who had had practical experience in immunizing troops against this disease in eastern Siberia.

11. These projects were carried out in the postwar period 1946–50 by the Neurotropic Virus Disease Commission (soon to become the Virus & Rickettsial Disease Commission), AFEB, under the auspices of the Public Health & Welfare Section of the Supreme Command for the Allied Powers in Japan, the U.S. Army, and the 406th Medical General Laboratory in Tokyo.

test the efficacy of a vaccine against Japanese encephalitis among children and adults living in the prefecture of Okayama, which had long been a hotbed of this mosquito-borne viral disease. Coincidently a program of vaccinating American troops against Japanese encephalitis was also inaugurated. In both projects an inactivated vaccine was used. Much to Sabin's dismay, after a trial of several years in army personnel, the program was abandoned by high military authorities largely on the grounds that it was expensive, apparently not needed, and did not seem to be particularly effective.

All in all, few people in the early 1950s had had more experience in trials in man of both *killed* and *live* virus vaccines in a number of infections than Albert Sabin. He was singularly well qualified to take an overall view of the vaccination field as it concerned viral infections in general. True, in his early efforts he had not been concerned with such large military populations of vaccinees as were used by Francis and Salk in their influenza immunization experiments, but Sabin made up for this in a variety of ways.

We have now caught up with Sabin's career and are able to return to 1954 and the cause of the live attenuated polioviruses. By this time Sabin was convinced that the oral vaccine was the lead to follow. At the New York meeting of the foundation's Immunization Committee in December 1954, he began eagerly on his favorite subject at the very point where he had left it more than a year earlier in Detroit.[12] It was enough to set off a full day of discussion.

Toward the end of this two-day meeting one item on the agenda was: If a noninfectious vaccine proves to be efficacious, should the NFIP continue to spend large sums of money to develop vaccines based on other principles? This proved to be a cause celebre, and one which caused the foundation endless trouble. Even at this early date, the question was indicative of the direction in which things were moving. Actually the NFIP was sufficiently interested in the new vaccine, even though in late 1955 it was in the beginning flush of success over the Salk-type vaccine, to form a small committee mostly under the guiding hand of Dr. Rivers to promote work and report progress of the live attenuated poliovirus vaccine. This committee only lasted for two years but was resurrected in July 1959 by another, a much larger one, which held one meeting and then issued the following news release:

New York, July 7 [1959]—The National Foundation's Vaccine Advisory Committee tonight praised the new Sabin oral polio vaccine

---

12. Item I (a–f) on the agenda of the Joint Meeting of the Vaccine Advisory Committee and the Immunization Committee of the National Foundation for Infantile Paralysis, New York, Dec. 18–19, 1954.

as "showing great promise as a potential vaccine." . . . [which has been] sponsored by $1,300,000 in National Foundation grants. . . .

". . . The capacity of these [attenuated] viruses to produce antibody is also reported to be good under most conditions, but their capacity to prevent paralytic poliomyelitis, while assumed, is at present not known." . . .

"The committee, therefore, believes it would be unwise to embark at this time upon mass vaccinations with live attenuated polioviruses in the United States."

This was a reasonable enough statement at the time, but for administrative authorities at the NFIP to have dropped the subject in the precipitous fashion they did in 1959 was less understandable. Two years earlier the WHO, sensing the flagging interest on the part of the NFIP in live attenuated virus vaccines took the lead.

For the NFIP this was perhaps a natural reaction; the inactivated vaccine had been the first to undergo significant trial and the first to reduce materially the incidence of poliomyelitis in this country—indeed in the world—and was anxious to hold to its gains. Furthermore the Salk-type vaccine apparently was well established, and the substitute oral vaccine held a certain number of unknown risks. So the argument was put forth that at least the inactivated vaccine should be given a proper long-term trial before any switch from "Salk" to "Sabin" was made. But the foundation had not reckoned with the enthusiasm and the determination that the champions of the cause of oral vaccines were to display.

To go back some years, eleven months after the December 1954 meeting, when most of the excitement over the launching of the Salk-type vaccine and the ensuing Cutter incident had abated, Sabin reported further progress with live virus immunization at a WHO meeting on poliomyelitis vaccination held in Stockholm in November 1955. By this time he had given each of his three types of attenuated oral poliovirus to approximately 80 volunteers.

At the same meeting, Koprowski had also sent in a working document on his oral vaccine. He had used a set of strains different from Sabin's and was able to give a favorable report on results in 150 subjects. He also stated that in children previously immunized with his vaccine "antibodies have persisted for five years after a single oral administration of this particular virus."[13]

Obviously Koprowski was further along than Sabin in terms of the numbers of vaccinees studied and the length of time that he had been able to follow some of them. Incidentally, the presentations of Sabin and Koprow-

13. World Health Organization: *Poliomyelitis Vaccination; A Preliminary Review.* WHO Tech. Rep. Series No. 101. Geneva, 1956.

ski marked the beginning of a protracted contest to achieve an acceptable live virus vaccine. Eventually Cox also entered the race, so there were not only two but three contenders.

In the immediately ensuing years, when the inactivated Salk-type vaccine was being successfully used in the United States and elsewhere, Sabin pursued his experiments with his customary vigor. He worked with prodigious energy and with an uncanny sense of keeping on top even when things went wrong for long periods of time. These preliminary studies involved tests on many thousands of monkeys, hundreds of chimpanzees, and hundreds of susceptible adult volunteers.[14]

Of great importance was Sabin's discovery by quantitative studies that the central nervous system of lower primates (rhesus and cynomolgus monkeys) was more susceptible to polioviruses than that of higher primates (chimpanzees)—and by epidemiologic analogy, man. The reverse was true for the alimentary tract particularly in rhesus monkeys; whereas the susceptible human intestinal tract was readily infected by doses of virus that were ineffective in monkeys. So the major task was to find or produce a strain of each type with the least neurotropism but which would multiply extensively in the human alimentary tract.

It is high time that the theoretical advantages of the oral vaccines over the inactivated Salk-type be considered in the light of knowledge of their respective properties in the mid and late 1950s. The subject was sharply controversial at the time for there were disadvantages as well. It was evident that inactivated vaccine stimulated antibody production and provided immunity sufficient to protect against the paralytic disease, but this immunity was not speedily induced, particularly in the very young, nor was it always long lasting. Revaccination—repeated annual booster doses—was essential, particularly for preschool children who had not had previous experience with polioviruses. In contrast, following ingestion of live virus vaccine (as a result of an actual infection) not only were circulating antibodies induced, but in addition a state of local resistance in the intestinal tract, subsequently shown to be due to stimulation of local secretory antibody, occurred. The immune state was thus more solid, comparable to to that following natural inapparent infection with "wild" virus. Furthermore, because of the speed with which immunity was achieved (often a matter of days instead of months) the live virus vaccine could be used to advantage in the face of an impending epidemic or even in the midst of one. Finally, oral administration instead of injection by needle was a boon, particularly to public health authorities in rural areas and in developing countries where facilities and public health personnel were limited. Yet

14. A. B. Sabin: Oral poliovirus vaccine. History of its development and prospects for eradication of poliomyelitis. *J. Amer. med. Ass., 194*: 130–34, 1965.

despite these considerations, in 1955–60 live virus vaccination was disparaged because of the risks involved. Few regarded it as a completely safe procedure.

For instance, at the very start all did not go smoothly with the Koprowski attenuated strains when a trial was put on in 1956 by a group in Belfast, North Ireland. In the course of their investigations Dr. George Dick and his collaborators noted that whereas the Type I SM strain and Type II TN strain had been attenuated when they were first fed to children, during the vaccine-induced inapparent infections that followed, these strains had reverted toward their former wild and virulent state.[15] This had been demonstrated by the fact that the virus excreted in the vaccinee's feces was found to cause severe paralyses when inoculated into monkeys. Here, according to the Belfast group, were the roots of a disaster! Dr. Dick was loud in his denunciation of the live virus principle, and as a result the whole group of attenuated poliovirus strains suffered a brief but undeserved eclipse. Dr. Dick clung to these implications, and more than two years later he said:

> . . . we must realize that once we have fed a population group with attenuated virus vaccines we have opened a Pandora's box. You may have stopped ten cases of paralytic polio but you may be responsible later on for paralyzing 100 children. I do not think this is likely, but it is our duty to consider the worst theoretical possibilities as well as the best.[16]

In 1957, the National Foundation for Infantile Paralysis was still supporting work aimed at solving the questions raised by Dick and his group, which were to plague proponents of the live virus cause for many years. But as mentioned before, the NFIP did not avidly pursue this particular preventive measure. Accordingly the World Health Organization quickly usurped this authority and called an important meeting of its Expert Committee on Poliomyelitis in Geneva, in mid-July 1957. It was an indication that although most of the research on poliovirus vaccines was carried on in the United States, interest in and control of the disease had by this time become an international affair.

At the WHO meeting, Sir Macfarlane Burnet was in the chair. The status of the killed vaccine was reviewed with satisfaction, but more attention

15. D. S. Dane, G. W. A. Dick, J. H. Connolly, O. D. Fisher, and F. McKeown: Vaccination against poliomyelitis with live virus vaccines. 1. A Trial of TN Type II Vaccine. *Brit. med. J., 1*: 59–64, 1957; and subsequent papers.

16. G. W. A. Dick and D. S. Dane: The evaluation of live poliovirus vaccines in *Live Poliovirus Vaccines; Papers presented and Discussions held at the First International Conference on Live Poliovirus Vaccines*. Scientific Publication No. 44, Pan American Sanitary Bureau, Washington, D.C., 1959, p. 10.

was paid to live virus vaccine. This emphasis was not surprising since seven years earlier the chairman had voiced his personal opinion that a live virus vaccine would eventually conquer poliomyelitis.

Subjects discussed included criteria for the selection of poliovirus strains and the degree of attenuation that was to be considered adequate; the effectiveness—capacity to "take"; and the safety of the oral vaccines. The committee also issued a plea that certain standards regarding scientific and statistical adequacy should be met if a trial of live virus vaccine was to be considered satisfactory.

This WHO committee, in short, took upon itself the duties of a steering committee and proceeded to specify certain principles or ground rules for the conduct of field trials which the various contenders were expected to follow. This was a necessary action if the trials and systematic evaluation of the various oral vaccines were to be comparable.

The wording of the statement was important:

> After careful consideration of the data at present available on the use of *live attenuated* polioviruses as immunizing agents against poliomyelitis, the Committee strongly recommends that controlled field trials be carried out for the purpose of testing further the value of these agents. . . . [These] have reached a stage in which trials in man on a larger scale than has been attempted hitherto are now indicated. This decision is based on the fact that preliminary tests on attenuated polioviruses in the hands of several investigators have failed to reveal signs of illness or harmful effects in the vaccinees or their associates. . . . The Committee strongly recommends that such trials be carried out in the near future within certain specified population groups and areas and under the most careful supervision.[17]

In addition to recommending that field trials should be under "the most careful supervision," the committee also enumerated the characteristics of strains which it considered fit for use in these vaccines. Six criteria were expected to be met. The suggestion was made that the properties of the strains "be measured in a number of different laboratories so that there can be more than one opinion as to their pathogenicity or the lack of it."

17. Expert Committee on Poliomyelitis. *Second Report. W.H.O. Rep. Series, No. 145.* Geneva, 1958, p. 25. Those in attendance at this meeting, which followed directly on the Fourth International Conference on Poliomyelitis, held in Geneva, Switzerland, were Drs. H. Bernkopf, Hebrew University, Israel; Sir Macfarlane Burnet, Walter and Eliza Hall Inst., Australia (chairman); H. K. Cowan, Dept. of Health, Scotland; S. Gard, Caroline Inst., Sweden; J. H. S. Gear, Inst. for Medical Research, South Africa; J. H. Hale, University of Malaya; P. Lépine, Pasteur Inst., France; F. P. Nagler, Dept. Nat. Health and Welfare, Canada; J. R. Paul, Yale Univ., U.S.A.; F. Przesmycki, State Inst. of Hygiene, Poland; A. B. Sabin, Univ. of Cincinnati, U.S.A.: V. D. Soloviev, Moscow, Inst. for Poliomyelitis Prophylactics, Soviet Union (vice-chairman). Invited but unable to attend was R. Murray, Nat. Insts. of Health, U.S.A.

It was in some ways a pity that Sabin happened to be a member of the WHO committee because it was subsequently charged that there was bias in establishing criteria for the selection of live attenuated strains, criteria which to all intents were fulfilled by the Sabin strains. Yet it was also true that he contributed enormously to the committee's deliberations by his grasp of the whole live poliovirus vaccine situation. Gradually, however, microbiologists and others throughout the world began to realize that the authority of Burnet as the committee's chairman made it clear that bias was not involved and that wise ground rules for live virus vaccine trials had indeed been set.

For the next two or three years the only section of the recommendations of the WHO report to which attention was paid by most of the interested parties was the one stating that the number of field trials should be increased. The two other groups besides Sabin (Koprowski and Cox), it would seem, were too far along in the preparation and use of their vaccines to make changes. They were all eager to see field trials carried out on their own strains under different environmental conditions and in various populations and were not to be deterred or influenced by the WHO recommendations. One prominent promoter of these vaccine trials in South America said to me that he was sick and tired of hearing about the WHO recommendations. The criteria of attenuation recommended for strains to be incorporated in the candidate vaccines were of particular unconcern. And yet by disregarding this very point the rival contenders in the race may have already lost the contest when it came to licensing the vaccine. But this is anticipating the story.

By December 1957 the Koprowski strains had already been tested on nearly 250,000 persons in Ruanda-Urundi and other communities in the Congo. Meanwhile the Lederle group[18] headed by Cox enlisted the support of Dr. Fred Soper, director of the Pan American Sanitary Bureau (a WHO subsidiary) in an effort to conduct trials of the Lederle strains in various Central and South American countries. The Lederle vaccine was also tested on pregnant women and their infants, under the auspices of the University of Minnesota.

By this time Sabin had given his strains to virologists in Leningrad and Moscow for trials in the Soviet Union where it was assumed that the WHO recommendations would be followed. By 1958–59 a total of twenty field trials using oral vaccines prepared by Koprowski, the Cox-Lederle group, and by Sabin had been conducted in no less than fifteen countries. These included the United States, northern Ireland, the USSR, Czechoslovakia, Poland, the Belgian Congo, and South and Central American countries.

At this point (in June 1959), unlike the carefully guarded events which

---

18. This group represented the Viral and Rickettsial Section, Research Division, American Cyanamid Co., Pearl River, N.Y.

surrounded the introduction of the Salk-type vaccine, the subject of live poliovirus vaccines had become "old hat" and was thrown wide open for discussion by those who either had worked with them in the laboratory or had conducted field trials and were willing to stand up and present their results and listen to the sometimes acrimonious criticism of fellow investigators. To this end a series of two international week-long meetings was staged in Washington, in 1959 and again in 1960. These were intensely interesting affairs, rivaling in many respects the international conferences of the National Foundation, but they were neither so heavily weighted with work and ideas which emanated from the United States nor with the usual polite kind of criticism that was exchanged in the latter conferences. Both Washington meetings were financed by that *other* foundation interested in poliomyelitis, the Sister Elizabeth Kenny Foundation of Minneapolis, and both were held under the auspices of the Pan American Sanitary Bureau (by 1960 called the Pan American Health Organization), which is loosely under the overall control of the World Health Organization.

These two conferences were extremely successful, as they should have been, considering that the subject was of such timely and absorbing interest. In the first one, impressive trials involving millions of persons were reported by Soviet scientists including Dr. Smorodintsev and his group and the husband and wife team of Drs. Chumakov and Vorosholova. Smaller and more carefully controlled studies were reported from Europe and the United States. As was to be expected, the degree of thoroughness with which orally vaccinated persons and their contacts had been observed for adverse effects had varied. However, no evidence was produced that any of the three live virus vaccines had been followed by either paralysis or ill-defined illnesses in vaccinees or their contacts, or among nonvaccinated people in the community at large. A cautious note was sounded in the summary of the first PASB international conference, echoing the recommendation made in the WHO report two years earlier that: "The desirability of standardization of the techniques was emphasized." This veiled criticism reminded some of the speakers who reported on live virus vaccine trials that neither the vaccines used nor the way the trials had been conducted had met WHO standards. To look into the second of these issues, WHO dispatched Dr. Dorothy M. Horstmann of the Yale Poliomyelitis Study Unit to the USSR in 1959 to determine whether the trials involving astronomical numbers of vaccinees had really gone off without a hitch and had been conducted under exacting principles. Her report[19] was guarded but favorable and, by and large, future events were to bear it out.

19. D. M. Horstmann: *Report on a Visit to the USSR, Poland and Czechoslovakia to Review Work on Live Poliovirus Vaccine, August–October, 1959.* Submitted to WHO. Unpublished.

The following year (1960) another successful international live poliovirus vaccination conference was held under the auspices of PAHO. From
this time on, issues soon resolved themselves into which strains were judged
to be acceptable for incorporation into a live virus vaccine. Considering
that all of the three vaccines were produced in the United States, their
promoters were subject to regulations of the U.S. Public Health Service,
which would be responsible for licensure. This meant that both the investigator who developed the vaccine and the company responsible for
its manufacture should demonstrate routine production lots that were not
only consistent in quality but were also potent, safe, and useful. Licensing
had become the final act in the research development of any new biological product. In the case of the live virus vaccine, unlike the hasty action
which transpired in a few hours at the meeting of the Licensing Committee for the Salk-type vaccine, deliberations of the USPHS Ad Hoc Committee on Live Polio Vaccine[20] lasted almost four years. This committee
had been organized in 1958 under the Division of Biologics Standards of
the National Institutes of Health and continued its meetings through 1962,
when all three of the attenuated poliovirus strains were licensed and released for manufacture. The vaccine was then at last given to the medical
profession for general use.

20. Membership in this NIH Ad hoc Committee for Licensing of Live Poliovirus Vaccine
consisted of: David Bodian of Johns Hopkins University; Joseph L. Melnick of Baylor University, Houston, Texas (who resigned after two years); Dr. W. McD. Hammon, University
of Pittsburgh; J. R. Paul, Yale University; Roderick Murray, director of Division of Biologics
Standards, NIH, Washington (chairman); and Joseph E. Smadel of the NIH. Drs. Murray
and Smadel both represented the Public Health Service.

CHAPTER 42

Controversies and Conclusions

The Ad Hoc Committee on Live Poliovirus Vaccines had been appointed by the U.S. Public Health Service within a year after WHO's second report on poliomyelitis had appeared. The committee was charged with the task of "remaining abreast of developments in the field of live attenuated poliovirus vaccines," and of assisting in the selection of attenuated strains for inclusion in a vaccine. Such a product could be licensed in the United States only if and when scientific experience indicated that it was safe and effective and that adequate biological controls could be maintained by the pharmaceutical houses which would be selected to produce it.

By 1958, some human trials with attenuated poliovirus strains were being conducted as if their use constituted regular established public health practice rather than as field studies of an experimental nature. Accordingly, the USPHS committee attempted to set standards. It maintained that there should be adequate and accurate documentation of events when a given strain was used in a vaccination trial of this kind; it also laid down criteria to be followed in testing the degree of attenuation of the three virus types and recommended that other things being equal, no strain was to be regarded as suitable for use in any trial unless one or more laboratories had shown that its neurovirulence was of the lowest order, comparable to that of the most attenuated strains known.

As the work of the committee progressed during 1959, it quickly became apparent that the candidate viruses displayed considerable differences in neurovirulence as measured by intracerebral and intraspinal inoculation of monkeys. On this basis the Sabin strains had an advantage over the others, but none of them proved to be completely avirulent when injected directly into the spinal cord. With this information in hand provisional criteria for acceptability of strains were set up. These criteria, modified in the cause of brevity were:

1. Minimal neurovirulence—as tested in the monkey
2. Absence of viremia, in man
3. Maximum genetic stability, i.e. absence of the capacity to revert to greater neurovirulence
4. Freedom from any harmful effects when administered to susceptible populations of approximately 100,000 individuals and where adequate surveillance of neurological illness had been maintained

5. Potency and effectiveness—namely the consistent production of specific antibodies and the capacity "to take," in 90 percent or more of susceptible vaccinees[1]

These five items were to undergo considerable modification as knowledge
increased,[2] particularly no. 2, which was to be eventually eliminated.

The efforts of the Ad Hoc Committee were aided to a considerable degree by the deliberations and discussions at the two international conferences on live poliovirus vaccines, the second of which had been held in
Washington in June 1960.[3] Among new features which were brought out
was a demonstration by the Melnicks of the usefulness in field trials of
Lwoff's temperature (T) marker for distinguishing between strains of low
and high neurovirulence.[4] This in vitro method depends upon the ability
of wild, virulent poliovirus strains to multiply in tissue cultures equally
well at 40° and at 37° C, whereas the attenuated vaccine strains grow at
37° but not at 40° C. As a result of this finding, monkeys were no longer
so essential for the complicated determination of the genetic stability of
vaccine strains, and this, to say the least, was a great relief for many a poliomyelitis laboratory.

Another new feature, which was of more than passing value, was the observation by John P. Fox and Henry Gelfand and their collaborators at
the School of Public Health, Tulane University, New Orleans, that the
infectivity or the degree of contagiousness of attenuated strains was also
greatly reduced as compared to "wild" strains, so that the risk of spread
was correspondingly less than with naturally occurring polioviruses.[5]

1. First, Second, and Third Reports of the Public Health Service's *Ad Hoc Committee on
Live Poliovirus Vaccine,* submitted to the U.S. Public Health Service, Washington, D.C. (unpublished), June 1, Aug. 1, Nov. 5, 1959.

2. Subsequently, it was to be shown that item no. 2 of these criteria could be disregarded.
At least viremia following the administration of Type II of the monovalent Sabin-type attenuated poliovirus vaccine proved to be a common, almost normal and nondangerous occurence.

3. *Live Poliovirus Vaccines; Papers presented and Discussions held at the Second International Conference on Live Poliovirus Vaccines.* Pan American Sanitary Bureau, Scientific
Publ. No. 44, Washington, D.C., 1960, pp. 1–713.

4. J. L. Melnick and M. Benyesh-Melnick: Problems associated with live poliovirus vaccine
and its progeny after multiplication in man. See n. 3, pp. 12–28.

Dr. Joseph L. Melnick had been among the early members of the Yale Poliomyelitis Study
Unit and had remained in that association for 16 years. Born in Boston, Massachusetts in
1914, he was educated at Wesleyan University and at Yale where he took his Ph.D. degree under Prof. C. N. H. Long in the field of biochemistry. He joined the Yale Poliomyelitis Study
Unit as an instructor in 1941, and his talents not only as a biochemist, a cell biologist, and an
epidemiologist immediately came to the fore. He was indeed a prodigiously able and independent worker. His departure from Yale came in 1957. For a year he was associated with the
National Institutes of Health in Washington, but eventually became professor of virology and
epidemiology at Baylor University Medical School in Houston, Texas.

5. H. M. Gelfand, L. Potash, D. R. LeBlanc, and J. P. Fox: Revised preliminary report on
the Louisiana Program of the natural spread within families of living vaccine strains of poliovirus. See n. 3, pp. 203–17, and many other subsequent papers by the same authors pertaining
to this subject.

As mentioned before, in the evaluation of the several candidate strains no evidence had as yet been presented indicating that any of them caused illness in the vaccinees, but the degree of thoroughness with which many of the observations had been made was limited. The question of strain reversion to previous virulence within the body of the vaccinee remained as the most important of the unsolved problems. Would vaccinated children excrete virus of increased virulence which might be dangerous to family contacts and to the community, as had been prophesied by Dick and Dane some years before? Or to the contrary, would the strain be *too* attenuated to immunize?

At the 1960 international meeting new vaccine trials were reported, bringing the total up to about forty or more. The Sabin strains had received extensive field tests in the United States, the Soviet Union, Czechoslovakia, Mexico, and Singapore; the Lederle-Cox strains had been widely used in Latin America; and the Koprowski Type I on a large scale in the Belgian Congo. Already in the USSR a first attempt had been made to abort an epidemic, which was already in progress, by means of a community-wide oral vaccination program. This was instituted at the peak of an outbreak in Tashkent, in the Uzbek Republic, and carried to completion within a few days.

In some small trials, involving not more than 500 people, there had been close clinical supervision, but in larger ones, some almost nationwide, ranging from several thousand to many million participants, this had not been possible. Still, in almost all instances, the opinion was universal that untoward reactions in the vaccinees or their families were either absent or insignificant. Nor had the progeny of the vaccine strains induced any harmful effects in the local community. This was true in the USSR even though the extensive programs there (far larger than anywhere else) had to be considered as massive public health campaigns rather than as carefully controlled investigations. In subsequent visits to Russia by United States microbiologists the question of the quality of supervision was to be a constantly recurring one. But following the Horstmann report, the verdict had been given that their results were indeed promising, and in fact, pioneer Russian efforts of 1958–59 have stood the test of time.

In addition to emphasis on practical aspects in the control of poliomyelitis by vaccination, by the late 1950s it was becoming abundantly evident to many clinical investigators that in the course of progress towards the main goal, many previously unknown facts about poliovirus infection had been brought out. Trials with attenuated strains made it possible to explore problems which had defied the experts for nigh onto fifty years; they also provided a unique opportunity to learn something of the ecology of polioviruses. What had heretofore been a dangerous agent had suddenly become tamed. Here was a safe way to study human infection and to observe the spread of the virus in different kinds of populations and environments, sociologic and climatic.

Along this same line of thought were observations by Fox, Gelfand et al., and those of the Yale Poliomyelitis Research Unit, which had already set up several small controlled trials in four different types of environments between the years 1957 and 1962. The first of the Yale studies (a) was in a closed institution, using Type III and Type I Sabin attenuated strains; the second (b) was carried out in 1958 using Sabin Type I in a somewhat isolated Arizona locale (Guadelupe Village); and the third (c) in 1959, in a subtropical village in Costa Rica, Central America, where the triple vaccine of the Cox-Lederle strains was already being used in a nationwide campaign initiated by the Pan American Sanitary Bureau and the Costa-Rican Ministry of Health. In addition, two oral vaccine trials with the Sabin strains (d) were conducted by the Yale group in Connecticut cities. Afterward, in 1964, there was a chance to explore the significance of viremia, and accordingly a study of vaccine-induced viremia was instituted in a foundling home in New York City (e). These were only a few of the cooperative efforts conducted by a single research unit.[6] They complemented many other vaccine trials conducted by others for similar purposes. So within the short space of six or seven years not only was the effectiveness of the attenuated vaccine tested but the natural history of poliomyelitis also was explored experimentally in a manner never before possible. The disease had given up some of its most important secrets at last.

A new and rather disconcerting discovery was reported at the 1960 conference on live virus vaccines by Dr. Maurice Hilleman of the Merck Institute for Therapeutic Research. This was the demonstration of a hitherto unrecognized contaminating virus in the tissue-culture substrate that was being used for production of live virus vaccines. This contaminating virus, tentatively called the *vacuolating agent,* appeared to be just one more of the troublesome agents that had to be screened out of tissue cultures in the course of the testing of the vaccine for safety.

Developments that followed this discovery were disturbing, for a while. Close upon the heels of Dr. Hilleman's announcement, Dr. Bernice Eddy and her colleagues at the Division of Biologics Standards of the National Institutes of Health made the discovery that the vacuolating agent, which had by this time received the name SV-40 (Simian Virus-40), induced malignant tumors when injected into hamsters—common laboratory animals! Here *was* a new cause for alarm, for it certainly was inadvisable to

---

6. Individual members of the Yale Poliomyelitis Unit shared in these studies to a greater or lesser degree. (a) *Trans. Ass. Amer. Phycns,* 70: 91–101, 1957; *J. Amer. med. Ass., 170*: 1–8, 1959. (b) *Amer. J. Hyg., 70*: 169–84, 1959; (c) *Bull. Wld Hlth Org., 26*: 311–29, 1962; (d) *J. Amer. med. Ass., 178*: 693–701, 1961; *Yale J. Biol. Med., 34*: 439–54, 1962; (e) *Amer. J. Hyg., 79*: 47–63, 1964.

to immunity, an immunity considered (but not yet proved) to be more lasting than that induced by the inactivated vaccine, and without the necessity of reinforcement.

Another asset was its effectiveness in halting incipient epidemics. Furthermore, the Sabin-type vaccine readily produced a marked state of resistance in the alimentary tract (so-called intestinal immunity), which greatly reduced the chances of reinfection by wild polioviruses. Thus not only were individual vaccinees protected, but they served as barriers to the spread of wild virus, and the community thus derived a certain amount of protection.

Besides, poliomyelitis was a disease with a worldwide distribution. In Italy, the South American republics, and many other countries there were insuperable problems not only of expense but also of the practicability of reaching young children with an inactivated vaccine which required so many injections. With live poliovirus vaccine the number of doses was limited to three, perhaps four (three monovalent in the first six months and one of a triple vaccine at one year), and there was the added convenience that it could be given orally. Any means of immunization that was so simple and did not suffer in the matter of safety or effectiveness had a great appeal to parents, physicians, pediatricians, and the public in general. In retrospect, sentiment shifted in America and elsewhere in favor of the oral vaccine. The cry has often been raised that the committee's decision was based on considerations of favoritism, even influenced by political motives.

At first glance one would suppose that it might have been a rather simple process for physicians and public health officers in 1962 to change from the inactivated Salk-type to the new oral vaccine. However, a gradual turnover did not hold the promise of bringing out the full potential value of the oral vaccine in terms of community-wide protection. This called for intensive mass vaccination campaigns conducted over a limited period of time and directed primarily to preschool and school-age children. In order to provide an effective barrier against the spread of wild poliovirus in the community it was considered that at least 80 percent of susceptible children in a given population should be immunized within a few days.

Licensure of Sabin's other strains followed: Type II occurred in October 1961, and Type III in March 1962. And it was not long before the oral vaccine also received approval by public health authorities in England. No fanfare, no popping of flashbulbs greeted these announcements in the United States or abroad. The decision had been so long in the making that when it came it was accepted perfunctorily.

Yet sad to say, in the summer of 1962, within a very few months of the time when the monovalent oral vaccines of all three types had been released, another new and formidable mishap occurred.

give children a vaccine made in monkey kidney tissue cultures which might contain a cancer-inducing agent and with perhaps other unknown potentialities. Not only did the problem exist with respect to live virus vaccines, but in early 1961 Dr. Norman Grist of the University of Glasgow discovered that the level of formalin being used for the manufacture of Salk-type vaccine was insufficient to inactivate SV-40 virus. By this time the Salk-type vaccine had been in use for some six years, but since the early Cutter incident there had been no sign of anything untoward in the millions who had been injected with it. Yet the question was immediately raised: Would complications occur in these vaccines ten or more years later? Here was another of the grave problems that were a source of worry in the unimpeded course of the Salk-type vaccine.

However, it came out that the potential dangers had apparently been exaggerated. Testing of inactivated poliovirus vaccine revealed that current lots from only two manufacturers contained SV-40. The data also suggested that most of the lots released in recent years by American manufacturers probably did not contain detectable amounts of the offending virus. An encouraging report was therefore issued by the Public Health Service in June 1961, to the effect that means were available for eliminating this recently recognized contaminating monkey virus from vaccines manufactured for general distribution and steps had to be taken to ensure in the future that both kinds of vaccines would be free from it.[7]

And so, with many sighs of relief, it seemed that another hurdle had been surmounted along the long road leading toward the ultimate control of poliomyelitis. Nevertheless, it still remains to be seen whether other contaminating viruses, oncogenic (related to tumor formation) or otherwise, may not be discovered in tissue cultures that are currently being used for poliovirus vaccine production.

In spite of early successes, all was not to be plain sailing for the oral vaccine. To retrace our steps once more to the international conference sponsored by the Pan American Health Organization in Washington in June 1960, one other feature that received but passing notice at the time should have been recognized. This was a prediction made with deadly accuracy by Sir Macfarlane Burnet of Australia, who had been a vigorous supporter of the principles of live poliovirus vaccination. He said:

> If we have reason to believe that a population undergoing immunization with a live vaccine contains a proportion of completely unimmunized individuals, and we are looking for possible cases of paralysis, then we should look for this among the young adults.[8]

7. Report of the Technical Committee on Poliomyelitis Vaccine. Submitted to the Surgeon General of the U.S. Public Health Service, by Dr. R. Murray, June 20, 1961, unpublished.

8. See n. 3, pp. 460–61; F. M. Burnet: "Poliomyelitis," chap. 7, in *Viruses and Man*, 2nd ed. Penguin Books, London, Wyman & Sons, 1955, p. 95.

The warning was based on the familiar principle that as age increased the clinical severity of poliomyelitis increased for susceptible individuals, i.e. in the persons who had previously escaped exposure and infection by any or even one of the three poliovirus types. Sir Macfarlane illustrated his discerning prediction by a graph (see fig. 61).

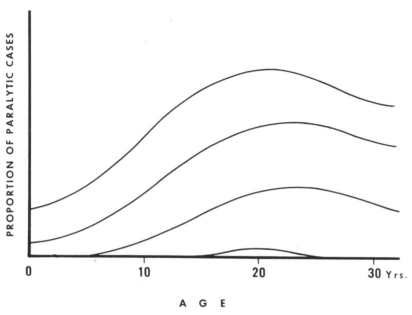

FIG. 61. Burnet's prophetic graph of the incidences of paralytic cases in a susceptible population undergoing live poliovirus immunization. The four different roughly parallel lines represent four degrees of response (from minimal to maximal) depending on dosages or degrees of virulence exhibited by the attenuated polioviruses being administered (see n. 8).

Meanwhile, however, during the period of 1960–61, the idea of an oral vaccine for poliomyelitis was receiving remarkable and increasing support. By this time the superiority of Sabin's strains had become apparent not only as to their safety ratings but also in their effectiveness in well-controlled trials. So in due time (March 1961) the Public Health Service committee decided to recommend the Sabin Type I as a reference strain to various American manufacturing companies. Also, mindful of the Cutter incident of some six years earlier, strict regulations were laid down, and technical details were spelled out as to how vaccines which fulfilled specifications should be made.

Later, on August 17, 1961, the surgeon general of the Public Health Service, Dr. Luther L. Terry, released the following statement to the press:

> The granting of a license to manufacture poliovaccine, live, oral type I, developed by Dr. Albert Sabin, was announced today. . . . The

vaccine will be marketed in the United States by Chas. Pfizer & Co., Inc., of New York.

The question had long been discussed, sometimes with inordinate heat, as to why the Salk-type vaccine, apparently doing "so well" in the United States and some other areas and with the prospect of further improvement in its potency, should be replaced by a live, attenuated poliovirus vaccine. Mr. Basil O'Connor himself came to an Atlanta meeting of the Public Health Service in February 1961 to protest this. The claim was that the massive "trial" of the Salk-type vaccine should be allowed to run its course for another one or two years in this country at least before any change in procedure was made.

Six months later an editorial appeared under the date of November 18, 1961, in the *Journal of the American Medical Association* announcing that:

> This has become a highly controversial and emotionally charged field, and it is difficult to get agreement, even in small groups, as to the indications for use of the oral vaccine under this or that circumstance. On the one hand, it would seem that in those countries where the killed Salk-type vaccine has not been widely or successfully used, there is little question as to the desirability of the immediate introduction of the oral poliovirus vaccine. On the other hand, in those countries where a well-established program entailing the use of the Salk-type inactivated poliovirus vaccine has been successful and is continuing to be successful, there may be a real question as to whether an immediate shift to the oral vaccine is indicated. Undue haste is always undesirable.
>
> Such highly controversial issues demand decisions by an official group. . . . At some point in the proceedings, the A.M.A., the Academy of Pediatrics, and perhaps other groups should be represented and together with the Public Health Service and its advisors should hammer out the vaccination policy and methods to be followed in the United States during this, the early stage of the introduction of the oral vaccine.

The questions raised by this editorial were by no means easy. Effort bring multiple administrative groups into the picture would hardly been useful unless the members were reasonably familiar with the cacies of the story of live attenuated poliovirus vaccines, which had more than a decade before.

To review the assets of the attenuated oral vaccine, besides ease ministration, one of these was its ability to induce resistance prom actually causing an immediate inapparent infection which could

By August 1962 the estimated use of oral vaccine in the United States had reached more than 21 million doses for Type I, 7 million for Type II, and 14 million for Type III. In view of the years of testing and the universal opinion that it was safe and effective, the expectation had been that this product would be spared the tragedy which had beset the Salk-type vaccine when it was first launched. But not so, for gradually evidence came to light that there had been a number of cases of poliomyelitis (62 on total count) which had followed within 30 days of immunization with live attenuated virus. The cases were largely in adults, and the majority were associated with the Type III strain. Early intimations were that the disease in these instances had actually been caused by the oral vaccine. A national committee,[9] immediately set up by Surgeon General Terry of the Public Health Service to review the situation, quickly realized that when millions of persons participate in an immunization program, any of a variety of events occurring subsequently or coincidentally are apt to be erroneously attributed to the vaccine. But it was recognized that a small number of the cases were possibly, quite probably, vaccine associated. On this basis, the committee soon narrowed its attention to 16 cases, all of which had been reported in nonepidemic areas within the period of January 1 to September 15, 1962; all cases had occurred after the administration of monovalent Type III vaccine; 12 were over the age of 15, and 8 of these were over the age of 30—clearly far different from the age group usually involved in naturally occurring poliomyelitis. On this basis the committee concluded: "There is sufficient epidemiological evidence to indicate that at least some of these cases have been caused by the Type III vaccines."[10] The old tragedy was with us once more.

This worrisome situation demanded prompt consideration of what measures were to be taken, but few were willing to hazard a guess. Events of this particular kind had not been recorded before in any of the previous live poliovirus vaccine trials. The accidents were particularly disturbing because the attenuated Type III poliovirus had been the one of greatest concern to the Licensing Committee and was the last of the series of three to be released as a monovalent vaccine. Some of the members of Dr. Terry's committee felt that the incident might burgeon into a national tragedy

9. Members of this committee consisted of: Drs. David Bodian of Johns Hopkins University; John P. Fox of the Research Institute of New York City; Archie L. Gray, Mississippi State Board of Health; William McD. Hammon of the University of Pittsburgh; Hugh H. Hussy of George Washington University; Alexander D. Langmuir of the Communicable Disease Center at Atlanta, Ga.; Roderick Murray of the National Institutes of Health; John R. Paul of Yale University; Albert B. Sabin of the University of Cincinnati; E. D. Shaw of the University of California; and Joseph E. Smadel of the National Institutes of Health.

10. L. L. Terry: *Association of Cases of Poliomyelitis with the use of Type III Vaccines; With the use of Type III Oral Poliomyelitis Vaccines.* A Technical Report. U.S. Department of Health, Education & Welfare. Sept. 20, 1962.

as alarming as the Cutter incident of 1955. Some felt that the whole program should be called off immediately. A few opponents of the live virus program were loud in condemnation, calling it a national scandal.

In subsequent meetings of Dr. Terry's committee it was found that although occasional suspicious cases continued to be reported, the maximum potential risk in the United States in 1962 of developing paralytic poliomyelitis after receiving Type I monovalent vaccine was one or less than one in a million, and that such a risk was not great enough to justify any restriction on the administration of the oral vaccine. For Type II, the committee found no measurable risk at all. The main question revolved about Type III, in older people.

Just as Burnet had predicted two years previously, this slight risk was far greater for adults than for children. It was not finally realized that the reason for such events occurring without precedent was that vaccination programs in the Soviet Union and elsewhere had all been restricted to the younger age groups. But in the United States things were slightly different. Here, so-called educational campaigns which had been in force for six or seven years with the Salk-type vaccine had so indoctrinated the public with the idea that *everyone*—man, woman, or child, regardless of age— should be vaccinated that naturally the same was thought to apply to the oral vaccine as well.

On September 15, 1962, the national committee pointed out that the need for immunization diminishes with advancing age, particularly for persons over 30, and since with the Type III there might be an infinitely small risk, the live virus vaccine should be restricted to preschool and school-age children under 18 years. It was significant that although this suggestion was made emphatically over and over again by some members of various committees, when it came to a vote it was repeatedly rejected with the argument that such a limitation might stop the oral vaccine program altogether. These objections would come from parents who would not be able to understand why they should not be vaccinated when the vaccine was freely given to their children.

In this confusing state the program went along for another two years. A new advisory committee met in July 1964 to review the situation and to report on a ten-year survey of the incidence of poliomyelitis, covering both the periods 1955–61, when only inactivated poliovirus vaccine had been given, and 1961–64, when oral poliovirus vaccine had come into use with increasing frequency. After 1962 the Sabin-type vaccine became the one of choice in the United States.[11] This new committee reported that since December 1962, a small number of additional cases of presumed vaccine-

11. Oral Poliomyelitis Vaccines. Report of Special Advisory Committee on Oral Poliomyelitis Vaccine to the Surgeon General of the Public Health Service. *J. Amer. med. Ass., 190:* 49– 51, 1964.

induced poliomyelitis had followed ingestion of the Sabin strains, but as before, they had occurred largely among adults. Yet the annual rate of vaccine-associated or vaccine-induced cases had not increased since 1962 but had even declined, whereas the popularity of the oral vaccine had increased enormously in the United States and elsewhere during the previous two years.

These experiences during the three-year period (1961–64) were considered at length in a study by Henderson et al.[12] The authors had been among the first to recognize that cases of this kind could occur and maintained stoutly that a minimum risk did indeed exist, particularly for the Type III monovalent vaccine. Langmuir, in particular, had the memory of the Cutter incident indelibly fixed in his mind. And to say the least he was not anxious to have repetition of this catastrophe. As time went on the apparent risk associated with oral vaccine was not considered sufficient reason to curtail its use.[13] The new committee, however, at long last as a body did recommend a change in emphasis, i.e. in stressing the desirability of continuing intensive immunization of *infants and preschool children,* who represent the largest and most important groups at risk, and a de-emphasis of oral vaccination for adults. Also, it was pointed out that as very young children were by far the principal disseminators of the natural infection within the community, any suppression of infection in this age-group would be an advantage to the total population by reducing the opportunity for exposure. With these procedures in force it remains to be seen what the coming years can bring. Nevertheless, occasional rare accidents can be expected, much as has been the case with vaccination against smallpox. It is a rare biological product with a high degree of effectiveness that exhibits complete safety. Poliomyelitis is not to be conquered everywhere without an occasional agonizing setback. But the overall outlook continues to remain bright.

Superficially, a glance at the figures listed in table 8 giving the decline in poliomyelitis rates in the developed countries of the world and the graphs showing the picture for the United States (figs. 58 and 59) show what a success story the vaccination programs have turned out to be. In spite of my efforts to tell the intricacies of the story in a different, even dispassionate, manner, it has been impossible to avoid ending on a note of triumph.

Yet it is far too soon to view in perspective, events which have befallen and will befall the oral vaccination program. In spite of a very minimal risk, the Sabin-type vaccine has gathered strength as the procedure of choice in the great majority of countries; not however, in all: Sweden,

12. D. A. Henderson, J. J. Witte, L. Morris, and A. D. Langmuir: Paralytic disease associated with oral poliovaccines. *J. Amer. med. Ass., 190*: 153–160, 1964.

13. C. C. Hopkins, W. E. Dismakes, T. H. Glick, and R. J. Warren: Surveillance of paralytic poliomyelitis in the United States. *J. Amer. med. Ass., 210*: 694–700, 1969.

TABLE 8.   Observations on the global incidence of
poliomyelitis in selected countries

	Average Annual No. of Cases	
Countries	*in 1951–55*	*in 1961–65*
United States	37,864	570
Australia	2,187	154
New Zealand	405	44
Austria	607	70
Belgium	475	79
Czechoslovakia	1,081	0
Denmark	1,614	77
Sweden	1,526	28
United Kingdom	4,381	322

Data collected under the auspices of the World Health Organization by W. C. Cockburn
and S. G. Drozdov: WHO/Vir/68./ Rev. 2: available from the organization on request.

which has continued to champion the Salk-type vaccine, has been a notable
exception.

It is somewhat of a pity that so much of the last five chapters, which
should have been taken up with the victorious conquest of poliomyelitis,
have instead been concerned with untoward reactions to the vaccines and
disturbing controversies which have punctuated the last dozen or so years
of the history of this disease.

But when all is said and done, once success in the conquest of poliomye
litis was in the wind, the great majority of American people—and no doubt
other peoples of the world—ceased to have any interest in how poliomyelitis is acquired, or the weapons to prevent it, which were forged in the
heat of controversy; or those distressing incidents which have led to many
lawsuits about the propriety of using this or that prophylactic agent, and
who is to be held responsible for such "criminal" action, or anything else
about it.[14]

However, as history is never finished, the story of poliomyelitis is not yet
over. True, there is a general belief that to all intents and purposes the disease has been conquered and is now done for; but actually in the developing countries of the world this is not the case, and it is clear that a new
array of techniques and approaches, administrative and otherwise, will
have to be found. We look thankfully to the NFIP and hopefully to the
World Health Organization to deal with the problems which now beset
many struggling nations. For, with vastly improved sanitary conditions,
paradoxically enough, endemic poliomyelitis is beginning to be replaced

14. Medicolegal aspects of poliomyelitis. *J. Amer. med. Ass., 205*: 185, 1968. See also Curran:
Law-Medicine Notes: Drug-company liability in immunization programs. *New Engl. J. Med.,
281*: 1057–58, 1969.

by periodic outbreaks and a rising incidence of paralytic cases in certain tropical and subtropical countries, just as happened in northern Europe and the United States at the end of the nineteenth century. The existence of such a precarious and unresolved situation is the reason why this history cannot claim to be a completely triumphant success story. The road will lead uphill for many years to come.

Subject Index

Name Index

Abercrombie, J., 30
Ackerknecht, E. H., 49 n
Adams, F., *12–14*
Addison, W. I., 42
Ager, L. C., 139 n
Agius, T., 354 n
Albutt, Clifford, 71
Amoss, H. A., 156 n, 157 n, 240 n, 241, 242, 253, 441
Andersen, E. K., 398 n
Anderson, Gaylord, 189
Anderson, J. F., 137, 140, 141, 143, 292
Andrewes, Sir Christopher H., 268, 431
Andrus, E. C., 390
Armstrong, C., 247, 272, 273 (fig. 38), *274–77*, 315
Armstrong, D. B., 305
Armstrong, Emma, 272 n, 273 (fig. 38)
Aschoff, Ludwig, 395
Aycock, W. Lloyd, 132, 144 n, 163, *177–87*, 179, (fig. 27), 189, 254, 282, 287, 306, 357, 390, 446

Badham, Charles, 40 n
Badham, John, 31, 33, *38–43*
Baker, A. B., 332
Baldwin, E. R., 301
Barker, L. F., 109–10
Barnett, V. H., 363 n
Barthez, E., 53, 69
Bayne-Jones, S., 414 n
Beecher, H. K., 410
Bell, Sir Charles, 18 n, 30, *42–45*
Bell, J. A., 422–23
Bell, John, 18 n, 44
Bell, W., 18 n
Benedek, T. G., 35
Benison, S., 114 n, 256 n, 272 n, 284, 305 n, 313, 406, 407 n, 420, 425 n
Bennet, B. L., 417 n
Benyesh-Melnick, M., 458
Bergenholtz, 72
Bernkopf, H., 421 n, 453 n
Bernstein, H. G. G., 354 n
Berry, G. P., 410
Beveridge, W. I. B., 372 n
Bigelow, Jacob, 61
Billick, Col. D. W., 351 (fig. 47)

Bishop, M. B., 293 n
Blackwell, Elizabeth, 66
Blake, F. G., 118 n, 414, 415, 430, 432
Blake, J. A., 302
Bodian, D., 6 n, *234–37*, 250, 251 n, 382, 388, 389 n, 407 n, 456 n, 465 n
Boldman, C. F., 139 n
Bosch, Hieronymous, 16
Bowen, Catherine D., 325
Boyd, Col. J. S. K., 351 (fig. 47)
Brebner, W. B., 390
Breed, R. S., 268 n
Breughel, Pieter, 16
Brodie, M., *254–61*, 270, 272, 406, 418
Brown, A., 248 n
Brown, G. C., 405
Brues, C. T., 137, 291, 292
Bull, A. C., 72, 73
Burnet, Sir Macfarlane, 1 n, 239, 269, 315, 316, 372, 383, 441, 452, 461, 462
Burrows, M. T., 246

Cadwalader, Thomas, 38
Cameron, V., 301 n
Campbell, A. W., 169
Carpenter, H. C., 390 n
Carrel, A., 370, 371
Carter, R., 407 n, 420
Caruthers, B., 328
Casey, A. E., 46 n, 293 n
Caughey, J. E., 348, 351 (fig. 47)
Caulfield, E., 17
Caverly, Chas. S., 79–80, *84–86*, 89, 120, 178, 241
Cecil, R. L., 1 n
Charcot, Jean-Martin, 5, 6, *54–58*, 63
Chase, H., 35
Chumakov, M. P., 455
Ciocco, A., 407 n
Clark, P. F., 115, 240, 243, 291 n, 292
Clarke, John, 26 n
Cleland, J. B., 169
Cockburn, W. C., 468
Cohn, A. E., 118 n
Cohn, E. J., 390
Cole, R. I., 119, 120, 430
Collins, J., 148, 149
Collins, W., 328, 332, 333